GENDER IN HISTORY

Series editors:
Lynn Abrams, Cordelia Beattie, Julie Hardwick and Penny Summerfield

The expansion of research into the history of women and gender since the 1970s has changed the face of history. Using the insights of feminist theory and of historians of women, gender historians have explored the configuration in the past of gender identities and relations between the sexes. They have also investigated the history of sexuality and family relations, and analysed ideas and ideals of masculinity and femininity. Yet gender history has not abandoned the original, inspirational project of women's history: to recover and reveal the lived experience of women in the past and the present.

The series Gender in History provides a forum for these developments. Its historical coverage extends from the medieval to the modern periods, and its geographical scope encompasses not only Europe and North America but all corners of the globe. The series aims to investigate the social and cultural constructions of gender in historical sources, as well as the gendering of historical discourse itself. It embraces both detailed case studies of specific regions or periods, and broader treatments of major themes. Gender in History titles are designed to meet the needs of both scholars and students working in this dynamic area of historical research.

Out of his mind

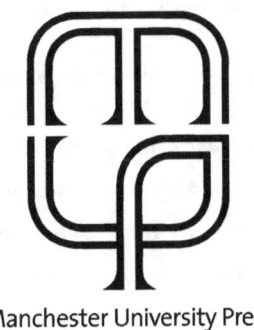

Manchester University Press

OTHER RECENT BOOKS
IN THE SERIES

The state as master: gender, state formation and commercialisation in urban Sweden, 1650–1780 Maria Ågren

Love, intimacy and power: marriage and patriarchy in Scotland, 1650–1850 Katie Barclay (Winner of the 2012 Women's History Network Book Prize)

Men on trial: performing emotion, embodiment and identity in Ireland, 1800–45 Katie Barclay

Modern women on trial: sexual transgression in the age of the flapper Lucy Bland

The Women's Liberation Movement in Scotland Sarah Browne

Modern motherhood: women and family in England, c. 1945-2000 Angela Davis

Women against cruelty: protection of animals in nineteenth-century Britain Diana Donald

Gender, rhetoric and regulation: women's work in the civil service and the London County Council, 1900-55 Helen Glew

Jewish women in Europe in the Middle Ages: a quiet revolution Simha Goldin

Women of letters: gender, writing and the life of the mind in early modern England Leonie Hannan

Women and museums 1850–1914: Modernity and the gendering of knowledge Kate Hill

The shadow of marriage: singleness in England, 1914–60 Katherine Holden

Women, dowries and agency: marriage in fifteenth-century Valencia Dana Wessell Lightfoot

Catholic nuns and sisters in a secular age: Britain 1945–90 Carmen Mangion

Medieval women and urban justice: Commerce, crime and community in England, 1300–1500 Teresa Phipps

Women, travel and identity: journeys by rail and sea, 1870–1940 Emma Robinson-Tomsett

Imagining Caribbean womanhood: race, nation and beauty contests, 1929–70 Rochelle Rowe

Infidel feminism: secularism, religion and women's emancipation, England 1830–1914 Laura Schwartz

Women, credit and debt in early modern Scotland Cathryn Spence

Being boys: youth, leisure and identity in the inter-war years Melanie Tebbutt

Women art workers and the Arts and Crafts movement Zoë Thomas

Queen and country: same-sex desire in the British Armed Forces, 1939–45 Emma Vickers

The 'perpetual fair': gender, disorder and urban amusement in eighteenth-century London Anne Wohlcke

Out of his mind

Masculinity and mental illness in Victorian Britain

Amy Milne-Smith

MANCHESTER UNIVERSITY PRESS

Copyright © Amy Milne-Smith 2022

The right of Amy Milne-Smith to be identified as the author of this work has been asserted by them in accordance with the Copyright, Designs and Patents Act 1988.

Published by Manchester University Press
Oxford Road, Manchester M13 9PL

www.manchesteruniversitypress.co.uk

British Library Cataloguing-in-Publication Data
A catalogue record for this book is available from the British Library

ISBN   978 1 5261 5503 0   hardback
ISBN   978 1 5261 7885 5   paperback

First published 2022

The publisher has no responsibility for the persistence or accuracy of URLs for any external or third-party internet websites referred to in this book, and does not guarantee that any content on such websites is, or will remain, accurate or appropriate.

Typeset
by New Best-set Typesetters Ltd

Contents

List of figures	*page* vi
A note on the text	viii
Acknowledgements	x
Introduction: madmen in the attic?	1
1 Men in care: the asylum	21
2 Men in the community: home care, doctors' care, and travellers	59
3 Personal shame: failures of morality and the will	98
4 Madmen out of the attic: reputation, rage, and liberty	140
5 Media panics: stories of violence, danger, and men out of control	183
6 Degeneration and madness: inheritance, neurasthenia, criminals, and GPI	221
Epilogue	263
Bibliography	270
Index	303

List of figures

1.1 Causes for attendant dismissal, 1872   page 42
Source: *Annual Report of the Commissioners in Lunacy*, 1872

2.1 Outcomes of male patients from Manor House Asylum, 1850–1914   64
Source: Manor House Asylum Casebooks, MS5725, MS6222, MS6223, MS6224, MS6227

2.2 Number and distribution of all reported lunatics, idiots, and persons of unsound mind residing with relatives or others   65
Source: *Annual Report of the Commissioners in Lunacy*, 1904

3.1 Intemperance in drink as formal cause of insanity (Yearly average number of instances in which each cause was assigned during the five years)   108
Source: *Fifty-second Annual Report of the Commissioners in Lunacy*, 1898; *Fifty-eighth Annual Report of the Commissioners in Lunacy*, 1904

3.2 Sexual intemperance as formal cause of insanity (Yearly average number of instances in which each cause was assigned during the five years)   113
Source: *Fifty-second Annual Report of the Commissioners in Lunacy*, 1898; *Fifty-eighth Annual Report of the Commissioners in Lunacy*, 1904

3.3 Drawing of 'Men' and 'Degenerates' in case notes of Rev. Arthur Henry Delmé Radcliffe   115
Source: Manor House Asylum Casebook, MS 6223

3.4 Drawing of 'Before Warned is to be Forearmed' in
 case notes of Rev. Arthur Henry Delmé Radcliffe 115
 Source: Manor House Asylum Casebook, MS 6223

3.5 Self-abuse as formal cause of insanity (Yearly
 average number of instances in which each cause
 was assigned during the five years) 119
 Source: *Fifty-second Annual Report of the
 Commissioners in Lunacy*, 1898; *Fifty-eighth
 Annual Report of the Commissioners in Lunacy*, 1904

5.1 Interior and exterior scenes of a violent encounter 189
 Source: 'Encounter with a Madman – Lambeth',
 Illustrated Police News (2 August 1884), p. 1

5.2 A lunatic in a railway train 196
 Source: 'A Madman in a Railway Carriage',
 Illustrated Police News (4 August 1877), p. 1

6.1 Percentage of recoveries vs admissions to asylums 226
 Source: Lunacy Commissioner reports

A note on the text

I use the term 'madness', along with 'insanity' and 'lunacy', not as a reflection of eighteenth-century terms and institutions, nor as any judgement on the actual mental health of Victorian actors. Rather, these phrases were most often used by lay and medical writers in the nineteenth century. 'Mad studies' set the tone for this nomenclature as a way to study those deemed mentally ill by their society without having to assess their actual levels of mental health or illness. Using terms like 'madness' reinforces the idea that the term itself is a cultural construct, and its boundaries were broadly defined. I also use the term 'alienist' as it was a neutral term from the 1860s until the twentieth century, and to differentiate the medical practitioners of the nineteenth century from modern psychiatry.[1]

I have chosen to use people's recorded names unless they were anonymized in the original source material or an archive requested anonymization. Concerns over privacy in psychiatric cases are linked to the idea that mental illness is particularly stigmatizing to patients and their families. And it is certainly key to always be sensitive to vulnerable populations. However, given that my topic is firmly rooted in the nineteenth century it is the perfect opportunity not to conceal names but rather reclaim patient voices and identities. As recent patients' rights activists point out, to shield names of those living three generations back or more risks reifying the stigma of mental illness.[2] The patients and families discussed in this text have nothing of which to be ashamed.

Notes

1 J. Oppenheim, *'Shattered Nerves': Doctors, Patients, and Depression in Victorian England* (New York, 1991), p. 27.
2 R. Saucier and D. Wright, 'Madness in the Archives: Anonymity, Ethics, and Mental Health Research', *Journal of the Canadian Historical Association* 23:2 (2012), pp. 81–82.

Acknowledgements

The inspiration for this book came from a strange incident I discovered in the early 2000s while researching the gentlemen's clubs of London. The *Pall Mall Gazette* reported on a man who entered his West End club and began stacking ice cubes on his head and letting them roll down onto the floor, the table, and other members. He roared at anyone who tried to intervene with his project. Scotland Yard was eventually called, but found they were unable to do anything as it was a members' club, and he was a member. Further inquiry revealed that the man had escaped a lunatic asylum and wandered straight to his club.[1] This incident stuck with me as it seemed to contradict the predominant narrative I knew about men and madness in the nineteenth century: insanity was a private matter and any public representation of madness was primarily female. Before I could investigate the topic any further, however, I had to finish my PhD dissertation, secure a permanent job, turn the dissertation into a book, get a new job, and then finally turn to the idea. This meant diving into an entirely new historiography that had only grown in the years since I originally developed an interest in the topic.

This book has taken even longer than my first book, and I am incredibly grateful to the wonderful historians who continue to publish fantastic, challenging, evocative works in my new-chosen sub-field. It is a much more crowded historiography than the world of clubland, but I believe I have become a richer scholar for it.

I am grateful to many people, and hopefully I don't leave anyone out of what has been a long and winding road. First, I have been lucky to be aided in small grants from Wilfrid Laurier University, both for research trips and to fund undergraduate researchers. Never underestimate the power of small grants! Thanks to student researchers Matthew Hargreaves, Stephanie Plante, Katelyn Leece. Thanks to Emily Nighman for some transcriptions when I couldn't type. Thank you to my colleagues in the Laurier writing group: Mark Humphries, Judy Fletcher, David Chan Smith, and Dana Weiner. Thanks to Andrew Haley and Jeff Bowersox who listened to many of the early tortured incarnations of this book, and to Ben Liu for the access. To Leandra Zarnow for her careful reviewing and to Allison Abra for hearing about this project forever and reading chapters during a global pandemic.

My research was greatly aided by various archives and libraries along with an increasing collection of digitized resources. Thank you to the librarians and staff at the Berkshire Record Office, the Liverpool Record Office, The British Library, the National Archives, and my new favourite archive, the Wellcome Library. I've benefited immensely over the years from a community of scholars who research Britain, including the Southern Ontario British seminar group (helmed by Stephen Heathorn, Stephen Brooke, and Catherine Ellis), the annual conferences of the North American Conference on British Studies, and the inspiring Diseases of Modern Life conference at Oxford. Many thanks to the *Journal of Victorian Culture* for permission to reproduce materials from my articles 'Shattered Minds: Madmen on the Railways, 1860–1880' and 'Work and Madness: Overworked Men and Fears of Degeneration, 1860s–1910s' in chapters five and six. Thank you to my editors Emma Brennan and Meredith Carroll at Manchester University Press, to my anonymous readers, and to Diane Wardle for editorial assistance large and small.

I am so grateful to be an academic who has a life outside of my research and teaching, and it is my friends who help keep me grounded. Thank you to my family for having way too much interest in my research, and to Nevin for having very little. And of course to my constant canine companion, who distracted me for thirteen years; yes, I'll step away from my computer now and sit on the couch with you.

Note

1 An Old Fogey, 'Clubs and Clubmen – iii The Eccentric', *Pall Mall Gazette* (28 January 1903), pp. 1–2.

Introduction: madmen in the attic?

> Many of the patients take no pleasure in any kind of amusement, but for hours will sit or stand alone wrapped in thought, some in the attitude of listening, some with sunken heads and hands clasped behind them; others with their arms pinned to their sides like recruits in the presence of the drill-sergeant. Others pace the long gallery incessantly, pouring out their woes to those who will listen to them, or, if there be none to listen, to the dogs and cats, or, just as frequently, to the air ... With an inward groan I murmured 'Let me be crippled, deaf, blind, paralytic, mutilated even to the negation of outward form, such by Thy will, but not Mad, O Lord, not Mad!'[1]

George Augustus Sala's description of the patients at Bethlem asylum in 1860 did not differ significantly from those who had visited nearly a century before.[2] The structure of the asylum had considerably improved, chains and manacles had long been removed, and humane methods of treatment had become the norm as the site transitioned from madhouse to hospital. However, the patients still presented a tragic appearance to Sala because madness was still a serious problem. The men he saw were just as ill as a century before, and they had no useful role in society. Sala was troubled by the experience and left shaken by the fear that he too might join their ranks. His fear of madness was neither an isolated nor an idiosyncratic concern in the nineteenth century. For men such as Sala, the spectre of madness was a truly terrifying prospect. While newly built asylums popped up across Britain, and specialist doctors investigated the breadth and width of lunacy, the reality was that experts had very few solutions for those who suffered a mental breakdown. And those solutions that were offered, even at the height of optimism about potential cures, always entailed a serious deprivation of liberty and autonomy. Men's authority in society was rooted in rule over dependants within their household and beyond; without that power the foundation of their manhood was in question.[3] As such, madness touched on a key tenet of nineteenth-century masculinity: control.

A primary definition of manhood was, from the early nineteenth century, a man's ability to demonstrate 'self-mastery, conscience and individual responsibility'.[4] This had long been a defining characteristic of respectable manhood, but in the nineteenth century it took on renewed importance.[5] As Joanne Begiato notes, a 'lack of self-restraint became more risky in the nineteenth century because persistent and extreme lack of control over passions, bodies, bodily appetites and feelings was increasingly pathologized as a cause of insanity'.[6] There was enormous variability between types of idealized manhood based on local norms, class expectations, and communication communities; self-control, however, resonates throughout most of these incarnations. The most extreme versions of Victorian manliness promoted absolute self-discipline, suppressing feeling and emotions of all sorts.[7] The ability to control oneself was a key marker of authoritative masculinity, and men were expected to repress and control their emotional expressions.[8]

A madman who had lost control of his emotions, his actions, or his intellect was therefore in many ways no longer a man. As such, insanity highlights the boundaries of masculinity, those who sought to police its borders, and those who contested these definitions. A madman was, by his very nature, a man who could or would not control himself; as such he could be a danger to himself and others and needed to be contained. The violent madman was seen as more of a beast than a man. Men whose symptoms were more self-contained, such as the melancholic or suicidal patient, were also understood as not being able to control their emotions. However, instead of being a threat, such a man was seen as effeminized. In some ways the madman resembled the male tuberculosis patient, as both were seen as unable to pursue a career and unsuitable to marry. Removed from commercial or reproductive success they were unable to live up to the male standards of the age, either their own or others'.[9]

Earlier centuries made space for some version of vulnerability in definitions of manhood.[10] This could always pose challenges. Some of the virtues of eighteenth-century masculinity were contradictory;

a man was to be both 'stoically self-controlled and an emotional man of feeling'.[11] And yet such tensions allowed a broad range of masculinities to be explored in public life. This even extended to public eccentrics and harmless lunatics. One author writing in 1859 bemoaned the loss of such characters like his old friend the 'General'. He was an eccentric man, whose delusions of military prowess brought him much joy; he was seen as a harmless character by his community. 'Such wanderers were not uncommon in former times, and everywhere their appearance was hailed as a sort of relief to the monotonous sobriety of sane life. The species must have died out, or their existence is hidden in asylums.'[12] Men like the General were no longer left to their own devices, and were increasingly sent to asylums, kept quietly in family homes, or sent abroad.

Before doctors had much experience treating the insane in large numbers, theories of madness were wide-ranging. Causes could be traced to medical, moral, or religious foundations.[13] In the early eighteenth century, most believed 'the mad were little better than wild beasts, requiring stern discipline while hoping that nature might perhaps work a cure'.[14] The moral treatment movement, inspired by medical and religious reformers in the latter part of that century, saw the humanity within their charges, and sought for better treatment and greater understanding. Institutions and asylums became curative sites in their purpose (if not always in practice).[15] Madhouse keepers were replaced with medical specialists who asserted their claim as the proper supervisors of mental disease in the nineteenth century.[16] While lunacy reform was championed as one of the Victorians' greatest achievements, scepticism of the alienists did not disappear overnight, nor did popular stigmas around madness.

In Andrew Scull's classic work *Museums of Madness*, he categorizes the nineteenth century as a period of enormous success for medical authorities in terms of their legitimacy and authority. He claims:

> Insanity was transformed from a vague, culturally defined phenomenon afflicting an unknown, but probably small, proportion of the population into a condition which could only be authoritatively diagnosed, certified, and dealt with by a group of legally recognized experts; and which was now seen as one of the major forms of deviance in English society.[17]

This might have been the goal of nineteenth-century lunacy experts, but this dream was highly contested.[18] Patients, legal authorities, families, and the culture at large continued to debate the definitions of insanity and its proper treatment throughout the century. Eighteenth-century ideas and practices were never so barbaric, nor were nineteenth-century practices ever so successful, as Victorian lunacy reformers liked to believe. And, as Scull notes, a lasting stigma of lunatics as deviants remained, particularly in the non-medical community. Lunacy was never just a problem for the doctors.

As Charles Rosenberg points out, disease is as much a biological fact as it is the creation of the society which names it. 'In some ways disease does not exist until we have agreed that it does, by perceiving, naming, and responding to it.'[19] The values and interpretive lenses that medical professionals bring to bear on a patient reveal as much about themselves and their culture as about the condition of the sufferer. Specialist narratives of insanity, and their various new structures of nosology, were only one of multiple understandings of madness, and do not reflect the full range of general medical practitioners, let alone the culture at large. Madness was as much a social construction as a medical fact.[20] I am inspired in this work by R.A. Houston's approach to the study of madness. He notes that 'the social constructions which sane people place on the behaviour of the insane may indicate their expectations about normality based on a condition they regard as "real," but pathological and worthy of care and treatment'.[21] This approach allows for recognizing that the term 'madness' incorporates both real disease and social constructions. There was no universally accepted test or standard to madness in the nineteenth century, and it was constantly negotiated by sufferers, families, medical authorities, and the public at large.

This book is a study of the consequences of a diagnosis of insanity for men who ascribed to the normative values of masculinity, and what this meant to their families, their friends, and the culture at large. As Jessie Hewitt notes in her French study, 'rereading the history of madness with an eye toward the inconsistencies inherent in gender, disability, and class ideologies … exposes the shaky foundations upon which dominant ideas about men, women, and irrationality rested over the course of the long nineteenth century'.[22] Studying the madman allows for an exploration of the cultural expectations of male behaviour, and how men responded to those norms in their lived experiences.[23] Authorities believed men who chose to indulge in violence, drunkenness, and debauchery threatened to succumb to their worst, bestial natures.[24] Those who completely suppressed their masculine virility, and surrounded themselves with deskwork, poetry, or domestic bliss, threatened to succumb to effeminacy and emasculation.[25] This is a multi-dimensional assessment of masculinity such as Ben Griffin calls for, where multiple kinds of masculinities were at odds with one another.[26] In the case of insanity, the ability to live up to social expectations of manhood did encounter a very concrete reality. Whether or not a man was mad was not simply a discursive exercise – it had real-world consequences. This is an example where institutions, courts, doctors, and families decided what forms of masculinity were acceptable, and which were beyond the pale. Madness is a compelling example to study the purchase of cultural models of masculinity.[27] Doctors, families, and individuals made decisions about when a man's behaviour had become pathological.

Each chapter examines how the study of madness reveals different tensions in the definition of masculinity. The first chapters of the book focus on the question of autonomy, and how men fought to maintain self-control in the face of a system that was designed to remove that control. Patients (when they were able) and families negotiated choices of care based on how best to preserve masculine integrity. The next chapters look at subjective experience and the voices of those who were deemed mad; some men internalized their shame while others fought against their diagnosis. They explore the value-laden field of medical diagnostics and advocacy groups fighting against the medical establishment. The final chapters explore the larger significance of public debates about madness. These chapters focus on the most public conversations about men's insanity. Representations of madmen pointed to deeper social anxieties about violence, modernity, degeneration, and the boundaries of Victorian masculinity.

Early trailblazers exploring Victorian women and madness did such a good job detailing feminist explorations of spiritualism and madwomen in the literary landscape that the historiography became lopsided.[28] While Elaine Showalter's focus in the nineteenth century was women, she does outline more generally how representations of madness can provide a key to understanding Victorian gender tropes and their lived realities.[29] Joan Busfield followed up, emphasizing that there were prominent female and male cultural narratives of madness in the nineteenth century.[30] This exploration of gender permeates the field of mental health research as social historians now regularly integrate gender as a key concept of analysis.[31] There were as many maniacs in the cellar as there were madwomen in the attic in Victorian sensation literature.[32] An examination of men is particularly important to emphasize the active policing of Victorian masculinity.[33] Recent historians and literary critics have shown that men's madness was far from hidden in the nineteenth century, and that it was rife for public discussion long before the dawn of shell shock.[34]

Scope

This book covers roughly the period between the Lunacy Act of 1845 to the First World War. This period is bookended by major events in the history of mental health, and yet this also highlights temporal ambiguities. Asylums did not become the universal care sites overnight in 1845; what changed was the official legislation deeming the asylum as the primary site of mental treatment. The 1840s and 1850s witnessed a wave of optimism that slowly slipped away. Alienists fought for recognition in the community, and new specialties like neurology attempted to firmly situate madness in the brain even as cure rates continued to stagnate.[35] This period witnessed both the normalization of the asylum system and repeated critiques from patients' rights groups, legal sceptics, and families of the mad. The war did not instantly transform mental health care, and the term 'shell shock' was not coined until 1915; yet the war certainly put mental health concerns in an entirely new context. The decades leading up to the war anticipated many trends of twentieth-century psychiatry while still playing out Victorian debates.

The geographical focus of this book is largely drawn from English archival sources. And yet it is impossible to maintain geographical divisions as popular culture transgressed national borders; English newspapers were as likely to report on a story from Dublin as Scottish papers were to relate a story of Manchester if they were sensational enough. Regional differences of law and custom were often explicitly discussed, and thus an English focus will not exclude relevant Scottish, Welsh, and Irish examples, and transnational perspectives. Very different national health systems coexisted within the same country, thus it is no surprise that authorities were always comparing and contrasting systems with each other. The Scottish system in particular was praised by English Lunacy reformers for its committal system that balanced medical and legal oversight.[36]

The focus of the book is on madness, broadly defined. This text largely excludes 'idiots' who increasingly had their own history in the second half of the nineteenth century. More importantly, 'natural born idiots' did not have any rights or freedoms to lose, as these were typically stripped in infancy. While idiocy was often dealt with by similar legal and medical processes, it existed in a different cultural context. A gendered study of idiocy is beyond the scope of this project.

There is a social power in naming disease, and nineteenth-century alienists were well aware of this fact. Psychiatry sought to define the boundaries of the normal, and to create standardized measures for mental health. Yet, as alienists sought to police these boundaries, their specialty suffered 'procedure envy'. They could not turn to the same kinds of specific, objective diagnostic categories of other sub-fields.[37] Diagnosis 'constitutes an indispensable point of articulation between the general and the particular, between agreed-upon knowledge and its application'.[38] And there was much debate on the agreed-upon knowledge of insanity in the nineteenth century. This project embraces the term 'madness' to reflect society's definitions of mental illness rather than strictly medical definitions. Madness is 'a linguistic black hole that (metaphorically) sucks in all peculiar human behaviour that society cannot digest or normalise but still feels compelled to explain in order to respond to it or control it'.[39] In no way do I assess whether or not those under care or certified as lunatics suffered what would today be considered a mental illness. Contemporaries themselves disagreed about diagnoses so commonly that it would be exceedingly difficult to effectively retrodiagnose people from the past. More importantly, such an assessment would have had no meaning to those who lived through being labelled a lunatic, those who were sent to an asylum, or those who faced friends and family that treated them as insane. It is far more important to see how madness was constructed and contested by those living in the nineteenth century. The Victorian madman was both a social reality and a cultural phenomenon, and loomed large in social anxieties about respectability, masculine self-control, and fears of degeneration.

Methodology and approach

My methodology is influenced by Peter Mandler's call to demonstrate the 'relative throw – the weight or significance' of culture on ordinary people in the past.[40] Christine Grandy underscores the need to ground our cultural history in an audience, to tackle the problem of perception, and bridge the gap between cultural representation and experience.[41] This monograph is doing just that, as the first half focuses on the social experiences of madness, and is a story of asylums, sufferers, and families grounded in lived reality. The second half of the book pushes outwards, looking at men who protested their incarceration or diagnosis, studying representations of madness in the media and popular fiction, and finally exploring how madness was central to broad social anxieties about sexuality and degeneration. It is a work of cultural history, but it borrows methods from social histories of asylums and mental health. This project interrogates the various framings of madness by medical and lay communities.[42] The cultural definition of madness had as much impact on Victorian society as laws and medical diagnostics ever did, and thus all need to be taken seriously.

This approach is ideal to study how normative codes of masculinity related to actual men's lived experiences. Here Michael Roper's call to pay attention to the lives that men lived, and how they did or did not manage their emotional impulses is key. This approach combines the biographical experiences of men whose stories were well documented with the cultural scripts produced by medical, legal, and cultural authorities.[43] Masculinity exists as a combination of lived experience and imagined ideals; the story of madness allows an exploration of how men navigated the cultural representations of ideals and their subjective identities.[44] Herbert Sussman challenged authors to 'consider male identity within the individual not as a stable achievement but as an unstable equilibrium, so that the governing terms of Victorian manhood become contradiction, conflict, anxiety.'[45] As Helen Goodman notes, there was a wide-ranging literary and social debate about what degree of emotional expression was appropriate in Victorian society; as she points out, there was no single answer to that question.[46] Even before the history of emotions was a recognized field, historians of medicine looked to the emotional lives of patients and families, and case histories can be used to investigate the 'emotional worlds' of historical subjects.[47] Asylum letters, when such sources exist, can aid in exploring both patients' and families' emotional reactions to incarceration.[48]

In this study, the impact of cultural tropes is evident in everything from men's personal memoirs to testimony captured in open court. As Michael McDonald has argued, 'Historians of insanity do not in the first instance study the insane at all: they study observations of the insane.'[49] The story of madmen is central, but it is just as important to place men within their familial and social contexts. This is where men's behaviour was first judged and found to be wanting; the family set and policed the norms of masculine behaviour.[50] Historians have worked to put families at the core of studies of mental illness for the past few decades, and this book follows that tradition.[51]

Out of his Mind builds on recent works by scholars exploring Victorian masculinity and disability. Mad studies set the tone as a way to study those deemed mentally ill by their society without having to assess their actual levels of mental health or illness.[52] As a society fascinated by physical and mental health, the ill body was a point of fascination fraught with meaning in the nineteenth century. Karen Bourrier notes that 'illness and disability are fluid states' and that 'illness, invalidism, and disability' provide important normative functions.[53] As Joanne Begiato notes, 'maimed or incapacitated men' did not see themselves achieving masculine standards, nor did their society.[54]

The middle- and upper-class man is the central figure of the cultural and social analysis in this text. While drawing on material from a number of asylums (including Broadmoor, Bethlem, and Glasgow Royal Lunatic Asylum), the most exhaustive asylum studied is Manor House, a private asylum based in Chiswick, for which 250 male case studies survive.[55] Charlotte MacKenzie's research on Ticehurst demonstrates just how rich such casebooks can be for understanding the experience of wealthy men.[56] And yet understandings of male madness only exist in a relational space. Pauper asylums held by far the greatest numbers of the insane; there has been admirable work exploring the gendered experience of the Victorian pauper asylum, and I do not try to replicate that intricate work.[57] However, the working-class madman was also an important cultural trope, as the fear of the violent, degenerate working-class insane was a pressing concern of governing elites. How insanity was diagnosed, and the experience of detention or constraint, was highly gendered, but just as significantly it was shaped by class-based assumptions.[58] Everything from perception of friends and family, lunacy certification, criminal insanity cases, treatment options, and potential outcomes were shaped by identity and class.

Asylum records form one part of the medico-governmental research in this project. Lunacy Commission reports reveal official narratives of lunacy, criminal trials highlight debates on responsibility, and Chancery records trace wealthy lunatics.[59] Medical sources for the project range from official medical textbooks and journal articles to fringe pamphlets and quack medicine. Newspaper reports demonstrate popular representations of madness and also highlight controversial lunacy trials. First-person narratives of madness, either as a form of protest or proof of recovery, highlight the patient's point of view. Finally, works of popular fiction are invaluable resources to explore the popular tropes of madness, and to see its representation in everyday life. The source base is thus quite extensive, if not exhaustive, to capture both representations and experiences of lunacy.

Chapter one, 'Men in care', traces madmen's place in a national network of asylums established across Britain in the second half of the nineteenth century. This chapter gives readers a brief overview of the structures of asylums and rules of admission for different classes and types of illness, and builds on the strong institutional histories of asylums. It provides information about the diversity of asylum experiences, from the elite institutions for the wealthy, to the large public asylums, to the criminal asylum, and highlights how men passed in and out of their walls. It tells the story of men such as Robert Clark, a pauper seaman, that the Inspector of Leith dismissed as a 'drunken fellow.' After being discharged from Morningside Asylum, a week later he ended up at Glasgow Royal Lunatic Asylum with hallucinations and a note claiming he attempted suicide.[60] The Victorian asylum was born out of optimism, flourished in an era of no better alternatives, and quickly became a symbol of failed expectations embodied by men like Clark who were in and out of asylums. I focus on the male experience of incarceration, and how this was particularly destabilizing for those used to being in control of themselves and their families. Men also proved particularly difficult patients to control if they were prone to violence. This chapter introduces the typical experience of madness in the Victorian era that saw the asylum as at least a part of most men's curative treatment.

'Men in the community' explores men who were treated at home, sent to travel, or lived in the community. Outside of any medical or government oversight, Lunacy Commissioners assumed patients would be mistreated. The Commissioners highlighted cases of abuse such as when two men were found naked and neglected in their family homes.[61] Yet, as this chapter explores, while some families hid their family members away in dark corners, victims of negligence and cruelty, others kept loved ones at home under expert care and keen attendance. Diversity is underscored both in patient experiences and the reasons for choices of treatment. Decisions of care were based on complex negotiations between patients, doctors, and families. While many madmen likely left no trace in the historical archive, there are many examples when single care went wrong, and families were forced to seek out authorities for help. This includes men at all income levels. The case of Henry Meux highlights the complex family dramas involved when a man of wealth and power refused treatment and would not be restrained. This chapter also explores the abuse that patients suffered outside of official legislation and sometimes within their own homes.

The third chapter puts the patient at the forefront of analysis and is deeply influenced by recent trends in the history of emotions to interrogate shame and stigma. Patients were often held responsible for their own breakdowns. This chapter outlines the intellectual framework of this culture of shame, and how patients struggled within this context. The ideal late-Victorian man was above all things in control of himself and his place in the world. A man who lost control of his mind and his emotions struggled to retain his sense of manhood. When men felt culpable for that loss, their shame added an extra layer of humiliation. In particular, when a man's madness was associated with alcohol or sex, internal and external pressures of shame intensified. Often patients were hardest on themselves, and doctors feared that guilt over indiscretions could be more damaging than the habits themselves.

'Madmen out of the attic' continues with the voice of the patient, but rather than focusing on those resigned and ashamed of their fate, these are cases of patients who fought back. Individuals and advocacy groups challenged diagnoses both inside and outside the asylum. This chapter explores how men fought back against certification and incarceration and attempted to restore their public reputations. Such disputes outline the boundaries of madness, and the debate over the line between eccentricity and insanity. Here contested Chancery lunacy cases take centre stage as they were widely publicized in the press as men of wealth and position battled to prove their sanity. Such situations were the worst-case scenarios for families of status and position, and demonstrate a complete breakdown in family coherence. The chapter ends with a discussion of the Windham case, the longest and most expensive Chancery lunacy case in history, where a man fought to secure his absolute ability to do as he pleased. This case was a very public airing of scepticism about the authority and legitimacy of lunacy 'experts'. This chapter also engages with long-running suspicions of private asylums.

'Media panics' places the cultural representation of madness as its central focus. Stories of madmen as perpetrators of violence made for sensational copy, and thus they are overrepresented in media coverage. These stories reveal larger anxieties of the modern age, and the fragility of established rules and norms of society. The fear that madness could strike at any moment, and that a man could suddenly fall victim to an irrational and violent breakdown, was particularly gendered as male. Madwomen were often portrayed as victims in the media whereas madmen were often portrayed as perpetrators of violence both within the home and within the asylum. These media panics are perhaps the most public expressions of underlying anxieties about the threat that madness posed to everyday people and highlights the deep stigma of men's mental illness. In assessing media trends, clear gender- and class-based panics emerge. In particular, the figure of the working-class madman who murders his family highlights fears of domestic instability. And stories of sudden madness emphasize deeper fears about the state of British manhood and the dangers of modern technology.

Introduction: madmen in the attic?

The final chapter explores why madness in particular could evoke so much social anxiety. Fears of perceived rising lunacy rates were used as proof of over-civilization. As the century progressed, cure rates seemed to plummet and degeneration literature flourished; insanity was a central point of argument in theories of national decline. Fear that madness was hereditary led to gloomy predictions about the deterioration of the British race paralleling conversations about urban decay and the criminal classes. Particular anxieties were linked to middle-class emasculated neurasthenics and working-class drunkards and criminals. A final focus on the diagnosis of General Paralysis of the Insane (GPI) demonstrates the social construction of medical thinking. GPI was often diagnosed through lifestyle as much as symptomology. The fact that GPI seemed to affect men more than women and led to almost inevitable death made it the embodiment of degenerationist fantasies that only increased as the century progressed.

The question of madness put many ideals of masculinity to the test in very public ways. The basic structure of nineteenth-century lunacy law assumed that anyone who was mad was best cared for in an institution.[62] For those who could or would not place their loved ones in institutions, they were expected at least to keep them well out of sight. Madmen were marginal figures, confined in private homes, hospitals, and asylums; and yet as a cultural figure the madman loomed large. Because men had the most power and authority in Victorian Britain, this also meant they had the most to lose should they be deemed a lunatic. The label of madness could instantly strip a man of his masculine privileges in a way unlike any other, and thus it is a particularly useful way to study definitions of masculinity.

In the midst of one of many public debates about lunacy policy in 1885, medical experts and members of the public dissected all of the problems of the existing and proposed system. People wrote into *The Times* about the legal technicalities of proposed legislation, about whether or not it would solve specific problems, and Lord Shaftesbury himself became so incensed he actually resigned as head of the Lunacy Commission for fear any new legislation would limit early treatment.[63] Such conversations were significant, and debates around lunacy law are vitally important and have been traced admirably by historians over the years. Yet, as a cultural historian,

I have tried to pay attention to the conversations happening in and around these big debates. In my research I have sought out not only the voices of the doctors and policy-makers, but the friends and relatives dealing with family members they feared were falling into madness. And finally, I try to be sensitive to the voices of those deemed mad themselves. As one doctor noted amid the 1885 debates, 'There is no reason, because a man is of unsound mind and has delusions on some subjects, that everything he says and does should be treated with contempt and sometimes with ridicule.'[64]

Notes

1 G. Augustus Sala, 'A Visit to the Royal Hospital of Bethlehem', *Illustrated London News* (31 March 1860), pp. 304–5.
2 It was also a longstanding fear; Harley's visit to Bethlem in *A Man of Feeling* was preoccupied with studying a group of men who were once scientists, teachers, investors, and men much like himself. H. Mackenzie, *The Man of Feeling* [1771] (London, 1886), pp. 47–50. As Michael Rowland notes, these men are particular examples of male shame; men who could not live up to their professional expectations, whose very work turned them to madmen. M. Rowland, 'Shame and Futile Masculinity: Feeling Backwards in Henry Mackenzie's *Man of Feeling*', *Eighteenth-Century Fiction* 31:3 (2019), pp. 540–41.
3 K. Chase and M. Levenson, *The Spectacle of Intimacy: A Public Life for the Victorian Family* (Princeton, 2000).
4 M. McCormack, *The Independent Man: Citizenship and Gender Politics in Georgian England* (Manchester, 2005), p. 2.
5 Although, as Alexandra Shepard notes, this was one facet of the male identity, and was balanced by youth codes of riotous living and alternative masculine codes that valorized violence. A. Shepard, *Meanings of Manhood in Early Modern England* (Oxford, 2003), p. 16.
6 J. Begiato, 'Punishing the Unregulated Manly Body and Emotions in Early Victorian England', in J. Parsons and R. Hehold (eds), *The Victorian Male Body* (Edinburgh, 2017), p. 51.
7 J. Tosh, *A Man's Place: Masculinity and the Middle-Class Home in Victorian England* (New Haven, 1999), p. 184.
8 J. Begiato, *Manliness in Britain, 1760–1900: Bodies, Emotions, and Material Culture* (Manchester, 2020), p. 5; M. Cohen and T. Hitchcock, 'Introduction', in M. Cohen and T. Hitchcock (eds), *English Masculinities 1660–1800* (London, 1999), pp. 1–22.

9   A. Tankard, 'Emasculation, Eugenics and the Consumptive Voyeur in *The Portrait of a Lady* (1881) and *The Story of a Nobody* (1893)', *Critical Survey* 20:3 (2008), p. 62.
10 J. Campana, *The Pain of Reformation: Spenser, Vulnerability, and the Ethics of Masculinity* (New York, 2012), p. 4.
11 S. Goldsmith, 'Nostalgia, Homesickness and Emotional Formation on the Eighteenth-Century Grand Tour', *Cultural and Social History* 15:3 (2018), p. 334.
12 A. Black, *Brown and His Friends* (Edinburgh, 1859), p. 30.
13 R. Porter, *Mind-Forg'd Manacles: A History of Madness in England from the Restoration to the Regency* (London, 1987), p. x.
14 R. Porter, 'Madness and its Institutions', in A. Wear (ed.), *Medicine in Society: Historical Essays* (Cambridge, 1992), p. 289.
15 E. Shorter, *A History of Psychiatry: From the Era of the Asylum to the Age of Prozac* (New York, 1997), pp. 8–9.
16 A. Scull, *Madhouses, Mad-Doctors, and Madmen: The Social History of Psychiatry in the Victorian Era* (Philadelphia, 2015), p. 6.
17 A. Scull, *Museums of Madness: The Social Organization of Insanity in Nineteenth-Century England* (New York, 1979), p. 49.
18 See for example: N. Glover-Thomas, *Reconstructing Mental Health Law and Policy* (London, 2002).
19 C. Rosenberg, 'Framing Disease: Illness, Society, and History', in C. Rosenberg and J. Golden (eds), *Framing Disease: Studies in Cultural History* (New Brunswick, 1992), p. xiii.
20 Porter, *Mind-Forg'd Manacles*, pp. 15–20.
21 R.A. Houston, 'Madness and Gender in the Long Eighteenth Century', *Social History* 27:3 (2002), p. 311.
22 J. Hewitt, *Institutionalizing Gender: Madness, the Family, and Psychiatric Power in Nineteenth-Century France* (Ithaca, 2020), p. 2.
23 Deviance from that norm had to be justified and rationalized so it did not become pathologized. Houston, 'Madness and Gender', p. 311; E. Stephens, 'Pathologizing Leaky Male Bodies: Spermatorrhea in Nineteenth-Century British Medicine and Popular Anatomical Museums', *Journal of the History of Sexuality* 17:3 (2008), p. 428.
24 J. Bailey, *Unquiet Lives: Marriage and Marriage Breakdown in England 1660–1800* (Cambridge, 2003); B. Capp, 'The Double Standard Revisited: Plebeian Women and Male Sexual Reputation in Early Modern England', *Past & Present* 162:1 (1999), pp. 70–100; E. Foyster, *Marital Violence: An English Family History, 1660–1857* (Cambridge, 2005); M. Rothery and H. French (eds), *Making Men: The Formation of Elite Male Identities in England c. 1660–1900: Sourcebook* (Basingstoke, 2012); D. Turner,

Fashioning Adultery: Gender, Sex and Civility in England, 1660–1740 (Cambridge, 2002).

25 H. Ellis, 'This Starting, Feverish Heart: Matthew Arnold and the Problem of Manliness', *Critical Survey* 20:3 (2008), pp. 98–102; J. Tosh, *Manliness and Masculinities in Nineteenth-Century Britain* (Harlow, 2005), p. 70.

26 B. Griffin, 'Hegemonic Masculinity as a Historical Problem', *Gender & History* 30:2 (2018), p. 378.

27 K. Harvey and A. Shepard, 'What Have Historians Done with Masculinity? Reflections on Five Centuries of British History, circa 1500–1950', *Journal of British Studies* 44:2 (2005), p. 277.

28 P. Chesler, *Women and Madness* (Garden City, 1972); S. Gilbert and S. Gubar, *The Madwoman in the Attic: The Woman Writer and the Nineteenth Century Literary Imagination* (New Haven, 2000); J. Kromm, 'Olivia Furiosa: Maniacal Women from Richardson to Wollstonecraft', *Eighteenth-Century Fiction* 16:3 (2004), pp. 343–72; H. Marland, *Dangerous Motherhood: Insanity and Childbirth in Victorian Britain* (Houndmills, 2004); H. King, *The Disease of Virgins: Green Sickness, Chlorosis and the Problems of Puberty* (London, 2004); A. Owen, *The Darkened Room: Women, Power and Spiritualism in Late Victorian England* (Philadelphia, 1990); W. Mitchinson, 'Hysteria and Insanity in Women: A Nineteenth-Century Canadian Perspective', *Journal of Canadian Studies* 21:3 (1986), pp. 87–105; H. Small, *Love's Madness: Medicine, the Novel, and Female Insanity, 1800–1865* (Oxford, 1996); J.M. Ussher, *Women's Madness: Misogyny or Mental Illness?* (Amherst, 1992); A.D. Wood, '"The Fashionable Diseases": Women's Complaints and their Treatment in Nineteenth-Century America', *Journal of Interdisciplinary History* 4:1 (1973), pp. 25–52.

29 E. Showalter, *The Female Malady: Women, Madness, and English Culture, 1830–1980* (New York, 1985).

30 She identifies three clear male icons: the mad genius, the criminal lunatic, and the sexual deviant. J. Busfield, 'The Female Malady? Men, Women and Madness in Nineteenth Century Britain', *Sociology* 28:1 (1994), pp. 269, 275.

31 See for example: J. Andrews and A. Digby (eds), *Sex and Seclusion, Class and Custody: Perspectives on Gender and Class in the History of British and Irish Psychiatry* (Amsterdam, 2004); L. Hide, *Gender and Class in English Asylums, 1890–1914* (Basingstoke, 2014); K. Rawling, 'Visualising Mental Illness: Gender, Medicine and Visual Media, c1850–1910' (PhD Dissertation, University of London, Royal Holloway College, 2011); A. Shepherd, *Institutionalizing the Insane in Nineteenth-Century England* (London, 2014).

32 While men are rarely confined to actual basements in literature, their madness was often fully on display in the private sphere. See H. Goodman, 'Madness in Marriage: Erotomania and Marital Rape in *He Knew He Was Right* and *The Forsyte Saga*', *Victorian Network* 4:2 (2012), pp. 47–71; W. Hughes, *The Maniac in the Cellar: Sensation Novels of the 1860s* (Princeton, 1980), pp. 45, 61.

33 S. Dudink, K. Hagemann, and A. Clark, 'Historicizing Male Citizenship', in S. Dudink, K. Hagemann, and A. Clark (eds), *Representing Masculinity: Male Citizenship in Modern Western Culture* (Houndmills, 2007), p. x.

34 See for example: J. Goldstein, 'The Uses of Male Hysteria: Medical and Literary Discourse in Nineteenth-Century France', *Representations* 34 (1991), pp. 134–65; H. Goodman, '"Madness and Masculinity": Male Patients in London Asylums and Victorian Culture', in T. Knowles and S. Trowbridge (eds), *Insanity and the Lunatic Asylum in the Nineteenth Century* (London, 2016), pp. 149–66; J.S. Hughes, 'The Madness of Separate Spheres: Insanity and Masculinity in Victorian Alabama', in M.C. Carnes and C. Griffen (eds), *Meanings for Manhood: Constructions of Masculinity in Victorian America* (Chicago, 1990), pp. 53–66; M. Kavka, 'Ill but Manly: Male Hysteria in Late Nineteenth-Century Medical Discourse', *Nineteenth Century Prose* 25:1 (1998), pp. 116–39; K. Makras, '"The Poison that Upsets my Reason": Men, Madness and Drunkenness in the Victorian Period', in Knowles and Trowbridge (eds), *Insanity and the Lunatic Asylum*, pp. 135–48; M. Micale, 'Charcot and the Idea of Hysteria in the Male: Gender, Mental Science, and Mental Diagnosis in Late Nineteenth-Century France', *Medical History* 34:4 (1990), pp. 363–411; V. Pedlar, '*The Most Dreadful Visitation*': *Male Madness in Victorian Fiction* (Liverpool, 2006); J. Shepherd, '"I Am Not Very Well I Feel Nearly Mad When I Think of You": Male Jealousy, Murder and Broadmoor in Late-Victorian Britain', *Social History of Medicine* 30:2 (2017), pp. 277–98; Stephens, 'Pathologizing Leaky Male Bodies', pp. 421–38.

35 M. Critchley and E.A. Critchley, *John Hughlings Jackson: Father of English Neurology* (Oxford, 1998).

36 L. Farquharson, 'A "Scottish Poor Law of Lunacy"? Poor Law, Lunacy Law and Scotland's Parochial Asylums', *History of Psychiatry* 28:1 (2017), pp. 15–28; R.A. Houston, 'Rights and Wrongs in the Confinement of the Mentally Incapable in Eighteenth-Century Scotland', *Continuity and Change* 18:3 (2003), pp. 373–94.

37 C. Rosenberg, 'Contested Boundaries: Psychiatry, Disease, and Diagnosis', *Perspectives in Biology and Medicine* 49:3 (2006), p. 411.

38 C. Rosenberg, 'The Tyranny of Diagnosis: Specific Entities and Individual Experience', *Milbank Quarterly* 80:2 (2002), pp. 239–40.
39 T. Gomory, D. Cohen, and S.A. Kirk, 'Madness or Mental Illness? Revisiting Historians of Psychiatry', *Current Psychology* 32:2 (2013), p. 122.
40 P. Mandler, 'The Problem with Cultural History', *Cultural and Social History* 1:1 (2004), pp. 96–97.
41 C. Grandy, 'Cultural History's Absent Audience', *Cultural and Social History* 16:5 (2019), pp. 643–63.
42 C. Rosenberg, 'Introduction: Framing Disease', in Rosenberg and Golden (eds), *Framing Disease*, pp. xiii–xv.
43 M. Roper, 'Slipping Out of View: Subjectivity and Emotion in Gender History', *History Workshop Journal* 59:1 (2005), pp. 58, 62–63, 67.
44 M. Roper and J. Tosh, 'Introduction', in M. Roper and J. Tosh (eds), *Manful Assertions: Masculinities in Britain since 1800* (London, 1991), p. 14.
45 H. Sussman, *Victorian Masculinities: Manhood and Masculine Poetics in Early Victorian Literature and Art* (Cambridge, 1995), pp. 14–15.
46 H. Goodman, 'Mad Men: Borderlines of Insanity, Masculinity and Emotion in Victorian Literature and Culture' (PhD Dissertation, University of London, Royal Holloway College, 2015), p. 42.
47 F.B. Alberti, 'Introduction: Medical History and Emotion Theory', in F.B. Alberti (ed.), *Medicine, Emotion, and Disease, 1700–1950* (Basingstoke, 2006), pp. xiii–l; Marland, *Dangerous Motherhood*; P. Stearns and C. Stearns, 'Emotionology: Clarifying the History of Emotions and Emotional Standards', *American Historical Review* 90:4 (1985), pp. 813–36.
48 A. Beveridge, 'Life in the Asylum: Patients' Letters from Morningside, 1873–1908', *History of Psychiatry* 9:36 (1998), pp. 431–69; A. Beveridge, 'Voices of the Mad: Patients' Letters from the Royal Edinburgh Asylum, 1873–1908', *Psychological Medicine* 27:4 (1997), pp. 899–908; J. Shepherd, 'Life for the Families of the Victorian Criminally Insane', *Historical Journal* 63:3 (2020), pp. 603–32; L. Smith, '"Your Very Thankful Inmate": Discovering the Patients of an Early County Lunatic Asylum', *Social History of Medicine* 21:2 (2008), pp. 237–52.
49 M. McDonald, 'Madness, Suicide, and the Computer', in R. Porter and A. Wear (eds), *Problems and Methods in the History of Medicine* (New York, 1987), p. 210.
50 The family is the place where men's physical and mental selves are formed. L. Davidoff, *Worlds Between: Historical Perspectives on Gender and Class* (Cambridge, 1995), p. 229.

51 C. Coleborne, 'Families, Patients and Emotions: Asylums for the Insane in Colonial Australia and New Zealand, c. 1880–1910', *Social History of Medicine* 19:3 (2006), pp. 425–42; M. Kelm, 'Women, Families and the Provincial Hospital for the Insane, British Columbia, 1905–1915', *Journal of Family History* 19:2 (1994), pp. 177–93; B. Labrum, 'Looking Beyond the Asylum: Gender and the Process of Committal in Auckland, 1870–1910', *New Zealand Journal of History* 26 (1992), pp. 125–44; M. Levine-Clark, 'Dysfunctional Domesticity: Female Insanity and Family Relationships Among the West Riding Poor in the Mid-Nineteenth Century', *Journal of Family History* 25:3 (2000): pp. 341–61; G. Reaume, *Remembrance of Patients Past: Patient Life at the Toronto Hospital for the Insane, 1870–1940* (Toronto, 2000).

52 Mad studies as a discipline is highly grounded in contemporary issues and influenced by the anti-psychiatry movement. My work is not grounded in those politics per se, but rather focuses on the lived experiences, histories, and cultures of those who were identified as 'mad', rather than self-identifying. B. LeFrancois, R. Menzies, and G. Reaume, *Mad Matters: A Critical Reader in Canadian Mad Studies* (Toronto, 2013).

53 K. Bourrier, *The Measure of Manliness: Disability and Masculinity in the Mid-Victorian Novel* (Ann Arbor, 2015), p. 17.

54 J. Begiato, 'Between Poise and Power: Embodied Manliness in Eighteenth- and Nineteenth-Century British Culture', *Transactions of the Royal Historical Society* 26 (2016), p. 127.

55 Over 340 records were sampled from Bethlem's casebooks. A smaller sample of 50 cases were chosen from Glasgow Royal Lunatic Asylum as a comparison with the Bethlem hospital. Over 20 cases from Broadmoor were studied that related to high-profile or controversial patients. This project is not an asylum history, but it is vital to understand the asylum archive as part of the larger context.

56 Manor House casebooks have been digitized by the Wellcome Archive (although after this research was completed) and thus should be of interest to even more scholars moving forward. C. MacKenzie, *Psychiatry for the Rich: A History of Ticehurst Private Asylum 1792–1917* (London, 1993).

57 Hide, *Gender and Class in English Asylums*.

58 Andrews and Digby commend scholarship in the early 2000s balancing research that solely focused on women's mental health, but called for more explorations of class among the incarcerated and their institutional settings. J. Andrews and A. Digby, 'Introduction: Gender and Class in the Historiography of British and Irish Psychiatry', in Andrews and Digby (eds), *Sex and Seclusion, Class and Custody*, pp. 18–19.

59 If a person had property worth over £1,000 or an annual income of more than £50, then their heirs or relatives could petition the Lord Chancellor for an inquiry into whether a person was of sound mind. As of 1845, proceedings in Chancery took place before two Masters in Lunacy, sitting with a jury of laymen who could preside at hearings. J. Oppenheim, *'Shattered Nerves': Doctors, Patients, and Depression in Victorian England* (New York, 1991), p. 71.

60 Admitted in 1884, he was released relieved in 1885. The case notes record he had a cousin who also died insane, and there seemed little hope or sympathy for his rehabilitation. House surgeon's notes for physician: Male, Records of Glasgow Royal Lunatic Asylum, HB 13/5/63.

61 *Copy of the Fifteenth Report of the Commissioners in Lunacy to the Lord Chancellor,* 1861, p. 70.

62 P. Fennell, *Treatment Without Consent: Law, Psychiatry and the Treatment of Mentally Disordered People Since 1845* (London, 1996), p. 5.

63 T.S. Clouston, 'Lunacy Law', *The Times* (3 January 1885), pp. 3–4; M.D., 'Lunacy Law', *The Times* (5 January 1885), p. 4; 'Supreme Court of Judicature', *The Times* (30 March 1885), p. 3; Lord Shaftesbury, 'Lord Shaftesbury and the New Lunacy Bill', *The Times* (9 April 1885), p. 12. The government fell; however, the Bill was withdrawn and Shaftesbury resumed his chairmanship of the Lunacy Commission. G. Finlayson, *The Seventh Earl of Shaftesbury, 1801–1885* (Vancouver, 1981), pp. 590–92.

64 M.D., 'Lunacy Law', *The Times* (5 January 1885), p. 4.

1

Men in care: the asylum

> The philanthropic views of the British Legislature and the British nation were at length realized. Harsh usage and irritating coercion gave way to mildness, forbearance, and indulgence, and the wretched inmates of this asylum of mental derangement were liberated from unnecessary violence, intimidation, and solitary confinement.[1]

John Haslam described the nineteenth-century asylum through rose-coloured glasses; the humane asylum doctor liberated patients from shackles into an era of enlightened and compassionate care.[2] While Haslam advocated a system of moral treatment, the realities at Bethlem were hardly the vision he painted in 1823. It would take decades to construct a system built on the hope and optimism that there was a humane and scientific way to treat the mad. While a nationwide system of asylums was built by mid-century, the next fifty years were devoted to figuring out the implications of this early work, including the fallout when asylums continued to expand while failing to meet their early promises.

While this text follows the recent historiographical shift to decentre the asylum from the history of mental health care, it is impossible to ignore asylums as they loomed large in both patient experience and the cultural understanding of madness for men and women. The rise of the asylum in the second half of the nineteenth century is astounding. At mid-century there were twelve thousand patients living in asylums as a result of the 1845 Lunatic Asylum and Pauper Lunatics Act, rising to a hundred thousand by 1900.[3] Most registered lunatics ended up spending at least some time in an asylum. The asylum was the medical and governmental response to the 'problem' of lunacy, and thus it plays an essential role in the culture of men's madness. Many opinions of the asylum are a microcosm of views of lunacy in general. This chapter does not attempt to be a comprehensive account, but rather explores issues that were particularly salient to men's gendered experiences.

Over the past decades, historians have unpacked Victorians' overly optimistic view of their asylums: from micro-histories of individual asylums to sweeping surveys of the changing nature of madhouses and the ideologies shaping institutionalization. In a recent review of asylum literature, Robert Houston offers a comprehensive, nuanced account of the asylum from the nineteenth and twentieth centuries.[4] Such overviews highlight the variety of approaches over time and by different disciplines, and the complicated negotiation between doctors, patients, and families over care. Other scholars have aptly described the medical rationalization of treatment and the shifting architecture and internal management of asylums.[5] The pauper asylum has been thoroughly explained both as part of larger government programmes and as part of institutional histories. Institutions that dealt with idiocy are the focus of their own thriving scholarly subfield.[6] Recent historical studies highlight the importance of gender and class in shaping all aspects of institutional life.[7] Gender is now an intrinsic part of many asylum studies, even when not the main focus.[8]

Research for this chapter is grounded in a variety of institutional, government, and medical sources. Annual Lunacy Commissioner reports were the official record of the asylum system, and often sparked public debate and comment. Experiences of asylum life are drawn from a number of hospitals and asylums to give a sense of the diversity of patient experiences; however, the richest asylum archival source is from Manor House, a private asylum based in Chiswick with no constraints of funding or size.[9] Manor House was, by its nature, exclusive and unique. Records of Bethlem and Glasgow Royal hospitals include men of a much wider range of economic backgrounds and provide relatively robust archives. Records from Broadmoor, the criminal lunatic asylum, add men from across the economic spectrum who were deemed dangerous to others. The archives of the pauper asylum have not been included but have been admirably studied elsewhere.[10] To connect the social history of the asylum to broader social and cultural representations, newspaper accounts, memoirs, and medical texts offer a window into the public discourse on asylum life.

The asylum is a microcosm of many larger questions about madness posed throughout the book. This chapter begins with brief overview of the rationale and philosophy of the asylum system. As work by Melling and Forsythe demonstrates, the asylum is part of the society that created it, 'a corridor between civil society and the state along which different groups met to negotiate'.[11] Men's particular place in that asylum system was significant, and in a highly gender-segregated system they were recognized as a distinct group in the asylum. Laws and policies surrounding confinement varied by nation, by class, and by type of mental distress. Men were taken out of their homes and workspaces, sometimes against their will, and placed in an enforced site of passive convalescence.

This chapter will briefly explore the institutional and legal frameworks of asylums, and men's standing within asylums across the nation. The focus of the chapter will be the particular challenges men faced in the asylum, and the particular negative associations of the asylum. While doctors and reformers attempted to destigmatize the asylum, these actions were undercut by larger social messaging. The next section focuses on how the experience of institutionalization challenged men's gendered identity on a personal level, and often destabilized family power dynamics. No matter the social background of the men involved, the decision to seek asylum care led to enormous tension and uncertainty. While few people enjoyed mandatory incarceration, for men the lack of control in determining their care undermined masculine authority across class boundaries. The final section details the issues of men and violence in the asylum. While media reports focused on madmen as sources of violence, the asylum also made patients the potential victims of violence. The asylum undercut men's gendered identity in a variety of ways, while demanding men live up to masculine ideals to prove recovery.

Paths to the asylum: laws and regulations of confinement

The roots of the nineteenth-century asylum system started in the eighteenth century. There were concerns that rich patients were being unjustly locked away in private madhouses by greedy relatives and corrupt owners. There was also a growing concern that the pauper insane were not being cared for in the hodgepodge system of workhouses, gaols, and lunatic hospitals, nor when they were left to wander the streets or be chained in private homes.[12] The asylums built in the first decades of the nineteenth century were set up to treat those with serious mental problems. People were singled out who were at serious risk of harming themselves, other people, or property. There were eventually four main types of institutions in Britain based on class and actions: private asylums, hospitals, pauper asylums, and criminal asylums. The large county pauper asylums took in the largest number of patients who needed care or were disruptive to the community.[13] The reformed Victorian asylum tried to ensure that only certified lunatics would be placed in asylums, and there was continual movement in and out of institutions. The ease of passing in and out of asylums was significantly shaped by wealth and family situation. Pauper asylums were most likely to discharge and private asylums least likely based on financial incentives. Other factors included severity of symptoms and the ability of families to care for ill relatives.

There were a number of significant national differences across the United Kingdom, both in the foundation of asylums and in their practice. Ireland was actually the first of the four nations to institute mandatory legislation providing asylums for the mad in 1817.[14] The 1808 County Asylums Act laid the groundwork of a system of publicly funded asylums in England and Wales that became mandatory in 1845. The county lunatic asylum system was quickly overwhelmed, and paupers continued to be sent to private systems for decades.[15] The Scottish were last to institute dramatic changes. Inspired by the 1855 Lunacy Commission Inquiry that revealed deplorable conditions for pauper lunatics, they introduced their own Act in 1857, although many counties resisted setting up their own district asylums into the 1870s.[16] Scottish asylums were in the 1860s the first to allow lunatics to be admitted on a voluntary basis; England and Wales only allowed the practice beginning in 1890. [17] However, it was rarely used outside Scotland until the Mental Treatment Act of 1930.[18] No system was without problems, and the differences between national systems could create substantial confusion for families navigating the system.

Specialists in mental ailments had increasing faith that the best place for the insane was in a well-regulated asylum.[19] In 1846, leading expert Forbes Winslow believed that most forms of insanity, if caught early, had a 90 per cent recovery rate in an asylum. It was only in cases of congenital disease, or physical damage to the brain, that there was little hope of cure.[20] Writing almost a decade later, Matthew Mather wrote that 'We cannot prevent insanity from making its inroads; but we can, by judicious treatment, allay its evils, and even produce a cure.'[21] While many authors have noted that few public asylums lived up to the ideals of moral treatment, for smaller asylums and those catering to the middle and upper classes, the dream of holistic and individualized treatment remained much longer.[22] And for doctors, though their optimism about cures may have diminished over the course of the century, they still had faith in the asylum over other alternatives.[23]

Asylums were sometimes discussed as if they were universal institutions; however, the experience of the asylum was highly dictated by gender, class, geography, symptoms, and family circumstances at every step. The system of asylums continued to be a patchwork solution to insanity. The Lunacy Commission oversaw most lunatics in asylums, but there was far more diversity in the system than they would have liked. The asylums themselves varied dramatically, from enormous institutions housing thousands of people, to small, private spaces that resembled country homes more than hospitals. Yet all patients who spent time in asylums shared certain experiences of institutionalization.

Men and the asylum

Elaine Showalter asserts that, by the 1850s, women made up the majority of the inmate population of asylums. While statistics are not central to her argument, she does emphasize the large number of women in asylums as part of a larger claim about the prevalent cultural connection of women and madness in nineteenth-century England.[24] Showalter is technically correct, in that women outnumbered men in most lunacy statistics. However, her statistics did not count military asylums or criminal asylums that were overwhelmingly male. With the addition of these populations, in 1849 certified lunatics were 48 per cent male and 52 per cent female. By 1903 they were 46 per cent male and 54 per cent female. As Joan Busfield notes, these figures did not consider population ratios, length of stay, cure rates and discharge, or mortality rates.[25] The actual difference in numbers is small, and not indicative of a plague of women being locked away by a misogynist culture as some early feminist scholars implied. This does not mean that some women were not unjustly detained, nor that husbands did not try to lock up their problematic wives.[26] Given the gendered power imbalance in Victorian society, it is perhaps surprising that there is not more of a difference in confinement rates. However, it is clear that male lunatics made up a substantial proportion of the asylum population.

The Commissioners in Lunacy were well aware of the gender imbalance of lunatics. All figures in their statistical enumerations of asylums, private care, types of insanity, and so on, were always broken down by sex. And in 1903 they could report that women had always made up a higher proportion of asylum inmates than men in relative and absolute terms. Yet, even then, the Lunacy Commissioners were aware that these numbers were more complicated than they first appeared. Total numbers under care are not as reliable as looking at number of annual admissions. From 1897 to 1901 admissions were 48.7 per cent male and 51.3 per cent female. They explained this discrepancy by the higher death rate among male lunatics, and that 'the excess of females in the insane population is mainly a matter of survival'.[27] Statistics gathered by the Lunacy Commission also consistently demonstrated a lower recovery rate for men vs women, averaging only 35 per cent to women's 43 per cent recovery rate between 1873 and 1903.[28]

The asylum system was highly regulated by gender, with separate wings and even separate institutions for men and women. In attempts to mimic domestic settings, men's and women's sections were given appropriate colourations, furnishings, and ornaments.[29] Asylum researchers have proven how and when people were sent to the asylum varied widely, influenced by factors as varied as gender, marital status, specific family histories, and living arrangements.[30] Men ended up in asylums through a variety of paths dependent on their actions, their symptoms, their family situation, and their level of wealth. Ideally for Victorian administrators for most of the century, asylums were also divided by class, as by the late 1850s the wealthy were insistent on the continued need for separate institutions for those who could pay.[31] But what all asylums had in common, from

Britain's largest lunatic asylum at Colney Hatch to the most luxurious private asylum at Ticehurst, was the confinement.[32]

The stigma of incarceration

While Victorian reformers tried to emphasize that mental disease was an illness like any physical illness, it was only the mad who were subject to 'compulsory and coercive medical treatment, usually under conditions of confinement and forfeiture of civil rights'.[33] The experience of being sent to an asylum, sometimes against their will, was particularly destabilizing for men who were used to being in control of themselves and their families. Many patients, and their families, were not ready to face the reality of a lunacy diagnosis, and thus hoped for any other solution. And while the broader connections of shame and lunacy will be outlined in chapter 3, the particular stigma of the asylum will be the focus of this section.

In the various debates about changing legislation for lunacy, the particular problems of the stigma of institutionalization had a direct influence on policy. Many commentators feared that if certification and confinement were in any way publicized, it would make wealthy families less likely to seek help. Any push to publicize lunacy proceedings always met opposition because of this desire to conceal insanity among wealthy families. The oft-suggested remedy to wrongful incarceration that suggested all patients needed to see a magistrate, court judge, or some public official before certification was met with absolute contempt by opponents:

> Any proceedings of this nature would be distressingly painful to the feelings of friends of a patient, if not of himself. The publicity incurred would cause many to shrink from the exposure, the consequence of which would be that dangerous lunatics would be suffered to be at large, and curable cases become chronic and hopeless for the want of proper treatment.[34]

The shame of a lunacy diagnosis made any further publicity anathema.

Asylum care for the poor was framed as a humane act of kindness. And while scholars have noted the intense shame that a mad relative could bring to a family, the focus has typically been on wealthy men.[35] However, recourse to the public asylum could bring just as much humiliation to a poor man. As Peter Bartlett notes, the pauper lunatic was the product of the Poor Law administrators who oversaw the identification, diagnosis, and commitment of lunatics.[36] The New Poor Law instituted the workhouse as a symbol of indignity.[37] One of the explicit goals of the county asylums' legislation was supposed to be the removal of lunatics from workhouses. Yet there was little discussion to end the practice of having pauper lunatics filtered through the workhouse infirmary, thus linking the two institutions.[38] Economically comfortable working-class men could feel an extra humiliation at the prospect of a public asylum that started in a workhouse. Doctor Joseph Mortimer Granville at least recognized this problem; he noted that for a respectable working man, the environment of a workhouse, 'if [he has] any wits about [him] what a depressing scene that must be, [and it] certainly wouldn't seem to help towards his recovery'.[39] Despite this, for those without means the workhouse was the typical first point of call. And in fact, later in the century, there was official acceptance that the workhouse infirmaries could be the appropriate place to deal with harmless and chronic lunatics permanently. The specific mortification of the experience of the workhouse-to-asylum pathway is worthy of note.

The workhouse was the ultimate proof of a man's failure in his role as provider and head of household. A man's ability not only to provide for, but also to control his family was paramount to a masculine identity in the nineteenth century. As Megan Doolittle notes, 'Providing for a dependent wife and children and exercising authority over them had long been a significant marker of adult masculinity and continued to be so during this period despite the many changes in nineteenth-century labour markets and family strategies.'[40] But a man who was confined to a pauper asylum was denied the ability to support his family, and instead was dependent on the support of the state as a pauper lunatic. Moreover, while the decision to enter a workhouse was typically a desperate one, it was typically the man's decision. When a lunatic was forced to enter an asylum, they often had little say in the matter, though they could have certainly had awareness and sometimes anger at the process happening around them.

Authorities advocated for separation by class in the asylum, believing it was necessary for recovery. In a society highly stratified in all forms of life, it must have seemed strange that the asylum offered two options (registered hospitals filled only a small portion of the gap between luxury and pauper accommodation). The Lunacy Commissioners noted that needs far outstretched existing resources for the middle classes. Some were housed in institutions with paupers, paying a fee for superior treatment and the ability to socialize among their own class. Yet these compromised solutions were routinely condemned.[41] Families would often pool as many resources as they could to try a private asylum for a few months, but without a speedy cure such patients ended up transferred to county asylums sometimes with their families reduced to ruin.[42] The county asylum was competent to deal with the mad labourer, but authorities truly believed the educated classes would find them a torture.[43] One physician wrote that mingling patients of different classes impeded treatment. He believed even if patients were kept separate, it would be 'galling' to the middle-class patients and damaging to their self-respect to live among paupers.[44] The stigma of the county asylum was even greater for middle-class men than their working-class peers.

Within the asylum, officials acknowledged that embarrassment was the natural sentiment of a man sent to an asylum, no matter his class. In fact, should a man not be somewhat humiliated by his condition, then this could be seen as a symptom of disease. On his admission to Manor House, John Price Carritt spoke quite directly about striking people in the street for no reason and he had no shame in his having done so. He admitted his mother had begged him not to act as he did, and while realizing he had been a great trouble to his friends, he was not bothered by his actions. He was happy to go where the medical staff told him and did not mind the asylum.[45] While doctors officially tried to lessen the stigma of insanity, even they believed men should feel some sort of discomfiture in being confined. There were few ways to fully reconcile the experience of forced institutionalization and masculine self-worth.

Families, asylums, and the loss of autonomy

Andrew Scull explains that families turned to the public asylum as the result of the modern demands of the workplace that left them neither the time nor the resources to provide such care.[46] The increasing number of pauper lunatics in workhouses and asylums across the second half of the century testifies to the financial burden a mad relative could place on a family. And yet while it may be true that some poor families welcomed the advent of the asylum as a way to relieve their burden, there was not a universal adoption of the asylum, and Scull's explanation does not describe the complex care decisions made by families. One cannot assume that the growth of asylum admissions across the nineteenth century reflects a universalizing power of the state, or an abrogation of familial connections.[47] Some turned to the asylum out of a belief it was the best site of care. And despite recourse to the asylum, many families were anxious to have their loved ones home as soon as possible, no matter the economic considerations.[48] The particularities of family dynamics, the quality of local care available, the particular symptoms and needs of the sufferer, and local public opinion would all have played as much of a role in decisions about patient care as the shifting patterns of industrial work.

For male patients, insanity radically upset traditional power structures within the family. Certification forms often reveal men protesting their family's assessments of their mental status. Those same documents demonstrate how family members most often started the process of institutionalization, and families gave relevant information as to symptoms. For example, Charles Boorman was admitted to Bethlem asylum in 1884. His doctors note he had a wandering mind, was marked by impulsivity, and would confuse people's names. It was family who provided the more troubling symptoms, as it was only his father who heard the young man's suicidal declarations and had witnessed his attempt to drown himself.[49] Admission documents were as much family documents as they were medical assessments.

Families often had very challenging choices on when and whether to send a loved one to an asylum. Physicians acknowledged that it was quite 'difficult to draw the boundary line between what are commonly considered purely nervous maladies, and diseases of the mind'.[50] In a conflict between patients and doctors, families could be awkwardly in the middle. William Knowles, a forty-five-year-old married man with eleven children, clearly fought the doctors and his family on care decisions. At the first sign of mental distress he insisted on travel instead of institutional care. After becoming violent and difficult to manage he was sent to Manor House, where he was furious at being detained. Knowles challenged his doctors at every turn and tried to remain the patriarch of his family.[51]

While doctors and family members were not willing to acquiesce to all of Knowles's demands, he was still kept within his social and familial circles as much as possible. His wife visited often, as did other members of his family and friends. Knowles sent his wife abusive letters and telegrams, pleading for his release. Men were often horrified to learn their mail was being monitored, or in some cases not sent out to its intended recipients. Knowles's desperation to communicate with his wife unobserved was so strong that he once threw a letter over the wall to be posted by a passer-by. Asylum authorities eventually had to restrict his movements after he sent a telegram to his wife instructing her to pick him up from the asylum and bring him his gun and ten cartridges (with instructions on where to find them). In this case, despite his incarceration, Knowles believed his power within the family remained unchallenged. He instructs his wife in one letter, 'Don't listen to what people tell you to do but do as I tell you if you still care for me at all.'[52] Knowles tried to retain his autonomy by attempting to threaten and harass his wife to bend to his will.

When attempting to trace patient autonomy within the Victorian asylum, historians face a particularly challenging task. Not only did lunatics face the normal power imbalance existing in any coercive institution, but most patients had the added disadvantage that they were suffering significant mental distress.[53] It is overly simplistic to view the patient as either a completely independent agent or an absolute subject of medical power.[54] Patients leave indelible marks within their communities and societies. 'The Foucauldian idea that madmen have always been "outside of history" is just one side of the story. In fact, we could even argue that patients have never talked more than after having been reduced to silence.'[55] Where patients' voices are recorded, it is even more clear that doctor–patient relations were always about negotiated treatments. This is even more true in private hospitals or asylums where doctors and patients had similar educational or class backgrounds.[56] Male patients in particular were expected to demand their independence as a healthy expression of manliness, no matter their level of illness. As John Home's letters as a patient at the Royal Edinburgh Asylum make clear, it was difficult to maintain autonomy when almost all elements of life were regulated.[57]

We know about individual patients in the asylums largely because case notes were required for every patient after 1845, forming a large 'discourse of practice'. Asylums were required at admission to record patients' name, age, marital status, sex, physical description, and an outline of symptoms. Entries were required once a week for the first month, and then once a month for cases deemed curable, and four times a year for the incurables.[58] Despite these requirements, casebooks often had numerous blank spaces because of a lack of information or clarity. Case notes could be cursory at best, often simply describing patients as the 'same' for years, or the cause of their illness listed as 'unknown'. Despite the illusion of standardization, case notes are hardly reliable or consistent archives of data.[59] Asylums varied their methods of entry, and vague or descriptive terms were common rather than exceptions. Case notes throw light on many things, but they can never be read as an objective truth.[60]

It was not uncommon for men to rage against their involuntary treatment because they believed they were not ill. Arthur Richard Wilde was admitted to Manor House Asylum in November 1884 at the age of twenty-one. He was a theology student whose family said his symptoms had been coming on for months after he received a severe shock walking in Switzerland. His parents worried he was suicidal and forced him into treatment. Yet Wilde would not admit suicidal intentions, despite proof he had bitten his own arms, secreted away a knife, and drunk a bottle of lotion marked poison. At Manor House he varied between seeming improvement and violent attacks on himself and others, often requiring two attendants to watch over him at night. He was desperate to return home, and clearly frustrated at being incarcerated. His only recorded explanation for his violence against the attendants was 'I must struggle.' After two months in the asylum his violence subdued to the point he was transferred to Bethlem asylum, relieved.[61] At Bethlem asylum he was incredibly withdrawn, and he strongly denied having any delusions or hallucinations to the doctors.[62] Clearly his anger remained, however. Case notes reveal that he tried to strangle an attendant after his transfer.[63] He was discharged as recovered on 30 September 1885.[64]

Case notes of Manor House record negotiations between patients and the medical staff over choices of treatment, the ability to go on temporary leave, and patients' own personal servants. While Alfred Hood had no choice in his family's decision to send him to Manor House, he did insist on hiring his own valet at a very high wage. It seemed that Hood was pleased not only to get his way, but also enjoyed 'perpetually watching the man' to ensure he did not do any tasks for other patients.[65] Many men remained keenly aware of their class position and were careful of any abrogation of their status. Henry Hadley was placed in Manor House on an emergency order in 1911. On admission he was described as unkempt, dirty, with filthy linens and black teeth. His few months at the asylum did little to change his habits, and he believed he was absolutely normal. He still had a clear sense of his own rank and station even as he refused to bathe. He agreed to a transfer to Brislington House Asylum only if he could travel in a first-class carriage.[66] Keeping up the appearances of class was a way to maintain a sense of personal dignity.

In some cases, complaints about private asylums more closely resembled complaints of bad service at a hotel or club rather than a lunatic asylum. Ernest William Radford was admitted to Manor House Asylum on an emergency order. He was initially violent and noisy. There are six letters from Radford preserved in the casebook, varying in levels of clarity and legibility. He complains about the circumstances of his admission to the asylum rather than the fact of being institutionalized itself. He wrote to his wife complaining about being forced to travel in a third-class train carriage to get to the asylum as 'The stink of the trains has made me sick.' Another note complains in the form of a prose poem about food and alcohol choices: 'And as for champagne he feels rather poor/ When he sees one small bottle divided in four.' Radford exercised his autonomy through his complaints, even as his wife was told to avoid visiting in person.[67] Radford clearly had a strong sense of his personal dignity intact, but saw the conditions of the asylum, rather than the incarceration itself, as the main personal affront. He was later released as cured and held no demonstrable ill will after the fact.[68]

Martin Jaffe was largely defined by his constant complaints. He was diagnosed with mania and involuntary acts of violence. He tried numerous types of treatment, including as a voluntary boarder, as resident of doctors' houses, and at six asylums within five years. Numerous times the police responded to his violent acts. Certificates were eventually signed in 1899 after he was arrested for an attack where he smashed the windows of a newspaper office and house. He complained frequently to the staff of Manor House and the Lunacy Commissioners, and wrote to the Lord Chancellor complaining he had been improperly institutionalized. He was a difficult patient, complaining of many issues but also attempting to bribe servants, playing on the delusions of other patients and encouraging them to escape. The case notes reveal the doctors' frustration as they complain 'His love of making mischief is remarkable and he does this under the name of philanthropy.' Yet such a note also demonstrates that Jaffe was aware of his actions and believed he was doing them for the betterment of other patients. Truly believing many were not insane, he was trying to advocate for his own and other patients' rights. Without having to make a judgement on the actual state of his mind, many of his actions were clear attempts to assert his autonomy.[69]

To what degree lunatics were conscious of their own fates was a matter of debate at the time. Medical author Alfred Swaine Taylor believed that only a small number of those suffering insanity were 'aware of their condition and lament it' unless it was in the early onset of disease, or when convalescent.[70] Yet others came away with a different impression. After a tour of Bethlem in 1860, where George Augustus Sala was generally impressed by the amenities and care on offer for the mad, the author was still left to lament the patients' fate.

> Save only when in an excess of frenzy, I believe that all mad people are conscious of, and possessed by, a sense of the unutterable wretchedness of their lot – of their doom to seek and search for continually that which, God help them! they seldom find on this side of the grave – their wits.[71]

One former asylum inmate insisted that most patients were well aware of their constrained status and understood their lack of freedom in spite of delusions and frenzy.[72]

First-person accounts testify to how being incarcerated was a blow to men whose minds were well enough to understand their situation. A former inmate of the Glasgow Royal Lunatic Asylum wrote his memoirs to make sense of his experiences, give himself some agency through the process, and try to lessen some of the stigma. The anonymous author asserts he recognized he had a problem when he began experiencing delusions, and that he sought help out of fear he would injure those he loved. Despite recognizing his position, it did little to allay the horror of the experience. 'It is a fearful thing for a man to be mad, and to be conscious that he is so.'[73] He acknowledges he was not in control of his disease at the Glasgow asylum, and that he needed to be incarcerated. His tale offers no apologies, nor does he try to pretend he was in control. However, he regains some sense of authority by his decision to seek help and offering advice to others on how to stave off madness. He includes detailed characterizations of types of madness he observed, and explains to his readers that there should be no stigma on either a mad person or their family. 'Lunacy, like rain, falls upon the evil and the good.'[74]

The voices of working-class patients in pauper asylums are even harder to find in the archive. However, scholars have found patterns of patient rebellion and disobedience in their actions, if not their words. The refusal to cooperate could take many forms, including not speaking, refusing to attend religious service, and resisting work. While some might have been symptoms of disease, doctors often noted cases of what they believed was plain obstinance.[75] The destruction of clothing was sometimes used as an indicator by medical authorities of the level of patients' mental distress. Baur and Melling contend that it might also be seen as a revolt against the conformity of the asylum system.[76] Jennifer Wallis uncovered evidence at the West Riding Lunatic Asylum of patients taking an active interest in their original histories recorded in the casebook, sometimes helping with an examination, or disagreeing with statements made. Such data demonstrate that patients were more aware of doctors' assessments than might be expected.[77]

Those most likely to see confinement in an asylum as an abrogation of autonomy, no matter their class, were those who did not believe they were significantly ill. One tailor was charged with threatening murder. At trial he was outraged that his counsel believed him to be insane. He wrote a letter outlining his grievances that was read aloud in court to prove his sanity. But to court reporters it seemed 'a rambling narrative of supposed wrongs, and [the] prisoner constantly interrupted, and was eventually removed from the dock'.[78] Men who felt themselves sane found the prospect of an asylum all the more galling. It is important to acknowledge that to many members of the general public, the asylum was seen as an essentially oppressive space and its patients as victims. According to one advocate, the lunatic had less rights than a criminal:

> [W]hereas, on the plea of insanity, he can be confined without at all knowing by whom this wrong is perpetrated, on what pretext, or by whose authority; and as the law has oddly provided that he can only be liberated by the order of the party who has been the means of depriving him of liberty, without any hope of ever being released except in his coffin, and until a man who is suspected of being a lunatic is allowed to claim a public trial of his sanity, these glaring abuses will still be perpetrated.[79]

No matter a man's mental distress, a significant anti-asylum discourse framed institutionalization as an absolute and unjust abrogation of autonomy.

Patients, doctors, and outsiders often had completely different impressions of what proved or disproved insanity. Observers were also prepared to admit that the utterances of the mad could prove a mix of entirely sound and unsound opinion. In the case of one man, 'a military gentleman, of an educated and elegant mind', doctors found he could write 'letters full of exquisite criticism on art, and just comments on topics of the day, with obscene ribaldry concerning the highest person in the land'.[80] To patients who believed their minds were sound, such judgements were infuriating, and the fact that they were placed in an asylum an affront. No matter to what degree a man may or may not have suffered mental distress, if he did not acknowledge he needed treatment, the asylum was injurious to his sense of power and control.

Institutionalization represented a significant loss of self-determination. This was particularly problematic for a man, as Victorian manliness was essentially rooted in self-control. The asylum denied a man the ability to determine his own destiny at every level from where he lived, to whom he saw, to what he ate. It would have been natural for men to chafe against a system that essentially controlled them. Authorities were accustomed to men protesting their incarceration. In some ways, they encouraged such natural 'manly' feelings, and worried if patients did not seek out their freedom. John George Logan was an engineer from Glasgow sent to an asylum after suffering some form of mental illness for five months. While authorities did not write an official diagnosis, they noted that he shunned his family, and 'does not exhibit anything like a proper interest in having been sent here'.[81] Logan's lack of interest in leaving the asylum was understood as a significant symptom, and to not desire self-control was an unmanly attitude at best, and a perturbing symptom at worst.[82] Asylum inmates who expressed outrage at their incarceration may have proven more difficult to manage, but doctors and families agreed it was a natural, masculine response.

Violence, suicide, and the asylum

The desire to send a family member to an asylum was sometimes done out of love and hope for a cure; it was also sometimes done out of fear. The men of Broadmoor were potent reminders that when an adult man lost control of his mind, he could be dangerous. Stories of lunatic men killing their wives and/or children were newspaper fodder and provided consistent copy across the second half of the nineteenth century.[83] In some cases, it was a violent act or threats of violence that triggered men into care. One of the strongest archetypes of the madman was as a source of violence. High-profile stories of male violence often obscured the fact that within the asylum men were as likely to be victims of violence as they were perpetrators. Popular stories reified visions of the violent male lunatic and yet Lunacy Commissioners' reports often reveal men as victims of violence. But there was no space in popular tropes for madmen as victims.

Levels of 'acceptable' violence varied significantly by class, yet most Victorians believed men's essential nature was ferocious.[84] Aggression as masculinity was prevalent in popular understandings, and non-criminal, controlled forms of violent expression were often seen as natural.[85] Historians disagree whether English society became less violent over the course of the nineteenth century; but it is clear that in terms of masculine ideals, control over such passion was essential.[86] And one way to establish respectable British masculinity was to define it against an aggressive other, whether that be a criminal underclass, a foreign national, or, in this instance, violent lunatics.[87] While violence might have been an inherent quality in man, Victorian codes of masculinity universally required that violence to be channelled and controlled. Lunacy was understood to release these barriers. A madman was a source of potential and unchecked violence; without the trappings of rationality, the darkest sides of masculinity were unleashed with dramatic consequences.

Families were often the first to notice violent behaviour and could be the subjects of that violence. Robert Moore Colling had attempted to kill his wife and himself. Arthur James Warry, house surgeon at the Great Northern Hospital, testified at Colling's trial. In his testimony, Warry stated that it was common for the mad to become deeply suspicious of their family and loved ones. Colling was known to occasionally lash out against his wife, which the doctor saw as a symptom of his depression. The doctor and the victim's son both mentioned having witnessed Colling crying before his eventual attack. His step-son in fact noted, 'I have noticed a strangeness about him several times', which included sudden mood shifts, lashing out at imaginary insults, and becoming very violent.[88] Often it was sudden emotion, and dramatic shifts in emotion, that were the tell-tale signs of a mind out of control.

Doctors note that James Robertson tried to murder his wife and child during an 'excited' moment; when he entered the asylum he had no memory of the events.[89] Some men's delusions were directly connected to their acts of violence. John Haggarty was troubled by evil spirits that caused him to lash out against others. While he lived in a 'state of dread', he spread that fear to all around him as he was constantly committing acts of violence against his wife, children, and any neighbours who came close before he was institutionalized. In the asylum he was plagued by voices that told him he had harmed his family.[90] William Gordon was a glass merchant whose madness manifested as delusions that led to acts of violence. Before admission to Glasgow Royal Lunatic Asylum he had threatened to shoot his elder son and sent threatening letters to the sheriff. His wife had been so terrified of him she refused to share a home with him.[91] Henry John Wiltshire was a fifty-eight-year-old 'corrector of press' who was sent to Bethlem in 1866 by his wife. While he complained that going to the asylum would destroy his family, he had also threatened to murder his wife.[92] Listed as recovered within a few months, doctors noted this was not his first attack. David Elderage was a pauper tailor who was admitted to Glasgow Royal Lunatic Asylum as a dangerous lunatic in 1867 after suffering for two weeks. He had been institutionalized in the past, and his lunacy was deemed to be hereditary. Before admission he showed symptoms of violence and rage, and he believed that people who approached him were devils. He threatened violence to those trying to restrain him and he seemed particularly threatening towards his mother.[93] Such symptoms made staying at home dangerous, and the asylum the logical solution. Incidents of men out of control were lamentable, but they adhered to Victorian gender stereotypes. A violent madman was simply an exaggerated, bestial version of inherent masculine forces.

Much less well publicized was the fact that serious violence was rare, and that patients were more likely to injure themselves than others, or be victims of others' rage. Medical professionals who worked most closely with the insane were well aware that not all lunatics were violent, and that when they were it was the result of a particular delusion or suspicion of a threat.[94] Suicide was a particular problem for men, as they were more likely to successfully end their lives than women.[95] And by the mid-Victorian period, suicide or suicidal attempts were markers of the clearest form of lunacy.[96] Most lay people agreed that self-murder was a clear indication of insanity; as one former inmate of the Glasgow Royal Lunatic Asylum confidently wrote in 1860, 'No sane man or woman ever committed suicide.'[97] Yet it was female suicides that often captured public fascination, with archetypal swooning maidens and fallen women.[98] The attempted male suicide found little space in the public imagination, and when it did it was often coupled with violence to others.[99]

The inability to recognize men's emotional distress could lead to ignoring serious symptoms of illness. One mother was distraught and shocked when her eighteen-year-old son, frustrated in his attempts to marry, took strychnine to end his life. His fiancée testified that the young man had been severely depressed, but the small family did not think of involving doctors or outside authorities.[100] Should families seek out help, doctors were more willing to at least acknowledge men could be ruled by their emotions just as readily as women. Robert Tempest Ricketts was admitted to a private asylum in 1870, six months after losing his young wife. He was excited, depressed, and experiencing delusions. In attempting to discover what caused his illness, the doctors simply wrote 'emotion'.[101] Doctors recognized that men's love could quickly turn to dangerous despair.

Most suicide attempts happened within the family home either as sudden acts, or as the final result of a family trying to deal with their loved one's depression. James Knox Talbot Wright was a widower admitted to Glasgow Royal Lunatic Asylum in 1895. He was epileptic, but had never suffered from an attack of insanity before his admission. He suffered for sixteen months before turning to the asylum, where he was noted as suicidal.[102] While attempted suicide could be clear cause for certification, many families and even doctors were reluctant to place suicidal and depressed relatives in the madhouse.[103] It was often only when there was a dangerous or violent attempt that families used the emergency order to have relatives confined to asylums.

The financial pressures of head of household could put enormous strain on men who failed at business. And yet their families did not intervene even as men's health spiralled. The family of a wealthy agriculturalist named Richard King felt they could not intervene in their relative's care even when he was damaging his financial interests. King suffered some losses in his business that seemed to trigger a mental collapse that led him to compound his financial troubles. It was only after a suicide attempt with a revolver that the family rushed to action. He was immediately placed in an asylum where doctors hoped for a speedy recovery.[104] Business failure could turn an upstanding leader of the community into a dangerous madman.[105] Henry Bessemer was plagued by delusions and fears and heard voices. He was afraid that he would commit suicide; doctors took the fear seriously as his mother had died by suicide.[106]

Doctors recognized the problem of male suicide as one of the more serious side-effects of mental disturbance. It was in keeping with a larger framework of male violence, as the act of suicide itself was a forceful act. An assumption of the inherently violent nature of men, and of madmen in particular, could lead to damaging results within asylums. While both men and women exhibited signs of violence while under institutionalization, there is evidence to suggest that attendants treated that violence differently. In two case studies of asylums, women clearly were treated with seclusion for violent outbursts, while men were treated with violence.[107] In the asylum, male patients were far more likely to be victims of violence than perpetrators. However, the figure of the madman as passive victim did not fit into existing norms of masculine behaviour.

Stories of men as victims of the asylum would rarely, if ever, reach public discourse. Occasionally there would be stories of patient-on-patient incidents; 'Murder at an Asylum' made for a good headline, and despite precautions it was an event that did happen from time to time.[108] More commonly, and much less publicized, were incidents of men who were victims of the asylum itself. The position of patients under confinement made them vulnerable. John Weston, a patient at the Bristol lunatic asylum, certainly believed male attendants were more cruel to their patients than attendants in the female ward. He cites the example of a night attendant who, frustrated with a harmless but endlessly muttering preacher, grabbed him out of bed, punching and kicking him for very little cause.[109] Yet such cases rarely made the newspapers.

The Lunacy Commissioners recognized that abuse happened to male and female patients. However, it tended to be violence towards female patients that generated the most controversy. Bethlem asylum was originally exempt from oversight by the Lunacy Commission, and they could only investigate on orders of the Lord Chancellor or Secretary of State who were charged as visitors to that hospital. After credible complaints about the treatment of one lady, they were granted access to visit in June of 1851 where they found numerous examples of abuse and neglect.[110] Lunacy Commissioners were frequently frustrated by what they saw as lax treatment of incompetent or violent attendants by both asylums themselves and the legal system. While male attendants were more likely to be dismissed than their female counterparts for all reasons, these cases only captured official dismissals and proven causes including cruelty (Figure 1.1). Commissioners assumed that even more might have been allowed to resign, erasing their misdeeds. The job of attendant was a largely thankless one that had a very high turnover rate and combined the roles of domestic servant, nurse, and security personnel.[111] Many attendants were simply dismissed by asylums rather than prosecuted for abuse.

While nineteenth-century reformers tried to banish abuse from the modern asylum, problems remained. The Lunacy Commissioners duly kept notes of every instance of abuse they investigated or prosecuted. Lunatics were particularly vulnerable as some could not report their mistreatment while others might not have been believed. In cases of nonverbal or non-communicative patients, it was often the injuries themselves that spoke for them. Moses James Barnes was a pauper lunatic admitted to Peckham House in 1850. The first

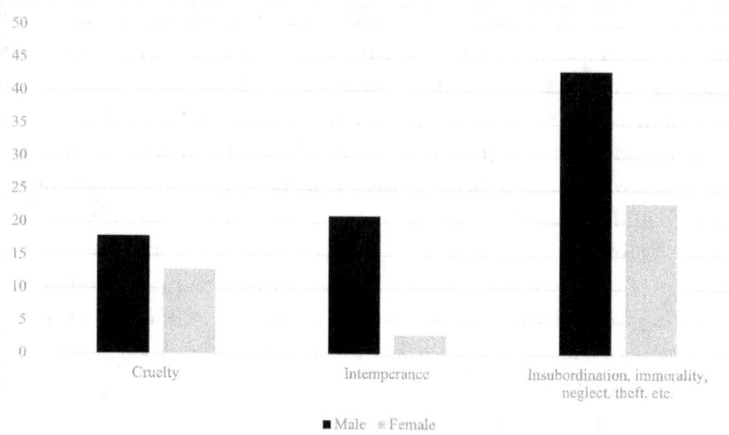

Figure 1.1 Causes for attendant dismissal, 1872

sign of a problem was when staff noticed he could not move his arm. His injuries were treated, and an investigation was started but the man died. Only later did investigators discover that a week earlier an attendant had thrown him to the ground after Barnes had refused to get into bed. He broke his arm and four ribs, which was the eventual cause of the man's death. The attendant was put on trial for manslaughter, but the only evidence came from another lunatic who witnessed the attack. It was only after much debate that the patient's testimony was accepted; his delusions were not felt to interfere in his ability to testify. The Commissioners were glad that the judges noted that in the asylum setting lunatics might often be the only witnesses, and that their testimony could not be discounted for fear of abusers running rampant.[112]

In deciding whether or not a lunatic should ever be able to give evidence at trial, one judge insisted they must be able to if they could understand the nature of the oath and could be cross-examined. Richard Donelly, a patient at a private lunatic asylum in Camberwell in the 1870s, was able to give evidence in a manslaughter case where an attendant was accused of causing the death of a patient. The judge remarked that should all lunatics be deemed unreliable witnesses, the management of lunatic asylums would be rendered incredibly difficult.[113] Not all authorities agreed you could trust testimony from a diseased mind.[114] For seriously ill patients, or patients whose delusions confused their realities, they might not have been able to reliably testify, potentially making themselves more vulnerable.

The Lunacy Commission did not see individual examples of abuse as undermining the asylum as an institution. They continued to detail examples of abuse every year, but were always careful to note they were rare, and this proved the system was working.[115] As attendants, nurses, and doctors were charged, Commissioners saw this as proof that 'bad apples' were being filtered out. A well-regulated lunacy system was seen as preferable to lunatics languishing in workhouses or living on parish charity with relations where, 'if they were not positively maltreated and abused, their mental disorder was utterly neglected'.[116] And in fact, it was unregistered or uncertified lunatics that the Commissioners worried about the most. Without official oversight, there was no one to ensure the insane were not being abused or neglected.[117]

Outside advocates could intervene in cases where they suspected abuse within asylums as well. This was particularly the case during the heyday of the Alleged Lunatics' Friend Society (ALFS). They wrote to the Home Office in 1861 about the death of a patient in care that had been dismissed as accidental. On investigation, two attendants were charged with manslaughter in 'a very grave case of cruelty and brutality'. The patient in question, William Swift, had tried to strangle the master of the workhouse where he was originally sent, and he got into a fight with two attendants a month after his admission. Swift died of a ruptured liver, a fractured sternum and ribs. The two attendants were dismissed for ill-using a patient. But it was only after notice from the ALFS that the Commissioners investigated that they were charged with manslaughter.[118]

The everyday violence of potential assaults or rough handling was much more challenging to track, or to prove. It was difficult to know whether patients' injuries were caused by abuse or by their own symptoms. Cases of cracked ribs leading to death were common enough that the Lunacy Commissioners sent out a circular to all asylums in 1868 to ensure a thorough exam of all patients coming in from workhouses, to ensure they did not enter the asylum with cracked or broken ribs.[119] Certain asylums had persistent problems with cracked ribs, and Commissioners put this down to the problem of not enough qualified attendants.[120] This was exacerbated by the fragile bone theory that purported that brittle bones were a symptom of mental disease. Such theories did not absolve staff from blame when patients cracked ribs, proving only that they needed to be more careful. But they could also be used to justify more patient restrictions such as padded cells, physical restraints, and constant surveillance.[121]

Tracing the exact aetiology of injuries was difficult with patients who were not always accountable for their actions. Before entering the asylum, Patrick Gallocher had tried to throw himself out of a window, suffered delusions, and was incoherent in his speech. Doctors suddenly noticed that he seemed to be having trouble breathing, and on examination they found ribs broken on his right and left sides. Inquiries as to the cause were inconclusive, although they noted he often did jump and tumble out of his bed when excited.[122] In 1877, when Lunacy Commissioners took a hard look at their practices, they only tracked eight cases where attendants were charged for abuse. The most serious was John Smith, who struggled with a patient, throwing him to the ground and kicking him several times. The assault was witnessed by two epileptic patients whose testimony was believed. Smith was found guilty and sentenced to three months in prison and a fine of twenty pounds.[123]

To determine cause of death of violent patients was often difficult. In one case at Durham asylum in 1874, the visitors and committee could not agree on who, if anyone, was to blame in the death of a patient suffering from mania. He was in a ward for refractory patients, but staff still had trouble controlling him. When he was transferred to the infirmary with an ankle injury it took three attendants to move him. When he could finally be examined, they discovered he had six broken ribs and a fracture of his breastbone along with the ankle injury. He died a few days later and at the post-mortem they found even more broken ribs and fluid in his chest. His ribs were found to be brittle, but there was no agreement between the coroner, visitors, and committee about whether attendants had used excessive force. What the Commissioners in Lunacy could agree was the asylum in general did not have an effective system to treat dangerous male patients.[124]

Some of these deaths were malicious or criminal, while others were the result of attendants struggling with violent patients. For all of the benefits of the non-restraint movement, without the use of physical restraints like straight waist jackets, attendants had little recourse to deal with violent or destructive patients other than to physically overpower and restrain them. One patient at Blacklands House was a tall, powerful man with mania who repeatedly assaulted attendants. His outbursts were so intense it sometimes took up to five men to control him. The morning of his death he tried to set fire to the door of his room. A lengthy coroner's inquest found his death was caused by heart disease and fractured ribs broken during one of his struggles with his attendants. The attendants were not charged with undue violence in their physical restraint, but two were asked to resign for the fact that they fastened him to his bed with sheets and towels after his arson attempt.[125]

Even in cases where the attendants were not abusive, but simply negligent, the Lunacy Commissioners intervened where appropriate. An attendant was fined one pound when the patient under his care committed suicide. The man had been working in the shoemaker's shop at the asylum and when the attendant left for the day he forgot to count his charges. The man snuck off to hang himself.[126] A case five years later played out a similar scenario. Henry Peters was charged with wilful neglect of his duties at Northumberland House in 1880. He was the head attendant in charge of a patient who died. The resident medical officer knew that the patient was at risk of suicide, and specifically charged Peters with looking after the despondent man. However, Peters was distracted by other duties and the man escaped and hanged himself. Staff blamed the proprietors for not employing enough people while the proprietor blamed the attendant for not following instructions not to leave the man alone.[127]

Lunacy Commissioners often complained that punishments were not strong enough to deal with violence and abuse. One attendant at Durham asylum was charged and found guilty of aggravated assault on a patient in 1869. Another, witnessed by the medical officer kicking a patient twice, was only dismissed and not charged. Commissioners were frustrated by the inconsistency.[128] However, the language of these reports sometimes belies that a certain amount of interpersonal violence was accepted on male patients, even by the Commissioners. They noted that this patient had done nothing to provoke the attendant to kick him; would they have seen the attendant as less culpable had the patient done something to 'deserve' such violence?

Government officials were dependent on medical staff to notice and report problems. At the Kent Asylum Dr Kirkman heard noises in the bath-room as a patient with epilepsy was struggling with two attendants.[129] They were holding him under the water despite the fact that there was a standing order not to bathe, dress, or interact with violent patients without the head attendant present. The patient died five days after this bath, and unfortunately no post-mortem was conducted. The Commissioners were frustrated by this and the fact that the casebook had not recorded enough information. But without more concrete evidence they could not prosecute.[130] Even the head doctor at this asylum could do little to stop mistreatment.

An attendant at Kent County Asylum wrote to the Lunacy Commission that some of his fellow attendants were abusing patients. As they investigated, one fled to America, one was warned, and two attendants were fined.[131] Sometimes it was only after multiple tragedies and the notice of other attendants that abusers were identified. And even then, it was difficult to know exactly how a patient had been injured, and who, if anyone, was culpable for an assault. A sixty-four-year-old patient died at Hanwell Asylum of unknown injuries. He had bruises from a struggle with his son before his admission to the workhouse and from pauper attendants at the workhouse, and died after he was transferred to the asylum, supposedly of pneumonia. In this case the son did not want a post-mortem, but the chief medical officer insisted and found that in fact it was ten fractured ribs that caused the man's death. There was not enough evidence, however, to determine when the man's ribs were cracked as he had never complained of pain in the asylum. It was only after a letter months later noting that the man in charge of the ward when this patient died had just been convicted of aggravated assault on another patient that doubts emerged about the cause of death at Hanwell.[132] But sadly, the man's multiple encounters with violence left it unclear which blow had been the fatal one.

That male lunatics were victims of violence in the asylum is beyond doubt. However, the level of that violence is difficult to assess as such complaints would often be underreported and easily dismissed. The non-restraint movement successfully lobbied for the end of strait-jackets and strapping to bedsteads and chairs in the

1840s.¹³³ In some ways this led to more physical confrontations between patients and attendants. Even the solution of the padded room for particularly unmanageable patients did not eliminate all violence. Reformer John Conolly believed a padded room was the solution to mechanical restraints or brute force to forcibly calm a patient; within the padded cell a patient would be protected even from harming themselves.¹³⁴ Yet patients still had to be ushered into those cells; they had to be fed and bathed in ways that always opened the door to struggle and violence. And the spectre of the violent madman justified the use of force, making it difficult to prove allegations of abuse.

Conclusion

Being admitted to a lunatic asylum could rarely be a positive experience, and it would be difficult for many men to accept the loss of control and admission of weakness it implied. To be placed within an extremely regimented institution was both frustrating and humiliating for men who did not think they belonged there, or for those who did not understand what was happening. It was an emasculating situation, as men were stripped of their decision-making and their working identity, and removed from their family setting. But the full male experience of incarceration was more than simply as passive victims of an authoritarian system; men found ways to negotiate elements of their care, keep in touch with families, and resist authority. Men also proved particularly difficult patients to control if they were prone to violence.

The goal of Victorian asylums was to provide a healthy and pleasing environment where inmates could enjoy clean surroundings, fresh air, healthy food, appropriate occupation, and regain their senses through constant surveillance. Moral reformers encouraged the building of small(ish) asylums to maintain some sense of the family atmosphere so lauded at the York Retreat.¹³⁵ However, by the turn of the twentieth century it was obvious that asylums were often not centres of cure and treatment, but simply places to warehouse the incurable. The Commissioners in Lunacy pointed out the problem of incurables overcrowding asylums in their reports from 1858, 1860, 1868, 1878, and, finally, in 1901:

There has, indeed, been a growing tendency to send persons suffering from all classes and degrees of mental unsoundness, whether the result of acute disease or of mere natural decay and failure, into Asylums, and in the last decade the process has been much accelerated, until now the Asylums are congested with aged, infirm, and broken-down persons, and vacancies for acute cases are difficult to secure.[136]

The Commissioners' proposed solution was to separate out the class of patient who could gain little from the expensive and specialized care of a moral treatment asylum. The old and infirm who had once been cared for in workhouses and private homes were now filling up space in institutions that were not designed for their needs.[137] Yet this was not exactly the case. Published results from six disparate asylums show that 40–60 per cent of patients were there one year or less. The perception that the asylum was filling up with chronic and incurable patients ignores the constant turnover of the other half of patient beds.[138] The reality of the asylum was that patients were more likely to move in and out of institutionalization than be institutionalized for life. While the asylum might have been the government's official response to lunacy, and it certainly loomed large as part of the cultural imagination, it was only one part of the patient experience.

Notes

1 J. Haslam, *Sketches in Bedlam, or, Characteristic Traits of Insanity as Displayed in the Cases of One Hundred and Forty Patients of Both Sexes, Now, or Recently, Confined in New Bethlem* (London, 1823), p. ix.
2 Haslam's writings had long advocated reform and moral treatment; however, the scandalous treatment of patients under his care at Bethlem at the turn of the century had damaged his early reputation. A. Scull, C. MacKenzie, and N. Hervey, *Masters of Bedlam: The Transformation of the Mad-Doctoring Trade* (Princeton, 2014), pp. 30–35.
3 This did not even include those housed in the infirmaries of workhouses or boarded out in licensed residences. S. Cherry, *Medical Services and the Hospitals in Britain, 1860–1939* (Cambridge, 1996), p. 50.
4 R.A. Houston, 'Asylums: The Historical Perspective Before, During, and After', *The Lancet Psychiatry* 7:4 (2020), pp. 354–62.

5 For example: J. Andrews, *The History of Bethlem* (London, 1997); A. Digby, *Madness, Morality and Medicine: A Study of the York Retreat 1796–1914* (Cambridge, 1985); M. Finnane, *Insanity and the Insane In Post-Famine Ireland* (London, 1981); C. Hickman, *Therapeutic Landscapes: A History of English Hospital Gardens since 1800* (Manchester, 2013); P. Michael, *Care and Treatment of the Mentally Ill in North Wales, 1800–2000* (Cardiff, 2003); J.R.B. Taylor, *Hospital and Asylum Architecture in England, 1840–1914: Building for Health Care* (London, 1991); L. Topp, J.E. Moran, and J. Andrews, *Madness, Architecture and the Built Environment: Psychiatric Spaces in Historical Context* (New York, 2007).

6 S. Eastoe, *Idiocy, Imbecility and Insanity in Victorian Society: Caterham Asylum, 1867–1911* (Houndmills, 2020); P. McDonagh, *Idiocy: A Cultural History* (Liverpool, 2008); D. Wright and A. Digby, *From Idiocy to Mental Deficiency: Historical Perspectives on People with Learning Disabilities* (London, 1996); D. Wright, *Mental Disability in Victorian England: The Earlswood Asylum, 1847–1901* (Oxford, 2001).

7 Hide, *Gender and Class in English Asylums*; Houston, 'Madness and Gender'; M.J. Kirata, 'Wrongful Confinement: The Betrayal of Women by Men, Medicine and Law', in K.O. Garrigan (ed.), *Victorian Scandals: Representations of Gender and Class* (Athens, 1992), pp. 43–68; Labrum, 'Looking Beyond the Asylum'; Marland, *Dangerous Motherhood*; W. Mitchinson, 'Gender and Insanity as Characteristics of the Insane: A Nineteenth-Century Case', *Canadian Bulletin of Medical History* 4 (1987), pp. 99–117.

8 See for example: J. Busfield, *Men, Women and Madness: Understanding Gender and Mental Disorder* (Basingstoke, 1996); C. Coleborne and D. MacKinnon (eds), *Madness in Australia: Histories, Heritage and the Asylum* (St Lucia, 2003); A. Mauger, *The Cost of Insanity in Nineteenth-Century Ireland: Public, Voluntary and Private Asylum Care* (Basingstoke and New York, 2018); R. Porter and D. Wright (eds), *The Confinement of the Insane: International Perspectives, 1800–1965* (Cambridge, 2003); B. Reiss, *Theaters of Madness: Insane Asylums and Nineteenth-Century American Culture* (Chicago, 2008).

9 Charlotte MacKenzie's research on Ticehurst demonstrates just how rich such casebooks can be, and for understanding the experience of wealthy men they are invaluable resources. MacKenzie, *Psychiatry for the Rich*.

10 For example: P. Bartlett, *The Poor Law of Lunacy: The Administration of Pauper Lunatics in Mid-Nineteenth-Century England* (London, 1999); R.H.S. Mindham, 'The West Riding of Yorkshire Pauper Lunatic

Asylum at Wakefield, 1814–1995', *British Journal of Psychiatry* 217:3 (2020), p. 534; R. Wynter, '"Good in All Respects": Appearance and Dress at Staffordshire County Lunatic Asylum, 1818–54', *History of Psychiatry* 22:1 (2011), pp. 40–57.

11 J. Melling and B. Forsythe, *The Politics of Madness: The State, Insanity and Society in England, 1845–1914* (London, 2006), p. 22.

12 W.L. Parry-Jones, 'English Private Madhouses in the Eighteenth and Nineteenth Centuries', *Proceedings of the Royal Society of Medicine* 66:7 (1973), pp. 659–64.

13 L. Smith, *Cure, Comfort and Safe Custody: Public Lunatic Asylums in Early Nineteenth-Century England* (London, 1999), p. 94.

14 M. Reuber, 'Moral Management and the "Unseen Eye": Public Lunatic Asylums in Ireland, 1800–1845', in E. Malcolm and G. Jones (eds), *Medicine, Disease, and the State in Ireland, 1650–1940* (Cork, 1999), p. 208.

15 W.L. Parry-Jones, *The Trade in Lunacy: A Study of Private Madhouses in England in the Eighteenth and Nineteenth Centuries* (Toronto, 1972), p. 21.

16 J. Andrews, 'Raising the Tone of Asylumdom: Maintaining and Expelling Pauper Lunatics at the Glasgow Royal Asylum in the Nineteenth Century', in J. Melling and B. Forsythe (eds), *Insanity, Institutions, and Society, 1800–1914: A Social History of Madness in Comparative Perspective* (London, 1999), pp. 202–3. The Scottish were the slowest to embrace institutionalization as the best or only solution to lunacy (or the pauper/workhouse paradigm). L. Walsh, '"The Property of the Whole Community": Charity and Insanity in Urban Scotland: The Dundee Royal Lunatic Asylum, 1805–1850', in Melling and Forsythe (eds), *Insanity, Institutions, and Society*, pp. 182–83.

17 R. Porter, 'Madness and its Institutions', in Wear (ed.), *Medicine in Society*, p. 293.

18 M.A. Arieno, *Victorian Lunatics: A Social Epidemiology of Mental Illness in Mid-Nineteenth-Century England* (Selinsgrove, 1989), pp. 30–31; Houston, 'Asylums', p. 357.

19 In practice, this was never realized. Many pauper lunatics ended up in workhouses for long or short periods of time, and in England the Poor Law and lunacy administration were linked. Even in Ireland, where discrete systems were maintained, asylums were always a part of pauper relief systems. C. Cox, *Negotiating Insanity in the Southeast of Ireland, 1820–1900* (Manchester, 2018).

20 F. Winslow, *On the Incubation of Insanity* (London, 1846), pp. 4–5.

21 M. Mather, *Thoughts and Suggestions Relative to the Management of Barony Parochial Board and Poor-House: Together with Hints on Monomania* (Glasgow, 1858), pp. 77, 164.

22 Smith claims that by 1850 moral management simply meant bending patients to administrators' will. Smith, *Cure, Comfort and Safe Custody*, p. 4.
23 A. Scull, 'The Social History of Psychiatry in the Victorian Era', in Scull, *Madhouses, Mad-Doctors, and Madmen*, p. 18.
24 Showalter, *The Female Malady*, pp. 17, 3.
25 Busfield, *Men, Women and Madness*, pp. 265–68.
26 For example, Rosina Bulwer Lytton was incarcerated by her estranged husband in 1858. R.B. Lytton, *A Blighted Life: A True Story* (London, 1880), pp. 35–36. And Georgina Weldon was almost placed in an asylum by her estranged husband in 1878 before turning the tables and becoming a public advocate for women's rights. J. Martin, 'Weldon [née Thomas], Georgina (1837–1914), campaigner against the lunacy laws and celebrated litigant', *Oxford Dictionary of National Biography*, 23 September 2004.
27 *Fifty-seventh Report of the Commissioners in Lunacy* (London, 1903), p. 8.
28 *Fifty-eighth Report of the Commissioners in Lunacy* (London, 1904), pp. 112–13.
29 The billiard room at Holloway sanitorium resembled that of a nice hotel with heavy leather furnishings, wood panelling, and an assortment of hunting trophies on the walls. J. Hamlett, *At Home in the Institution: Material Life in Asylums, Lodging Houses and Schools in Victorian and Edwardian England* (London, 2014), p. 44.
30 R. Adair, J. Melling, and B. Forsythe, 'Migration, Family Structure and Pauper Lunacy in Victorian England: Admissions to the Devon County Pauper Lunatic Asylum, 1845–1900', *Continuity and Change* 12: 3 (1997), p. 391.
31 Parry-Jones, *The Trade in Lunacy*, p. 23.
32 R.A. Hunter and I. Macalpine, *Psychiatry for the Poor: 1851 Colney Hatch Asylum-Friern Hospital 1973* (Folkestone, 1974), pp. 11, 162; MacKenzie, *Psychiatry for the Rich*, p. 137.
33 R. Porter, 'Madness and its Institutions', in Wear (ed.), *Medicine in Society*, p. 277. This statement requires some tweaking, however, as asylums were not the only example of coercive medicine in the nineteenth century. England's increasingly strict compulsory Vaccination Acts (1853, 1867, 1871) are another such example. M. Fichman and J.E. Keelan, 'Resister's Logic: The Anti-Vaccination Arguments of Alfred Russel Wallace and Their Role in the Debates over Compulsory Vaccination in England, 1870–1907', *Studies in History and Philosophy of Biological and Biomedical Sciences* 38:3 (2007), pp. 586, 604. A precedent-setting medical malpractice suit near the end of the century also established a broad definition of patient consent; the jury trial

affirmed doctors' broad discretionary powers for treatment. 'Beatty v. Cullingworth', *British Medical Journal* (21 November 1896), pp. 1546–48. The most famous Victorian experiments in forced treatment, however, were the Contagious Diseases Acts that for two decades allowed the police to detain and examine suspected prostitutes and to force treatment in lock hospitals. E. Liggins, 'Prostitution and Social Purity in the 1880s and 1890s', *Critical Survey* 15:3 (2003), p. 39.

34 A Physician [pseud.], 'Lunatic Asylums and the Lunacy Laws', *The Times* (19 August 1858), pp. 8–9.
35 A. Suzuki, *Madness at Home: The Psychiatrist, the Patient, And the Family in England, 1820–1860* (Berkeley, 2006), p. 121.
36 Bartlett, *The Poor Law of Lunacy*, p. 32.
37 As Marjorie Levine-Clark notes, it was specifically designed to penalize men who were no longer economically self-sufficient. Paupers had to give up their right to vote when they accepted relief. M. Levine-Clark, *Unemployment, Welfare, and Masculine Citizenship: 'So Much Honest Poverty' in Britain, 1870–1930* (New York, 2015), pp. 4–5.
38 *Sixth Annual Report of the Commissioners in Lunacy* (London, 1851), p. 6; *Twenty-third Annual Report of the Commissioners in Lunacy* (London, 1869), p. 27; *Twenty-fourth Annual Report of the Commissioners in Lunacy* (London, 1870), p. 68; *Twenty-sixth Annual Report of the Commissioners in Lunacy* (London, 1872), p. 52.
39 J.M. Granville, *The Care and Cure of the Insane: Being the Reports of the Lancet Commission on Lunatic Asylums*, vol. 2 (London, 1877), p. 154.
40 M. Doolittle, 'Fatherhood and Family Shame: Masculinity, Welfare and the Workhouse in Late Nineteenth-Century England', in L. Delap, B. Griffin, and A. Wills (eds), *The Politics of Domestic Authority in Britain since 1800* (London, 2009), p. 85.
41 *Eighth Annual Report of the Commissioners in Lunacy* (London, 1854), p. 23.
42 *Ninth Annual Report of the Commissioners in Lunacy* (London, 1855), p. 35.
43 Philanthropos, *A Voice from the Wilderness: Being A Plea for a Lunatic Asylum for the Middle Classes on Self-Supporting Principles* (London, 1861), pp. 5–6.
44 A Physician [pseud.] 'Lunatic Asylums and the Lunacy Laws', *The Times* (19 August 1858), pp. 8–9.
45 Manor House Asylum Case Notes, Male Patients, MS 5725, pp. 437–42.
46 Scull, *Museums of Madness*.

47 This is in keeping not only with recent studies of families and social services in the nineteenth century, but also with even broader studies of modernity pushing back against the idea that industrialization resulted in universal atomization and the breaking down of family ties. J. Vernon, *Distant Strangers: How Britain Became Modern* (Berkeley, 2014).
48 Smith, '"Your Very Thankful Inmate"', pp. 248–49.
49 Male Patient Casebook, Bethlem, CB-124, p. 7.
50 D. Noble, *Elements of Psychological Medicine: An Introduction to the Practical Study of Insanity, Etc.* (London, 1853), p. xii.
51 Manor House Asylum Case Notes, Male Patients, MS 6224, pp. 125–27, 131, 163, 165.
52 Telegram from James to Mrs. Knowles, Manor House, MS 5726/4.
53 T.E. Brown, 'Dance of the Dialectic? Some Reflections (Polemic and Otherwise) on the Present State of Nineteenth-Century Asylum Studies', *Canadian Bulletin of Medical History* 11:2 (1994), p. 277.
54 L.S. Jacyna and S.T. Casper (eds), *The Neurological Patient in History* (Rochester, 2012).
55 A. Bacopoulos-Viau and A. Fauvel, 'The Patient's Turn: Roy Porter and Psychiatry's Tales, Thirty Years On', *Medical History* 60:1 (2016), p. 13.
56 S. Chaney, '"No 'Sane' Person Would Have Any Idea": Patients' Involvement in Late Nineteenth-Century British Asylum Psychiatry', *Medical History* 60:1 (2016), pp. 47, 52.
57 M. Barfoot and A.W. Beveridge, 'Madness at the Crossroads: John Home's Letters from the Royal Edinburgh Asylum, 1886–1887', *Psychological Medicine* 20 (1990), pp. 263–84.
58 L. Ray, 'Models of Madness in Victorian Asylum Practice', *European Journal of Sociology* 22:2 (1981), p. 230.
59 However, some historians have been able to pull remarkable insights from these fragmentary sources. For example, Rory du Plessis and Laure Murat's studies of delusional content and its connection to national events. L. Murat, *The Man Who Thought He Was Napoleon: Toward a Political History of Madness*, D. Dusinberre, trans. (Chicago, 2014); R. du Plessis, 'A Hermeneutic Analysis of Delusion Content from the Casebooks of the Grahamstown Lunatic Asylum, 1890–1907', *South African Journal of Psychiatry* 25 (2019), pp. 1–7.
60 S. Swartz, 'Asylum Case Records: Fact and Fiction', *Rethinking History* 22:3 (2018), pp. 293, 297.
61 Manor House Asylum Case Notes, Male Patients, MS 6222, pp. 31–35.
62 Male Patient Casebook, Bethlem, CB-126, p. 7.
63 Manor House Asylum Case Notes, Male Patients, MS 6222, p. 35.

64 Discharge and Death Registers, Bethlem, 1885–1890, DDR-06, p. 29.
65 Manor House Asylum Case Notes, Male Patients, MS 5725, p. 211.
66 Manor House Asylum Case Notes, Male Patients, MS 6224, p. 176.
67 She called daily for updates on her husband's condition. After more than two months she was able to visit with him and visited him daily along with many friends. Manor House Asylum Case Notes, Male Patients, MS 6222, pp. 333–43.
68 His discharge as cured was a 'very satisfactory result of the case [even though to] some extent unexpected'. The following year he and his wife paid a visit to Chiswick, and he met his former doctors a few times in the years following. Manor House Asylum Case Notes, Male Patients, MS 6222, p. 344.
69 Manor House Asylum Case Notes, Male Patients, MS 6223, p. 569.
70 A.S. Taylor, *The Principles and Practice of Medical Jurisprudence* (London, 1865), p. 1025.
71 G. Augustus Sala, 'A Visit to the Royal Hospital of Bethlehem, pt. 2', *Illustrated London News* (31 March 1860), p. 304.
72 J. Weston, *Life in a Lunatic Asylum: An Autobiographical Sketch* (London, 1867), pp. 10, 15, 34.
73 *The Philosophy of Insanity, by a Late Inmate of the Glasgow Royal Asylum* (London, 1860), p. 20.
74 *The Philosophy of Insanity*, p. 91.
75 E. Halliday, 'Themes in Scottish Asylum Culture: The Hospitalisation of the Scottish Asylum 1880–1914' (PhD Dissertation, University of Stirling, 2003), p. 127; O. Walsh, 'Lunatics and Criminal Alliances in Nineteenth-Century Ireland', in P. Bartlett and D. Wright (eds), *Outside the Walls of the Asylum: The History of Care in the Community 1750–2000* (London, 1999), p. 147.
76 They also note that authorities were most concerned with the destruction of women's clothing versus the cleanliness of men's clothing. N. Baur and J. Melling, 'Dressing and Addressing the Mental Patient: The Uses of Clothing in the Admission, Care and Employment of Residents in English Provincial Mental Hospitals, c. 1860–1960', *Textile History* 45:2 (2014), p. 165.
77 J. Wallis, *Investigating the Body in the Victorian Asylum: Doctors, Patients, and Practices* (Basingstoke, 2017), p. 88.
78 'Judge and Madman', *Daily Mail* (20 January 1905), p. 6.
79 *Public Opinion on Private Lunatic Asylums, Giving an Account of the Frightful Mortality in Them, Disclosed by the Report of the Commissioners in Lunacy* (London, 1890), p. 13.
80 'Parliamentary Intelligence', *The Times* (12 March 1862), pp. 5–6.
81 House surgeon's notes for physician: Male, Glasgow Royal Lunatic Asylum, HB 13/5/63, p. 381.

82 Begiato, *Manliness in Britain*, p. 5.
83 Sadly, wife murder was a common feature in general, and the story of a man who killed his wife and was then taken to the asylum was far too common. See chapter five for a full account of violence and media panics.
84 A definite marker of middle-class status became the ability to restrain and control that violence; yet still it was seen as an inherent masculine trait. J.C. Wood, *Violence and Crime in Nineteenth Century England: The Shadow of Our Refinement* (London, 2004), p. 37.
85 J. Middleton, 'The Cock of the School: A Cultural History of Playground Violence in Britain, 1880–1940', *Journal of British Studies* 52:4 (2013), pp. 903, 906.
86 E. Godfrey, *Masculinity, Crime and Self-Defence in Victorian Literature* (Basingstoke, 2011), pp. 128–30; M. Wiener, 'The Victorian Criminalization of Men', in P. Spierenburg (ed.), *Men and Violence: Gender, Honour, and Rituals in Modern Europe and America* (Columbus, 1998), p. 198; Wood, *Violence and Crime in Nineteenth Century England*.
87 C. Emsley, *Hard Men: Violence in England since 1750* (London, 2005).
88 Robert Moore Colling, 31 July 1882, t18820731-779, Old Bailey Proceedings online, hereafter OBP.
89 House surgeon's notes for physician: Male, Glasgow Royal Lunatic Asylum, HB 13/5/58, 1868, p. 243.
90 House surgeon's notes for physician: Male, Glasgow Royal Lunatic Asylum, HB 13/5/61, 1875, p. 389.
91 House surgeon's notes for physician: Male, Glasgow Royal Lunatic Asylum, HB 13/5/63, 1881, p. 65.
92 Admission registers 1865–1869, Bethlem, ARA 26, 1866.
93 House surgeon's notes for physician: Male, Glasgow Royal Lunatic Asylum, HB 13/5/58, 1867, p. 1.
94 P. Prior, *Madness and Murder: Gender, Crime and Mental Disorder in Nineteenth-Century Ireland* (Dublin, 2008), p. 91.
95 H.I. Kushner, 'Suicide, Gender, and the Fear of Modernity in Nineteenth-Century Medical and Social Thought', *Journal of Social History* 26:2 (1993), p. 468.
96 Death by suicide carried the stigma of lunacy, but no longer held the additional shame of an unconsecrated burial. A. Shepherd and D. Wright, 'Madness, Suicide and the Victorian Asylum: Attempted Self-Murder in the Age of Non-Restraint', *Medical History* 46:2 (2002), p. 178.
97 *The Philosophy of Insanity*, p. 11.
98 V. Bailey, *'This Rash Act': Suicide Across the Life Cycle in the Victorian City* (Stanford, 1998), p. 184.

99 One short story recalls the tale of a man who lost his fortune in an ill-fated copper mine. His son hears of this by telegraph while studying at university, and he rushes home to find his father dying and his mother dead. He explains 'the loss must have driven him mad, for he shot himself, and his violent act killed my mother'. The man survived and was sent to an asylum. F.M. Foster, 'Slaves of Fate', *Leicester Chronicle and the Leicestershire Mercury* (24 January 1891), p. 4.

100 'Love, Madness, and Suicide', *Daily News* (30 December 1897), p. 7.

101 Manor House Asylum Case Notes, Male Patients, MS 5725, p. 6.

102 House surgeon's notes for physician: Male, Records of Glasgow Royal Lunatic Asylum, HB 15/5/130, pp. 17–18.

103 Bailey, *'This Rash Act'*, pp. 1, 54.

104 'Commission of Lunacy', *Daily News* (16 August 1850), p. 6.

105 The desire to provide for a family was not limited to the middle class, though for the working classes it was a tougher challenge. But even among working-class men, a failure in being able to provide for the family was interpreted as a personal failure. J. Shepherd, '"One of the Best Fathers until He Went Out of His Mind": Paternal Child-Murder, 1864–1900', *Journal of Victorian Culture* 18:1 (2013), p. 19.

106 Manor House Asylum Case Notes, Male Patients, MS 5725, pp. 595–601.

107 Hide, *Gender and Class in English Asylums*, p. 162; P. Tobia, 'The Patients of the Bristol Lunatic Asylum in the Nineteenth Century, 1861–1900' (PhD Dissertation, University of the West of England, 2017), p. 121.

108 'Murder at an Asylum', *York Herald* (11 December 1886), p. 4; 'Murder by a Madman', *Leicester Chronicle and the Leicestershire Mercury* (15 April 1882), p. 4; 'Murder by a Madman', *Illustrated Police News* (7 May 1887), p. 4.

109 Weston, *Life in a Lunatic Asylum*, p. 135.

110 *Seventh Annual Report of the Commissioners in Lunacy* (London, 1852), pp. 15–19.

111 C. Chatterton, '"Always Remember that you are in your Senses": From Keeper to Attendant to Nurse', in Knowles and Trowbridge (eds), *Insanity and the Lunatic Asylum*, pp. 88, 93.

112 *Sixth Annual Report of the Commissioners in Lunacy*, pp. 17–18.

113 F. Wharton, *A Treatise on Mental Unsoundness Embracing a General View of Psychological Law* (Philadelphia, 1873), pp. 248–51.

114 J. Eigen, *Unconscious Crime: Mental Absence and Criminal Responsibility in Victorian London* (Baltimore, 2003), p. 93.

Men in care: the asylum

115 *Thirty-third Annual Report of the Commissioners in Lunacy* (London, 1869), p. 110.
116 *Ninth Annual Report of the Commissioners in Lunacy*, p. 33.
117 *Twenty-first Annual Report of the Commissioners in Lunacy* (London, 1866), pp. 35–36.
118 *Fifteenth Annual Report of the Commissioners in Lunacy* (London, 1861), pp. 55–57.
119 *Twenty-third Annual Report of the Commissioners in Lunacy*, p. 12.
120 *Twenty-fifth Annual Report of the Commissioners in Lunacy* (London, 1871), p. 32.
121 Wallis, *Investigating the Body in the Victorian Asylum*, pp. 129–30.
122 It was easy for patients to be injured or injure themselves, but treating those injuries proved more difficult. The following month doctors noted they were still having trouble keeping Gallocher's bandages on his ribs and keeping him in bed. House surgeon's notes for physician: Male, Glasgow Royal Lunatic Asylum, HB 13/5/61, 1875, p. 207.
123 Six of the eight cases involved male attendants of male patients.
124 *Twenty-Eighth Annual Report of the Commissioners in Lunacy* (London, 1874), pp. 30–31.
125 *Seventeenth Annual Report of the Commissioners in Lunacy* (London, 1863), pp. 18–19.
126 *Twenty-ninth Annual Report of the Commissioners in Lunacy* (London, 1875), p. 35.
127 In the end Peters was found guilty of gross negligence and fined fifteen pounds. Testimony also revealed that during the five years that Mr Wright had been in charge of the asylum, two patients had committed suicide and 3–4 had escaped. This hardly provided much confidence in the institution. 'At Bow Street', *The Times* (29 October 1880), p. 9; *The Times* (5 November 1880), p. 10.
128 *Twenty-third Annual Report of the Commissioners*, p. 14.
129 In the nineteenth century, epilepsy was explicitly understood as a mental disorder. Without effective treatment, it could produce serious fits, mood changes, and even death. Tobia, 'Patients of the Bristol Lunatic Asylum', pp. 164–69.
130 *Twentieth Annual Report of the Commissioners in Lunacy* (London, 1866), p. 36.
131 *Forty-third Annual Report of the Commissioners in Lunacy* (London, 1889), p. 111.
132 *Sixteenth Annual Report of the Commissioners in Lunacy* (London, 1862), pp. 54–59.
133 Smith, *Cure, Comfort and Safe Custody*, pp. 248–59.

134 L. Topp, 'Single Rooms, Seclusion and the Non-Restraint Movement in British Asylums, 1838–1844', *Social History of Medicine* 31:4 (2018), pp. 772–73.
135 B. Franklin, 'Hospital – Heritage – Home: Reconstructing the Nineteenth Century Lunatic Asylum', *Housing, Theory and Society* 19:3–4 (2002), pp. 171–72.
136 *Fifty-fifth Annual Report of the Commissioners in Lunacy* (London, 1901), pp. 8–9.
137 *Fifty-fifth Annual Report of the Commissioners*, pp. 8–9.
138 D. Wright, 'Getting Out of the Asylum: Understanding the Confinement of the Insane in the Nineteenth Century', *Social History of Medicine* 10:1 (1997), p. 143.

2

Men in the community: home care, doctors' care, and travellers

[He] miscalled her like a dog, and raged at her dreadful, and at last, what with love, and fury, and despair, he had the terriblest fit you ever. Fell down as black as your hat, he did, and his eyes rolled, and his teeth gnashed, and he foamed at the mouth, and took four to hold him, and presently as white as a ghost, and given up for dead. No pulse for hours; and, when his life came back, his reason was gone ... And now he lies in his own house, as weak as water.[1]

In 1871 novelist Charles Reade described the mental breakdown of Sir Charles Bassett in empathetic and graphic detail. Bassett's spurned mistress communicates details of his mental collapse after his mind increasingly slipped out of his control. His family, his staff, and even his former mistress tried to help him. His family was motivated by two desires: to provide him the best possible care, and to keep him out of an asylum.

The last chapter outlined the most well-documented treatment of insanity in the nineteenth century: the asylum. And yet many men and women who suffered mental distress never saw the inside of an asylum, or were only institutionalized as part of a broader network of treatment options. Even at the height of the asylum century, thousands of registered lunatics lived outside of institutions.[2] And Lunacy Commissioners were convinced that an even larger number of unsupervised men and women suffering various levels of mental distress were unregistered and living outside of government oversight.[3]

The reasons patients avoided the asylum varied wildly. Some families kept sufferers at home to preserve family secrets; some families attempted to exploit their ill relatives; others believed they were doing what was best and fulfilled their loved one's requests.

This chapter explores the variety of care men and their families sought out to deal with insanity beyond the asylum. Treatment options were largely dictated by gender and class contexts in concert with family dynamics. As men were breadwinners, families were more likely to spend resources to restore their health. And yet men's power and privilege allowed them to pressure medical and family contacts to avoid the asylum. Men were able to maintain their autonomy outside of the asylum system and keep control within their families; it is no surprise that many resisted being placed in an asylum. When designated as mad, however, men and women of all socio-economic levels were vulnerable.

Since the 1990s, there has been a growing interest in studying patients outside the asylum. As Akihito Suzuki notes in his study of eighteenth-century lunatics in London, social structure, the particular composition of households, economic and emotional dynamics, and the number of breadwinners and dependants all dramatically shaped decisions around home versus asylum care.[4] Historians studying Ireland, Australasia, the United States, Canada, and around the world note the complex power relationships between medico-governmental authorities and families. Such work places agency back with families, emphasizing the continuing importance of families in the care of the insane.[5] Care decisions were rarely made by doctors alone and were far more likely to be a negotiation between patients, families, and medical authorities.[6]

Discovering men outside of the asylum requires crafting an oblique archive of information. As Catherine Coleborne notes in the Australasian context, asylum records can be surprisingly rich about care beyond their walls.[7] Asylum records capture men whose treatment before and after arrival included living within the home, travel, or private care. While many experts pointed to the asylum as the single point of care, medical authorities in their practice and in broader works acknowledged alternative methods according to circumstances. While reading against the grain of the archive can be a useful way to trace the voices of the mad, it is also important to pay attention to how the official archive is constructed, and the power relations it embodies.[8] The most in-depth stories of men outside the asylum come from Chancery lunacy cases, limited to families of means. The records of the court itself are quite scant, but when cases were contested press accounts relate detailed testimony and reveal the minutiae of care decisions. Government inquiries and Lunacy Commissioners tried to get to the heart of private care and investigated allegations of abuse, in particular of the poor. Press accounts tend to favour sensational stories of abuse, violence, or family breakdowns outside of the asylum, but stories of more banal examples of private care can be uncovered with careful excavation.[9] And finally, the world of fiction gives a key context for broader understandings of lunacy, and insight into general beliefs about patterns of care. All of these sources form an incomplete, but telling, archive.

The social historian will be frustrated in getting any firm understanding of the actual numbers of people who lived with mental distress outside of the asylum, and what percentage was male or female. If patterns of unregistered lunatics followed those on the record, madwomen would have been slightly overrepresented outside the asylum.[10] Outside of the asylum, it is only possible to trace an imperfect, anecdotal, and circumstantial picture. Yet tracing anecdotal experiences and cultural understandings does give a more complete picture of men's experience of care. And while this chapter is an act of reconstruction, it acknowledges that many stories remain secret because families, and sufferers themselves, actively sought to keep their stories out of any official record. Privacy was an overarching desire for the Victorian family, and in particular for the middle or upper classes.[11] However, it would be wrong to assume this secrecy was always motivated by shame.[12] As this chapter demonstrates, personal and family decisions to avoid the asylum were based on a complex and interrelated set of emotional and practical decisions.

This chapter will explore both the commonplace and exceptional stories of madmen outside of asylums. Treatment was dependent on financial circumstances, the particularities of symptoms and needs, and the wishes of patients and their families. Men, on the whole, seem to demonstrate more control over their care choices than women, and this ability intensifies for the wealthy. For those sceptical of the efficacy of the asylum, or who wanted to keep their loved ones' struggles secret, there were other options. Families made decisions sometimes on the advice of doctors, and sometimes against that advice. Many men remained at home or were sent as single patients to be cared for in a domestic environment; this was done either as a way to maintain family secrets or as a deliberate choice for the best possible care. Travel was another popular option for those seeking to avoid the asylum, or for those who would not admit the extent of their disease. While many of these extra-asylum solutions worked well, the chapter ends with the failures of extra-asylum care. Outside of official oversight, madmen could fall victim to egregious abuse. Just as stories of asylum care ranged from qualified success to abysmal failure, so too did outcomes for sufferers outside of asylums vary considerably.

Lunatics at home

The novel that began this chapter, Charles Reade's *A Terrible Temptation*, explores how care in the home could offer an attractive option for wealthy patients who wanted to avoid the asylum. Lady Bella Bassett is horrified to see her husband slowly descend into madness as his jealous cousin tries to destroy him. Sir Charles has no heir, and he is consumed by the fear that his property might revert to his cousin Richard and his nephew. After a serious epileptic fit, he becomes raving mad. His wife and her loyal maid try to shield him from the world, and more particularly from his grasping cousin. When neighbours hear about an apparent fall and a mental breakdown, they come to visit and try to get a sense of the nature of his illness. His wife guards her husband's condition fiercely, and 'they got nothing out of her except that Sir Charles's nerves were shaken'.[13] She employs a doctor to care for her husband, but is fearful to send Sir Charles to an asylum lest his cousin use it as an excuse to take control of the property. This proves to be true, as Charles is eventually secreted away to a private asylum against the will of his wife and his personal doctor's orders with the express intent to make his illness worse.

Reade's fictional account underscores a very real anti-asylum sentiment in popular culture. Even with the rise of the asylum, and doctors' increasing interest in the treatment of the mentally ill, decisions on care almost always started in the family. The state did not go out seeking the mad to detain; men ended up in asylums due to family decisions or an encounter with the law.[14] Families could legally keep lunatics at home without the need for any outside intervention or notice. However, the income of a wealthy person could not be maintained unless under the authority of the Chancery

Court, and the relative overlooking their care could not receive payment.[15] The government would only intervene in cases of suspected abuse. Reade's story also highlights a less well understood concept; families themselves were complex groups that could have radically different motivations. One of the hardest decisions that sufferers, family members, and doctors had to face was deciding when eccentricity, irascibility, forgetfulness, or anxiety veered into actual madness. Home care provided an alternative where the severity or type of illness could be left ambiguous and where families could keep their relatives' conditions private so long as they did not prove any threat to themselves or others.

One way to track families' desire to keep loved ones at home is through the common practice of discharging men to their families after brief stays in asylums, even before they had recovered.[16] Asylums had several categories of patients they discharged, including those who were cured and those who were simply 'relieved'. This assessment could cover a multitude of outcomes, but generally indicated that a patient was considered stable enough to be transferred, though not fully sane. It is often unclear why some patients left asylums to return home before they had recovered.[17] Even private asylums with rich records provide fragmentary evidence about the fate of their patients (Figure 2.1). Between 1870 and 1914, Manor House Asylum released forty-eight 'relieved' male patients back to their homes and families, sometimes against the wishes of the doctors.[18] In such cases the institution certainly had a vested financial interest to keep the patient, and it is possible families had to bring patients home because they ran out of funds. Yet there is evidence that the reasons many families wanted mad relatives at home were more complex.

Private care within the home could be a compromise in cases where parties disagreed about the nature of a man's illness. John Wild was a respectable man whose business speculations turned into delusions. His brother George had him charged at the Mansion House police court for being a lunatic at large.[19] George Wild explained he had not wanted to take such proceedings but did so after his brother John had terrified agents of a mining company with a revolver. They, in turn, threatened to charge John Wild as a dangerous lunatic if his brother did not intervene. He produced a dozen similar letters from friends demanding he take charge of his brother. If John Wild was such a public menace, why did his brother

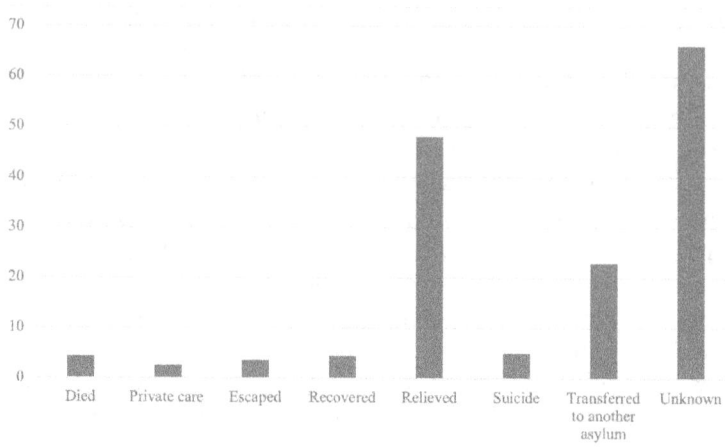

Figure 2.1 Outcomes of male patients from Manor House Asylum, 1850–1914

not intervene sooner? John's defence team explained why; John had his own supporters who believed him perfectly sane. His lawyers provided their own version of events. H.A. Butler-Johnstone, a former Conservative MP, testified that he and John were co-directors of a gold mining company. They dined and met frequently, and he found his friend to be neither mad nor even eccentric.[20] A man who could appear to be a dangerous lunatic to some and a completely rational individual to others made for a complicated case. The rather perplexed alderman who had to declare a ruling agreed to a compromise whereby John Wild would be sent to the care of his brother rather than to an asylum.[21]

Such a case garnered much debate around breakfast tables, consulting rooms, and clubrooms. Dr W.M. Morgan wrote to the *Western Mail* with an explanation as to how a man could seem sane to some, and a lunatic to others. He clarified that cases like John Wild were typical of the early stages of a severe form of paralytic mania. He warned that it was a fast-moving disease and agreed with the outcome of the trial.[22] Incipient or periodic madness was hard to identify and quantify, and thus home care offered an alternative to formal certification and institutionalization. When families and patients could agree, home care avoided the issue of a formal declaration of lunacy and determining the extent of mental disturbance.

Men in the community 65

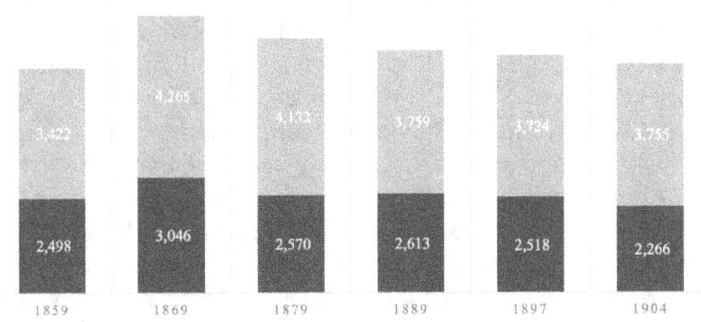

Figure 2.2 Number and distribution of all reported lunatics, idiots, and persons of unsound mind residing with relatives or others

While acknowledging many patients were never registered officially, there were still a significant number of registered lunatics living with relatives outside of asylums (Figure 2.2).[23] The gender breakdown of these numbers might be surprising, as men had more power within households yet were less likely to be residing with relatives. Men consistently made up no more than 42 per cent of the total number of registered single lunatics staying with relations or others. This could be a reflection of the general gender imbalance in lunacy statistics, or the fact that men were physically stronger and harder to manage, or the fact that families were willing to invest funds in men's private care.

Families of limited means could and did make sacrifices to care for their loved ones at home. The working-class family unit had a complex and fragile connection to the middle-class ideal of male dominance over his household. The family as a whole typically contributed to the economic and domestic labour of the household.[24] While the employment of a private attendant was a financial burden, it was within reach of artisans and members of the middle classes. One lithographic engraver, Joshua Armitage, suffered an attack of madness and was kept at home under the supervision of an attendant. His family did not take him to an asylum nor did they have him formally certified as a lunatic; they maintained him within the home with an attendant either at their choice or his own.[25] The cause of his insanity was supposed to be the death of a beloved daughter and anxiety over his professional life. He suffered delusions and violent episodes, and yet the family still kept him at home until a crisis forced their hand.[26] It is important to note that families kept men at home even when it was inconvenient, and even when it was potentially dangerous.[27] While the motive for such choices is not known, the action speaks to an active choice to avoid the asylum.

As Akihito Suzuki demonstrates, many families tried every means at their disposal to keep their insane loved ones at home.[28] While some families likely wanted to avoid the scandal and publicity of a mad relative, in other cases families believed that an asylum would be detrimental to a man's recovery. Sometimes it is clear the sufferer themselves dictated their treatment (or lack thereof) in the home. When a man stayed in his home, either independently or under the care of family or medical experts, it is difficult to know if it was his or his family's choice.[29] Real-life stories are difficult to access unless something went wrong.

The more independence and financial resources a man had, the more likely he could avoid the asylum should he choose. If a man were single, of independent means, and caused no disturbance, his choices were largely his own. Edwin Granville Ley was a retired army surgeon who served many years on the West Coast of Africa before living a life of travel. He maintained lodgings in London, where his landlady had thought him eccentric for many years. After a trip to the Mediterranean in 1886, he was discovered in his lodgings suffering from a fit. The result was partial paralysis, and yet he refused treatment and continued to independently recover. Rejecting medical care, he was able to rely on his servants to carry out his whims. In the autumn of 1890, he suffered another attack in his London club, and he had to be removed to his Weymouth Street home. He continued having epileptiform fits, once as many as seventeen in a single day. For three months he continued at home under outside care. While his fits eventually subsided, his mental health deteriorated. He began to suffer delusions, and he refused to eat. And yet still he lived at home. His level of autonomy can be deduced from his subsequent acts, where he abused his relatives in public and wandered the streets without his hat. At some point he was convinced to move into his brother's house until he was finally transferred to an asylum.[30] He was showing serious signs of illness for a long time and was clearly seriously ill for the better part of a year before certificates were sought for his institutionalization.

Staying at home could allow men to become quite ill should their family not be able to control them. And when family situations shifted, all plans could be thrown into disorder. The case of the Earl of Eldon demonstrates the complex and fluctuating decisions in caring for a mentally ill patriarch. When a doctor was first called in to help, Eldon was on the verge of starving himself to death. Dr Sutherland examined Eldon in June of 1851 and found the forty-six-year-old man was emaciated, tremulous, and inarticulate. The doctor was able to feed his body and his mind improved. After that point, Eldon was prone to fits of excitement, and the family and the doctor took turns reading to him to calm his temper. Diligent care and attention helped improve his situation, and yet he was never truly well. Moments of excitement could strike him at any time, such as when he was riding and he would tear at his clothes and throw his cap in the water.[31] Despite being disruptive, Eldon stayed in his own home, and was able to maintain his old pursuits including riding in the neighbourhood.

The family kept Lord Eldon out of an asylum, but his mental status would not have been secret given his neighbourhood rides and the number of servants involved in his care. His story might never have been widely publicized, however, had Lady Eldon not died in November 1852. She had been taking care of her husband and managing his estates. Her care for her husband was demonstrated by her 'great affection and tact', and there was no critique of her choice to keep him at home when his condition became public.[32] It was only her death that rendered any outside intervention or notice necessary. It was with 'extreme reluctance' that the family turned to the exigency of a formal Lunacy Commission.[33] Eldon was quickly found of unsound mind with little debate, preserving his £60,000 a year at the expense of the family's secret.[34] He died, still in the family home, almost two years later.[35] The Eldon family preferred to deal with their mad relative at home, bringing in medical and state authorities only when needed. There is no mention of asylum care, as they established workable alternatives that were easily available to wealthy families.[36]

Whether all of these decisions were unanimous, and what role Eldon played in these consultations are largely missing from reporting of the Chancery case. One might hope that for families with extensive private archives such conversations would become explicit. However, even then, some families kept their secrets well. Perhaps it should come as no surprise that in an increasingly modern information culture, the pressures on privacy led to a reactive tendency to protect secrecy even within the domestic sphere.[37] Sometimes these secrets extended even to private family archives. Charles Molyneux, known to the family as 'Mull', was the eldest son of the Earl of Sefton. He was a typical young sporting man, engaged to be married. His diaries are brief accounts of hunting, social events, travels, and riding steeplechase.[38] The latter was a pursuit he most enjoyed, although he did not have much skill in that area.[39] But in 1894, when he was twenty-six, the diaries abruptly end. Charles Molyneux was riding the steeplechase when he was thrown and injured his head. When first reported, it did not seem a serious injury. Whether this was due to wishful thinking or a failure to understand the true gravity of the event is unclear.[40] Within a few months, however, his prospects looked bleak, and the family ended his engagement on his behalf.[41]

The Sefton archive contains diaries of several family members who recorded regular interactions with the young heir. And yet most scarcely mention his accident, and there is no trace of the family decisions in his care.[42] Molyneux lived largely at Croxteth Hall, the country estate of the Sefton family, and the family tracked the young man's deteriorating condition in their diaries sporadically, and with few details.[43] His sister-in-law, Lady Helena Mary Molyneux, gives perhaps the most complete account of the young man's fate. She noted interactions with her ill brother-in-law just as she would any other social engagement.[44] As Charles Molyneux's symptoms seemed to vary, he was able to occasionally play billiards and go out driving with the family.[45] While many doctors recommended patients be removed from their old environment, this was sometimes deemed neither practical nor desirable.[46]

Molyneux's father, the Earl of Sefton, died in 1897.[47] The new Earl was quickly declared a lunatic by commission with no trial.[48] By the following year, the press was reporting that not only was his condition considered hopeless of recovery, but there were fears he could die at any point.[49] Such immediate worry was premature. In the summer of 1901 he was still visiting friends in the neighbourhood, but his health did deteriorate in the autumn.[50] He died at the family home in 1901, his obituary revealing little beyond the fact that his mind and physical health had failed after an accident.[51] To his family, he had been 'Poor Mull' for many years.[52] Why his family decided to keep him at home was never discussed; but he remained a part of the family until he died.

Molyneux's family drama left few traces even in a rich archive. Because his family did not challenge care decisions, the details of his life are lost to the historian. When Chancery cases were contested, the trial revealed medical decisions in ways private correspondence rarely did. In the case of Sir Henry Meux, he was kept at home because he would not heed his doctors' warnings, and clearly did not believe that he was mentally ill. Meux exercised his strong paternal will over his young wife and household. While his sisters later stated they could have done more, his wife claimed she was powerless to place him under restraint. Sir Henry Meux left no archive, and yet being a man of means and political prominence, much of his life was on public display. He was an active sportsman and was known as a man who 'rents largely and spends liberally in the North every year'.[53] One can easily draw a timeline of Meux's history around the time of his protracted mental collapse through newspaper reports of his political and social activities. Medical observers agreed his illness was not quite as sudden as any side wished to admit, with symptoms as early as 1855. However, the evidence was conflicting as to when his unsoundness of mind could reliably be dated.

He certainly had a scare of sorts in the winter of 1856, as the family called in four medical men to discuss the state of the baronet's mind after an epileptic seizure. The family doctor, James Allen, advised Sir Henry he needed to take better care of himself. There was no Lunacy Commission held at the time, and none of the doctors felt compelled to write up certificates. According to Allen's later testimony at trial, Meux was suffering from a brain disease at the time and was advised to live quietly as the only way to recover. Sir Henry, however, was of a different opinion, as he had no intention of changing his lifestyle. He and his wife welcomed an heir in 1857 and there were grand celebrations at his country estate.[54] Much like a man with a heart condition might ignore a doctor's orders to modify his diet and exercise, Meux ignored his doctors' advice to lead a quiet life for the sake of his sanity.

In the summer of 1857, Meux suffered some transitory physical ailments, and might also have demonstrated some mental aberration; however, he remained completely in control of his life and his affairs. He continued to engage in various complex business deals that no parties disputed; as late as August 1857 he signed a cheque for £14,000 with his brewery partners.[55] More controversially, Meux executed a codicil in July 1857 that gave the whole of his fortune to his wife should she outlive any children of the marriage.[56] The couple had only one son, Henry Bruce Meux, whose survival would have made the codicil moot. But should the young boy not survive infancy, Lady Meux would inherit the entirety of the estate, to the exclusion of all of his other family. His sisters, once very close to their brother, called for the Lunacy Commission to contest the codicil the following year. As counsel for one of the sisters pointed out, the nature of Sir Henry's actions and in particular cutting his sisters out of his will and handing his entire fortune over to his wife, itself indicated unsoundness.[57]

At the time of the Chancery trial in 1858, all parties agreed Sir Henry was not in his right mind. No one disputed Meux's current care, or the choice to keep him out of an asylum. His address at the time of the commission was the family home at Theobald's Park.[58] Instead, the court was asked to decide when exactly Meux's lunacy began, and if the codicil could be considered valid. As the local newspaper reported, however, 'The point where insanity begins and reason ends is a psychological problem most difficult to determine.'[59] Without direct, detailed knowledge of the events, and without lunacy certificates, the Commission's attempt to backdate Meux's lunacy was doomed from the start. In the end, none of this legal wrangling mattered. Meux lived on for many years, enough to ensure that his son Henry Bruce survived to maturity and succeeded to the Baronetcy at the age of twenty-seven. Henry Meux died at his home in Grosvenor Square in January 1883 with a large estate.[60] Had his sisters never intervened, his experiences would have been absent from the historical record.

Home care could prove challenging if a man were stubborn or the only member of a household; yet there were clearly a number of families who quietly and successfully kept their mentally troubled loved ones at home. Glimpses of more detailed accounts like Charles Molyneux and Henry Meux indicate how successful care was dependent on family consensus. It was only because of a disputed will that any record of Meux's sordid family drama was preserved. Molyneux's illness is only mentioned in fragments of family diaries, with no indication as to why decisions were made. To lunacy reformers, the benefits of privacy were outweighed by the need for supervision, protection from abuse, and their faith in the curative powers of the asylum. Many families clearly disagreed.

Single care: on and off the record

Not all families could or would accept a lunatic within their home, but they still might have wanted to keep them out of an asylum in a domestic environment. Lunacy Commissioners oversaw all single patients who were required to be certified as lunatics.[61] Pauper lunatics were boarded in the community: in Scotland as a matter of course, in England and Wales when asylums were scarce. For families who had resources to pay for some level of care, an ill person could be sent to live with a medical man, a respectable family, or a licensed home care provider.[62] These people were supposed to be certified and housed with registered providers; however, evidence suggests there was a much larger unregistered practice going on. Some trained doctors took on patients whose certification might have been doubtful or controversial, while quacks advertised in the newspapers under the guise of treating 'nervous' patients.

The largest number of registered lunatics housed outside of asylums in the United Kingdom were likely experiencing some kind of community care in Scotland. In the Scottish system, a patient showing signs of lunacy could be sent to private care for a six-month trial without certificates.[63] In fact, quiet or easier to manage cases were regularly boarded out from asylums into the countryside to live with families. The story of boarding out 'harmless' lunatics is well known in the Scottish historiography.[64] In what was praised as a successful system, medical and government officials regularly visited these pauper patients who made up close to 20 per cent of the total pauper lunatic class.[65] Such cases also existed in rural and under-resourced areas in England, where lunatics were boarded out to families.[66] In the English context, however, such examples were seen as failures.[67] Whether malfunctions of an overstretched system or the result of planned care, there were far more lunatics purposely living outside of the asylum, both pauper and private, than Commissioners might have wanted.

Some doctors sought out wealthy single lunatics as private patients, to the great frustration of private asylum owners. Not only did this represent a direct competition to their services, but some lunacy reformers also worried that the practice was open to abuse. According to Dr Lyttelton Forbes Winslow, owner of the private Sussex and Brandenburgh House asylums in Hammersmith, asylum patients were always better off than single patients in private care in every way. During committee hearings in 1877, the chairman questioned Winslow's absolutism, noting that some patients were known to do better in private care than in the asylums. Winslow disagreed, in particular in cases of men who could afford private care; he strongly believed that Chancery patients needed the extra protection of the private asylum.[68] According to Winslow and his supporters, it was only with the added supervision of impartial observers that abuses could be avoided. The fact that the owner of a private asylum would reject single care as an option is not surprising. But clearly his inquisitors had personal or anecdotal evidence of successful home care.

Many patients drifted in and out of official care. In the case of George Edmunds, his family removed him from a private asylum in Hammersmith to live under the care of a medical man in Islington.[69] Families took patients out of the asylum either due to financial constraints or simply because their loved ones seemed to show no improvement. Even Lord Ashley, later Lord Shaftesbury, chair of the Lunacy Commission from 1845 to 1884, preferred single care for his own epileptic son.[70] While scandals might have reached the newspapers, it is plausible that many families quietly boarded their mad relatives with caring and benevolent individuals who treated them well.

Even some doctors who specialized in lunacy wondered if private care might be preferable to the asylum in some cases; such scenarios removed them from their home environments but kept them within a domestic scene. William Richard Gowers was a leading neurologist, teacher, and author on mental disease.[71] And yet even he acknowledged that law and practice did not overlap; and in fact, perhaps the law did not always best suit the patient's interest in terms of private care. He writes of one patient in particular who was suffering from the last traces of a delusion. His friends were quite anxious about the situation, and Gowers sent the man to live with a doctor and his wife for a while. By doing this and sending a delusional patient to a fee-charging doctor while not under certificates, he acknowledged he skirted the law. And yet he also believed it was the best choice, as the man was fully restored within a few weeks. Gowers stated that had he followed the letter of the law and had the man certified, it would have impeded his recovery.[72] As he explained to the Medico-Psychological Association, 'Many who are on the brink of insanity are distressed intensely by the haunting question, and its constant pressure on the quivering mind – "Shall I go mad" and the process seems to give them the answer – you are mad.'[73] In such cases, the asylums became the opposite of their curative intent. Gowers was not prosecuted, but rather praised for his actions.[74]

The fact that lunacy existed outside of the asylum was well recognized. Family doctors likely had the greatest contact with the mad, often for long periods while they recovered or before they were sent to institutions.[75] One of the greatest challenges in the Victorian medico-legal system was that the law required a hard line between madness and sanity. And yet, to the medical community, mental soundness was not an absolute.[76] Mr Thomas Merchant Taylor was a well-respected medical man who was charged with harbouring an unregistered lunatic in his home. His defence explained that the man in question suffered from melancholia but had been discharged as cured from an asylum; the man subsequently relapsed. This time a family doctor suggested that private care might be a better treatment and the patient agreed to the course of treatment.[77] So concerned were the Lunacy Commissioners and the justice system to stamp out any claims of unlawful confinement, even technicalities could appear as severe breaches.

Unofficial care of the mentally ill was well known enough to appear in popular novels. In Charles Dickens's *David Copperfield*, young David encounters an odd man named Mr Dick. He quickly suspects that Mr Dick was 'a little mad' due to his 'childish delight' on being praised and his generally 'vacant manner'.[78] Betsy Trotwood, a distant relation, took Dick and his small income into her own household, insisting he was perfectly sane, if somewhat peculiar. Trotwood makes very clear that Dick's own brother was embarrassed to keep him, despite that being their late father's wish.[79] Technically, such an arrangement could have been skirting the lunacy laws. Mr Dick's small income might have made him a likely candidate for Chancery oversight.[80] And yet in practice, it is likely many families avoided this step and set up single care alternatives.

Individual medical men advertised taking on private patients without the need for certificates.[81] Doctors could not legally offer their services to the truly insane unless they ran licensed establishments. However, advertisers did use coded language to appeal to those with mental disorders without actually using the word 'lunatic'. A medical man or gentleman could legally take in someone who was behaving erratically but did not quite meet the threshold for certification, just as they could any other kind of invalid. Advertisements couched nervous or mental weakness among other bodily diseases.[82] One medical man advertised for any patient who could benefit from the bracing seaside air, including those suffering from chest complaints, scrofula, or 'nervous debility'.[83] Whatever the law might have proscribed about keeping single lunatics in private homes without a licence, it is clear that the law was regularly violated either consciously or in ignorance. In one instance, a woman was fined for keeping a patient suffering from melancholia with delusions in her home. Her defence was that the patient's own medical advisor had recommended against any kind of institutional care, advocating instead a private home.[84] The practice of private care was common enough that a brisk trade in keeping one or two unlicensed lunatics continued throughout the nineteenth century.

Periodic arrests and convictions for keeping single patients without a licence did not seem to greatly limit this income-generating practice.[85] For instance, Henry Baker was a former attendant at Bethlem hospital who translated his experience there into a profitable, if illegal, side-business. He kept three uncertified lunatics in his home in 1851 without a licence. The patients were well treated, and Baker had discovered a niche market, both taking patients into his home and attending them in their own homes. Some of these patients were awaiting removal to an asylum, some were transitioning out of the asylum system, and some were avoiding it altogether. The Commissioners in Lunacy decided to pursue prosecution and he was sent to trial because he had violated the law, even though there was no charge of abuse; he was found guilty but with the sole penalty of not continuing in his actions. In fact, on a follow-up visit, they found another lunatic within his home.[86] There was obviously a demand for such services, and they did not always end in the mistreatment of patients. Baker provided a good level of care and even employed a doctor to look after his charges' medical needs. The practice did not seem to diminish over time, even as the capacity of asylums expanded.

Patients in single care, both on and off the record, were a frustration to Lunacy Commissioners and private asylum owners. While most officials believed asylums to be the best treatment, it is obvious that many patients, families, and even medical practitioners did not agree at the individual level. More than that, this section highlights the diversity of reasons that people sought out private care, and the multiplicity of treatments received. The reasons that families chose to keep their loved ones out of asylums were varied, and often left unexplained to medical authorities and unrecorded in family histories.

'Taking the waters': travel to ease a troubled mind

Another option to avoid the asylum was to quit Britain altogether. Wealthy men could choose travel as a way to seek treatment without necessarily acknowledging the seriousness of their illness. Some men did so on the advice of doctors, others against that advice, and in some cases families used travel to get lunatics out of the country. Health manuals offered vague advice that travel could be a panacea for almost any illness. As one brochure for Southern California boasted: 'Convalescents from any acute disease will hasten their complete recovery by coming here, and will be restored to perfect health much sooner than is usual at home.'[87] Such hopeful promises from places as disparate as Italy, Australia, and Egypt were tempting to those looking to bypass tough conversations with men who would not admit insanity but could accept a vague nervous debility.

There was a strong, genuine belief that foreign travel could be a useful choice in both medical and popular culture. The idea of foreign travel for health was a common trope in popular fiction.[88] The potential curative powers of a different climate or environment offered more hope than the definiteness of an asylum stay, in particular for those in the early stages of a disease. Asylum records demonstrate that men commonly travelled under the supervision of medical men or attendants before turning to the asylum. The option of travelling, going to a water spa, or taking a long sea journey also allowed patients a sense of agency over their treatment. Taking charge of their care, men in the early stages of mental collapse could hope to rejuvenate themselves and did not have to place themselves at the mercy of a doctor or asylum superintendent.[89] Thus it is no surprise to find men trying travel, and to find their male support networks backing up that decision.

While doctors often complained that patients were not sent to asylums early enough, it was often family doctors who recommended foreign travel.[90] The reason for this was simple: most patients with early mental symptoms would have first met with local doctors, not specialists. Few doctors received specialized training in mental disorders, and alienists did not find widespread acceptance of their theories in general practice. Most medical men believed in the curative power of a change of air, a new way of living, and an enhanced exercise routine as a general panacea for ailments of all sorts.[91] And the early symptoms of mental distress could be indistinguishable from many physical illnesses.

Another reason doctors might suggest travel is that they had a much greater chance of patients heeding their advice. The suggestion to travel was an easy proposition and there was an extant infrastructure to support health travel both domestically and internationally. Aristocratic people of delicate health or vague malaise had long entertained and strengthened themselves through leisure travel, including those suffering from nervousness or hysteria.[92] Hydropathy and hydrotherapy centres were popular destinations to treat the Victorian semi-invalid, men and women alike. Either for pleasure or medical cure, such water treatments permeated the upper and middle classes.[93] Some sites advertised not only restoring health and vitality, but even obliquely referenced a renewed manly vigour.[94] Such vague descriptions could be appealing to men with nebulous mental symptoms. But it was not simply water spas, but full-fledged grand tours of resort towns across the continent and around the world that were marketed as respites for invalids, complete with specialized guides that highlighted trails to follow depending on the type of ailment.[95] Families and medical professionals could cling to the hope that a patient was suffering from a minor nervous debility rather than actual incipient lunacy.

The semi-invalid health crisis seemed a *sine qua non* for Victorian intellectuals.[96] John Stuart Mill suffered two mental breakdowns in his life, and his reaction to his different treatment options are revealing. In 1826 he suffered his first major crisis, but as he was able to continue working he was largely left to his own devices.[97] Middle-class masculinity was grounded in a work identity, and thus a man who could continue working was less likely to solicit doctors' help or listen to outside advice.[98] Mill related the story of this breakdown in depth in his autobiography and had little shame about the event. However, when his father died Mill had a far more serious illness that he did not publicise. This time he stopped working and was sent to Brighton to recover. Finding no relief, doctors recommended he travel the continent. His doctors saw his inherent nervous temperament mixed with overwork as the perfect storm for a mental breakdown.[99] Mill's experiences would have been interpreted by contemporaries as a success story, proving that travel alone could restore a worried mind. Yet Mill himself did not write about it – giving a sense that for some men any reduction of their productivity was a story best kept private.

European spas and health resorts offered curative options, but they were not designed for treating actual insanity.[100] And travel would not always guarantee a man could avoid an asylum. For instance, after suffering from symptoms for three years, John Dyer travelled to Germany for his 'health'. German authorities quickly found he was not nervous or exhausted but insane, and he was sent to an asylum.[101] His wife then had to initiate a Lunacy Inquiry in England.[102] In Dyer's case, it is not clear if his family knew how serious his condition was before he travelled to Germany. While water cures could be the first line of treatment for mild illnesses, they could also be used as a last resort when all hope was seemingly lost.[103]

While travel had its medical supporters, some doctors were scathing of the practice.[104] Thomas Stretch Dowse was particularly contemptuous of the idea of travel as a cure-all. Dowse cautioned that simply getting to fashionable resorts and hotels on the continent could actually exacerbate fractured nerves, believing railway journeys could trigger a mental breakdown.[105] The only travel he could recommend was an extended sea voyage.[106] Dowse's credentials were solid: he was a fellow of the Royal College of Physicians in Edinburgh, had served as physician-superintendent at the London Sick Asylum in the 1880s, and had experience working at a London hospital specializing in epilepsy and paralysis.[107] And yet in practice it appears that men of means often tried travel of various sorts as their first attempt at cure, and general practitioners had no problem recommending it to their patients.

While travel might have worked for some sufferers, official records tend to capture the failures. Such chronicles also outline the lengths some men would go to to avoid institutional care. Even in cases where the patient was quite ill, he might defy doctors' recommendations and choose travel over the asylum.[108] John Whaley, a hotel manager, had been advised by a doctor to alter his lifestyle and travel at his first signs of physical and mental debility. The idea that middle-class men could restore exhausted nerves by getting away from the home and the demands of work simply by change of air was widespread.[109] Whaley's first destination was to Norfolk, hoping perhaps the sea air would help. His move did little good, so he travelled on to Lowestoft, where he seemed to further deteriorate. He was then sent to the other coast at Cornwall under care of attendants. His behaviour became even more extreme; his general rowdiness was so intense it created a 'public scandal'.[110]

At this point, it would be hard to imagine a woman would have been allowed to continue unchecked by her family, friends, or even public authorities. However, for Whaley, this simply inspired an even greater distance of travel. He embarked on an overseas journey to France, where he eventually became so unmanageable that hotels refused to take him as a guest. In fact, he would have been arrested had not attendants been sent by friends to ferry him home. When he arrived at the railway station in England, he was finally certified under an urgency order as a lunatic.[111] Whaley had the means, and the independence, to try a variety of destinations in his quest for health until he was actually threatened with imprisonment. His peripatetic lifestyle finally ended in Manor House Asylum as a last resort.[112]

Another major impetus to foreign travel was clearly its ability to remove an embarrassing relative from the family scene. When a man's behaviour became uncontrollable, he risked losing his reputation and his status in society.[113] The Australasian governments believed that English Poor Law authorities were encouraging emigration or simply shipping off lunatics in order to reduce their financial responsibilities.[114] One doctor writing about New Zealand claimed the problem of sending hopeless lunatics to the colony had become so extreme that Parliament had to intervene. This author believed that while most of these lunatics temporarily improved during the sea voyage, they became more insane than ever after a month or two in the stimulating air of New Zealand.[115] The situation was serious enough that in 1899 the colony enacted legislation to deport certain types of undesirable immigrants including the insane.[116] Another handbook written for medical travel mentioned the unfortunate practice of sending seriously unwell people of various sorts from England to 'Buenos Ayres', with only the vaguest instructions.[117] Whether out of a desire to avoid responsibility of care, or to avoid the stigma of a mad relative, foreign travel could be a way for heartless families to dispose of madmen.

A multitude of reasons likely motivated foreign travel and spa culture, inspired both by families and the patients themselves. For families, the formal requirement for admission to a private asylum was high, demanding two independent doctors' certificates. There was no process for voluntary admission until 1890, and thus foreign and domestic spas could step into this institutional middle ground. Should a man recover overseas he could simply return to his normal life. For sufferers, the choice to travel or to seek out hydrotherapy gave them autonomy over their cure, and more control over the definition of their illness.[118] Some men might not have wanted to admit the seriousness of their symptoms, while others might not have recognized they were ill at all. Evidence also suggests that travel was used as a way to get rid of troubling, embarrassing, or truculent family members. As a panacea treatment, travel reveals the wide possibilities that families of means had when considering care for men on the borderlands of insanity.

Violence and terror: the dangers of private care

In all of the above examples of treatment outside the asylum, all parties tried to humanely manage or treat the mentally distressed. However, the very lack of oversight that made extra-asylum treatment appealing could leave lunatics in danger or put the community at risk. Accordingly, one of the markers officials used to determine lunacy was whether a man was dangerous to himself or others. While cases of lunatics in the community were typically uneventful, media stories highlighted the potential disaster of madmen outside the asylum. Such media representation reinforced stereotypes of the violent madman and, more importantly, reinforced the idea that male lunatics needed to be kept in asylums for the protection of their families.

Sometimes men were kept from the asylum and looked after by family because they had no other choice. John Patten's family were able to control him for sixteen years after he had a mental attack. The had consulted medical men over the years and they were eager to reach out for care. However, as his lunacy was episodic, doctors found that he did not quite meet the threshold for certification as he could answer questions reasonably, despite showing clear signs of lunacy. He managed to live quasi-independently, even keeping a job as an agent. After sixteen years, however, he finally came under the notice of the authorities. He was arrested trying to enter officers' quarters in Buckingham Palace, evidently inebriated. His sister testified that he was prone to 'illusions and to fits of violence, which rendered him dangerous to his family'. Patten's family did not choose to keep him at home; they simply had no other option. Even this incident did little to change the situation as the magistrate accepted Patten's apology and his statement that he never meant his family any harm. He was discharged with a warning that if the court saw him again, he would once and for all be dispatched to jail or to an asylum.[119]

It is not clear why the family of Captain Andrews kept him at home. Perhaps he did not meet the technical threshold of madness. Perhaps he still had enough patriarchal control to cow his wife into not sending him away. Perhaps the family felt he had the best chance of recovery at home. However, it was a dangerous choice as the family lived for years in 'continual dread' of Andrews as he alternately attempted violence on himself and his family.[120] Early one morning his daughter woke to her father bashing in her mother's head. The Inquest found wilful murder and that the man was not in control of his actions at the time of the crime.[121] Sometimes it was only with an unprovoked act of violence that a man's madness was fully established. After Broadmoor opened to male patients in 1864, there was an increasing willingness to use it for violent lunatics.[122]

While shame, bullying, or desperation could be motivators to keep violent men in the home, some families genuinely wanted to care for their loved ones. Even men who demonstrated violence towards their families, and whose presence would likely cause a financial burden, could still be welcomed in their homes. John Aitken, a chairmaker, was indicted for attempting to murder his five-year-old great-niece. His daughter at first refused to give evidence against her father, who could afford no legal counsel. Eventually she agreed, and she testified that she witnessed her father attack the young girl for no reason. He had attacked the girl with a razor; witnesses testified they believed he was losing his mind. In his defence, the seventy-year-old Aitken stated he had no memory of the event and that he suffered from depression that led him to drink.[123] The judge found him not guilty on the grounds of insanity.[124] He was sent to Broadmoor, but his family continued to hope for his return. His wife wrote to the asylum a few years later asking that her husband be sent home. She and his friends believed he had regained his sanity, or at the very least was no longer dangerous to anyone, and he should be set at liberty.[125]

The place of a man within his home, even when he had lost control of his mind, was paramount in some families. There are numerous examples of families removing their loved ones from institutions against doctors' orders, sometimes with tragic results. Insanity was a significant factor in domestic murder cases; from 1841 to 1900, in cases where the husband was found to be the killer, 17 per cent of those verdicts found the killer to be insane.[126] A madman was a source of potential and unchecked violence, and without official control could be a danger to his family and the community.

Neglect and abuse: the dangers of private care II

Stories of violent madmen were tragic but not surprising. The violent madman was a longstanding trope that did not fundamentally challenge masculine norms. Well-known cases of madwomen as victims of abuse also reaffirmed the fragile nature and inherent vulnerability of women. The Lunacy Commissioners framed their opposition to single care for both sexes as a problem of vulnerability, but stories of helpless women being abused struck a particular nerve with the general public. In particular, stories that touched on wives confined by scheming husbands connected with broader concerns about the failures of marriage.[127] Surrounded by caring people, a lunatic might be well protected even if not registered. However, any unregistered lunatic could easily be the victim of abuse or coercion. And while Commissioners tried to address cases of abuse of both men and women, invariably stories of women held more cultural weight. Unlike stories of violence towards men in the asylums, however, there were some notable stories of abused men that did break through to a public scandal.

Novelists understood the potential tensions men's madness could wreak in the family, especially when men could not exercise their self-control.[128] However, it was more unusual to find madmen as the victims of abuse in popular fiction. Wilkie Collins, the master of sensation, understood this. He explained his process of choosing settings and characters; on deciding to write about a lunatic asylum, he instantly thought about the idea of false incarceration through the use of a double. For 'The victim to be interesting [she] must be a woman, to be very interesting she must be a lady.'[129] Sympathies for the madman were not as natural as for the madwoman, and many feelings lingered that families had every right to lock up their mad relatives however they saw fit.

Sensational stories of abused madmen were dutifully reported by the Lunacy Commission, and sometimes reached the newspapers, even if they did not spur the same kind of moral panic as stories where vulnerable women were the victims. Nor did such tales reach the prominence of stories where madmen were perpetrators of violence. But these stories did allow opportunities for medical men to assert their power and underscore why oversight was necessary when even men could be locked away by scheming or abusive relatives.

Experts in lunacy were concerned with lunatic men and women's vulnerability to abuse. In 1854 the Lunacy Commissioners noted that while they were not looking to prosecute poor people who tried to provide care but did not know all of the rules, they did want to ensure all lunatics were being well cared for.[130] They focused their attention on cases where there were reports of abuse.[131] One instance of an abused unregistered lunatic was revealed only after a man jumped out of the window of a home. He was a blind madman, kept in a third-floor attic by his supposed friends.[132] Writing for the *British Medical Journal* in 1870, one author noted that if lunatics were not in asylums they were likely to be abused and neglected because of lingering stigmas around insanity. The harmless wandering lunatic was likely to become 'a driveling and repulsive being, half-starving on his Poor-law pittance and the fruits of his begging, pelted and tortured by the village schoolboys, worked like a galley-slave by inhuman taskmasters, privileged only in the matter of kicks'.[133]

The behaviour of William Roberts was so 'aggravated and disgraceful' towards his lunatic brother that in 1853 the Commissioners felt the need to intervene. William Roberts had been keeping his brother Evan in a nine- by six-foot room with no fire or ventilation that one could only access through a dark scullery. He was well fed and clean but was chained by both ankles to the bed. Evan was forty-eight, the eldest son of a farmer, and he had suffered periodic fits of mania since reaching adulthood. According to his brother, the attacks became increasingly severe, culminating in one where he threatened his father and brother. He was then locked up in a small room on the upper floor of his father's house (a literal madman in the attic). He was never allowed to leave or go outside. When his father died three years later, his younger brother took over his care and built his current prison. What was most shocking about this case was that Evan was not a dangerous or raving lunatic when he was discovered; in fact, he quite frequently had long periods of lucidity.[134]

Dr Lloyd Williams visited Evan in his room, lying on his wooden bed. He found the man completely coherent, and devoid of hallucinations or delusions. After this discovery, he was transferred to the North Wales Lunatic Asylum, where he continued to demonstrate long periods of rationality; even in moments of insanity, he was never violent. The question in this case, because he was kept by a family member, was whether excessive restraint was used: more than was necessary to the security and care of the lunatic. The actual manacles used were produced in court.[135] The jury found there had been excessive force; William was found guilty of unlawfully confining and imprisoning his brother and sentenced to one month in prison.[136] The Lunacy Commissioners believed the sentence had been too lenient in the case; however, they acknowledged it likely reflected the fact that William's action 'was regarded as the usual course in North Wales in similar cases'.[137] At the time, the non-restraint movement was well established and the use of strait-jackets, let alone leg irons, was becoming anathema to medical practitioners; yet clearly the local community did not always agree.[138] Such stories could be used to educate the public on expected care.

Ten years later, Theodore Edgar Byrne, a physician from Falmouth, was still deeply concerned about the state of single lunatics living outside of the asylum system in family care. After hearing local gossip of a lunatic being held in inhumane conditions, he uncovered that Robert Porter was being kept in a horrible state in his brother's house. Byrne was shocked to discover that here, 'covered by a portion of wet and filthy sacking, was Robert Porter, engaged [in] *eating his own excrement*'.[139] The man was deformed, filthy, wounded, and had clearly been kept in that state for years. The Lunacy Commissioners were alerted to the case and launched an investigation. Samuel Porter was a prosperous builder, living in a respectable house with his wife and family. The room they kept his elder brother in was purpose-built and disconnected from the home with no heat or ventilation. Robert Porter had been a mason himself until the age of twenty, when he drifted into melancholia. He lived with his father until his death in 1850, when he moved in with his unmarried sister before she left for America in 1853. Since then, he had been with his younger brother Samuel. For twenty years he had not seen a doctor, and for over ten years the only human contact he had had was with his brother, sister-in-law, and their child. His living conditions were well known in the neighbourhood, and yet no action was taken until Byrne intervened. The Commissioners found that Robert had for many years been treated with 'the grossest neglect and cruelty'.[140]

The details of the case were horrific in and of themselves, and the case received widespread newspaper coverage.[141] The defence team's attempt to argue based on technicalities also received little press sympathy.[142] While the jury found Samuel Porter guilty, they also recommended mercy due to his ignorance of the law. One reporter found the whole situation reprehensible, but not unexpected. He blamed the prejudice of the 'poorer classes' who feared sending their relatives to asylums. He believed popular opinion and the legal system were out of step. 'But, according to old notions, lunatics are no more than wild beasts, and these notions must be eradicated before juries can take a reasonable view of the obligation incurred by the sane to the insane.'[143] Papers framed these stories to educate people on the need for asylum care.

Byrne did not see his exposé of the Porter case as an isolated incident. Rather, he stated that within fifty miles of that place he found five lunatics privately confined in homes, and two of those under horrible conditions. He believed the law needed to change to better protect private lunatics.[144] Authorities saw these men as harmless victims; but clearly their families saw them as bestial figures that needed to be locked away and controlled. Yet such families still chose to keep them at home rather than send them to the asylum. Whether they were motivated by the shame of sending a family member to the pauper asylum, or fear that sending him away would increase his visibility to the neighbourhood, the family's treatment of Robert was clearly out of step with medical advice.

By the end of the century, communities were more vigilant in seeking out potential cases of abuse. In the case of the Hutton family, someone notified the police about a lunatic living in the stables of the family home. The scandal of the case increased as his keeper was not only his brother, but also a doctor. John Hutton was charged with keeping a lunatic in an unlicensed home. His brother Robert, then thirty-six years of age, was a congenital idiot. He lived most of his life at home, apart from a stay at the Royal Albert Hospital for four years around the age of seven. He was discharged with no improvement and lived the rest of his life with his brother. On the surface, the case looked like one of cruelty as Robert lived in a six- by four-foot pen with a single wooden seat. And yet he was clean and well dressed, showed affection to his brother, and when transferred to Earlswood Asylum, died within four days.[145]

Detailing his life with his brother, John spoke of how they could not keep servants as they refused to work in a house with a lunatic. Robert had a heart condition, and his isolation was his own choice as he was frightened of strangers. The reason he slept outside was because at night he constantly made noise and woke the house. Claiming that he and his wife had given the best years of their lives to his brother, the court broke into supportive applause for John.[146] Charges of abuse were dropped and eventually even the charge that the doctor kept his brother without the oversight of the Commissioners in Lunacy broke down. In fact, an affidavit from 1892 was produced showing that the Master of Lunacy approved of the arrangement and had known of it since 1889.[147] Dr John Hutton still believed that keeping his brother at home in an isolated state was his best option for care and had acted accordingly.

These cases demonstrate a longstanding public acceptance that families could look after mad relatives; and yet neighbours were increasingly attentive to the level of care provided. While such episodes are anecdotal, they suggest that the practice of confining men within the home did happen. These cases also demonstrate that the likelihood of a male relative being locked up in the proverbial attic dramatically increased when there was a male head of family. Wives found it a challenge to control a mad husband in the home against his will. The paterfamilias was the unquestioned head of the household.[148] A woman would have had less capability to hide her husband, and a breadwinner's absence from the public world would have been marked. While the practice of keeping family members confined in the home did not seem to change much over time, public acceptance of the practice waned in the latter decades of the century if the lunatic were not being treated humanely.

Conclusion

While tales of violent and destructive madmen in the community consumed public representations, that should not cloud the fact that there was a great deal of diversity in private care. Madmen were kept out of the asylum for various reasons. Sometimes families sought out improved or alternate treatment methods or wanted a family member kept within the home no matter their condition. As this chapter demonstrates, men also established a remarkable level of autonomy to make decisions against medical, family, or even government advice. For those who still knew their own will, madmen could assert a surprising level of legal authority over themselves and their families. In the balance between family stability and mandated care, maintaining family power structures was typically favoured over what may have been the best method of treatment. Men's ability to dictate their own treatment was dependent on a

Men in the community 87

variety of factors including wealth, severity of symptoms, or even their tyrannical relations over their family. These situations could work out to everyone's benefit; yet these are the tales least likely to survive in the historical archive.

The previous two chapters have explored the various care options to treat the mentally disturbed. However, they have generally treated lunacy as a monolith, as if all forms of madness were equal, with only a variation in family and personal circumstances. Not only did symptoms of lunacy vary greatly, but so too did people's reactions to those various forms of lunacy and their supposed causes. If shame cannot be located on the asylum/private care axis, that does not mean it was not important. The next chapter puts shame at the forefront of analysis and interrogates the value judgements inherent in Victorian diagnostics.

Notes

1 C. Reade, *A Terrible Temptation: A Story of the Day* [1871] (Paris, 1900), p. 67.
2 According to the Lunacy Commissioners there were 44,695 patients officially recognized as insane in England and Wales in 1864. Forty-eight per cent were in county asylums, 21 per cent in workhouses, 12 per cent lived with relatives, 9 per cent in licensed houses, 5 per cent in licensed hospitals, and the rest boarded out in lodgings or lived as single patients. *Eighteenth Report of the Commissioners in Lunacy* (London, 1864), p. 108.
3 See, for example: *Fourth Annual Report of the Commissioners in Lunacy* (London, 1850), p. 10; *Seventeenth Annual Report of the Commissioners in Lunacy*, p. 25; *Thirty-ninth Annual Report of the Commissioners in Lunacy* (London, 1885), p. 112. Only after the 1890 Lunacy Act were the Commissioners convinced the problem had finally abated. *Fifty-fifth Annual Report of the Commissioners in Lunacy*, p. 55.
4 A. Suzuki, 'The Household and the Care of Lunatics in Eighteenth-Century London', in P. Horden and R. Smith (eds), *The Locus of Care: Families, Communities, Institutions, and the Provision of Welfare since Antiquity* (London, 1998), pp. 168–69.
5 N. Tomes, 'The Anglo-American Asylum in Historical Perspective', in C. Smith and J. Giggs (eds), *Location and Stigma: Contemporary Perspectives on Mental Health Care* (Boston, 1988), pp. 14, 19; N.

Tomes, *The Art of Asylum Keeping: Thomas Story Kirkbride and the Origins of American Psychiatry* (Philadelphia, 1994), p. xix; M. Finnane, 'Asylums, Families, and the State', *History Workshop Journal* 20:1 (1985), p. 135; S. Garton, *Medicine and Madness: A Social History of Insanity in New South Wales, 1880–1940* (Kensington, 1988), p. 189; Kelm, 'Women, Families and the Provincial Hospital for the Insane, pp. 177–93; Levine-Clark, 'Dysfunctional Domesticity'; P. Prestwich, 'Female Alcoholism in Paris, 1870–1920: The Response of Psychiatrists and of Families', *History of Psychiatry* 14:3 (2003), pp. 321–36.

6 Chaney, '"No 'Sane' Person Would Have Any Idea"'; A. Borsay, *Disabled Children: Contested Caring, 1850–1979* (London, 2012); Marland, *Dangerous Motherhood*.

7 As Coleborne notes, Australian public records are much richer than their counterparts in the United Kingdom. However, private British asylums contain a wealth of such data. C. Coleborne, *Madness in the Family: Insanity and Institutions in the Australasian Colonial World, 1860–1914* (Basingstoke, 2010), p. 4; C. Coleborne, *Why Talk About Madness? Bringing History into the Conversation* (Basingstoke, 2020), pp. 15–28.

8 Much like with the colonial archive, with the asylum it is tempting to read the asylum against the grain and focus on patients from the ground up. This project must be placed against a concurrent study of the institutional powers themselves, and men's patriarchal power to resist state and medical authorities. A.L. Stoler, 'Colonial Archives and the Arts of Governance', *Archival Science* 2:1–2 (2002), p. 101.

9 Such research might have been frustratingly difficult in an era before digitized newspapers, but due to the efforts of the British Library's Nineteenth-Century newspaper database you can easily search for what often amount to little more than one-sentence descriptions in small, regional papers.

10 In the case of single patients that were registered with the Lunacy Commission, there were more women than men. However, the difference was not inordinate. For example, between 1876 and 1898 there were 547 more registered women than men out of a total of 5,192.

11 D. Cohen, *Family Secrets: The Things We Tried to Hide* (New York, 2013), p. xiv.

12 As Albert D. Pionke points out in his study of secrecy in Victorian fiction, the 'bewildering range of secrets and motives for keeping them exerts tremendous pressure on any hermeneutic deployed to make sense of Victorian secrecy as a general cultural practice'. A.D. Pionke, 'Victorian Secrecy: An Introduction', in A.D. Pionke and D.T. Millstein (eds), *Victorian Secrecy: Economies of Knowledge and Concealment* (Aldershot, 2010), p. 10.

13 Reade, *A Terrible Temptation*, p. 181.
14 Suzuki, *Madness at Home*, p. 2.
15 A.W. Renton, *The Law of and Practice in Lunacy: With the Lunacy Acts 1890–91* (Edinburgh, 1897), p. 87. Alexander Wood Renton was a respected jurist, and this work was long held as the key reference text on law in lunacy in the United Kingdom. 'Obituary: Sir A.W. Renton', *The Times* (19 June 1933), p. 19.
16 Coleborne demonstrates the porous boundary of public asylums in Australasia, as patients often went home on trial leave. Coleborne, *Madness in the Family*, pp. 122–42.
17 The reason Suzuki turned to Chancery lunacy cases is that they provide rich and detailed accounts of exactly these kinds of discussions. Suzuki, *Madness at Home*.
18 Walter Whitehead was allowed to go to Brighton for a change of air with an attendant and had his certificates lapse. His new attendant would not sign new certificates, nor would his family intervene. The asylum was forced to discharge him as relieved. A few months later he jumped out of a window to his death. Manor House Asylum Case Notes, Male Patients, MS 5725, pp. 238–39.
19 'Singular Case of Alleged Lunacy', *Monmouthshire Merlin* (20 October 1882), p. 3.
20 In his testimony, he went so far as to state that if John Wild were sent to an asylum, there was 'not a man in London who would be safe from being placed in a similar position'. 'Extraordinary Charge of Lunacy', *Daily News* (14 October 1882), p. 2.
21 'An Alleged Lunatic at Large', *St James's Gazette* (14 October 1882), p. 12.
22 W.M. Morgan, letter to the editor, *Western Mail* (20 October 1882), p. 4.
23 These numbers are likely a dramatic underestimate of the number of lunatics kept at home in England and Wales.
24 Y.S. Lee, *Masculinity and the English Working Class: Studies in Victorian Autobiography and Fiction* (London, 2007), pp. 13–14.
25 His wife told Broadmoor officials her husband had been insane for eight years. Berkshire County Record Office, Broadmoor asylum, D/H14/D2/2/1/709/4.
26 Armitage attacked his attendant, John Howard and killed him. He was brought to the Leeds Assizes and put on trial, where he was found insane and transferred to Broadmoor. Berkshire County Record Office, Broadmoor Asylum, D/H14/D2/2/1/709/1. Schedule A. Admitted May 1871.
27 The stigma of being a pauper lunatic surely influenced this reluctance to have recourse to the asylum. While it was not the same as sending

a family member to a workhouse, to be a patient at a county asylum did make them dependent on poor relief. Melling and Forsythe (eds), *Politics of Madness*, p. 23.
28 Suzuki, *Madness at Home*, pp. 90–147.
29 P. Bartlett and D. Wright, 'Community Care and its Antecedents', in Bartlett and Wright (eds), *Outside the Walls of the Asylum*, pp. 4–5; Levine-Clark, 'Dysfunctional Domesticity', pp. 341–61; J. Melling, 'Family Matters? Psychiatry, Kinship and Domestic Responses to Insanity in Nineteenth-Century England', *History of Psychiatry* 18:2 (2007), pp. 247–54.
30 It is not clear what Ley suffered from, and his subsequent asylum admission does not report a diagnosis. His symptoms, however, were both physical and mental. They included paralysis, delusions, and the refusal of food. Manor House Asylum Case Notes, Male Patients, MS 6222, pp. 307–16.
31 *London Evening Standard* (15 January 1853), p. 3.
32 *The Times* (17 January 1853), p. 4.
33 'Commission of Lunacy on the Earl of Eldon', *Daily News* (17 January 1853), p. 3.
34 *Hampshire Telegraph and Sussex Chronicle* (15 January 1853), p. 5.
35 'Death of the Earl of Eldon', *Morning Post* (16 September 1854), p. 7.
36 C. Mackenzie, 'Social Factors in the Admission, Discharge and Continuing Stay of Patients at Ticehurst Asylum, 1845–1917', in W.F. Bynum, R. Porter, and M. Shepherd (eds), *The Anatomy of Madness: Essays in the History of Psychiatry*, vol. 2 (London, 1985), pp. 147–74.
37 A. Welsh, *George Eliot and Blackmail* (Cambridge, 1985), pp. 13–15.
38 His forefathers were deeply involved in racing and helped to bail the Grand National at Liverpool out of financial difficulties in 1839. J. Pinfold, 'Horse Racing and the Upper Classes in the Nineteenth Century', *Sport in History* 28:3 (2008), p. 417.
39 Diary of 5th Earl of Sefton, Charles Molyneux, 920/SEF/2/3.
40 Early reports that the injury was slight and that he joined the evening's dinner party were obviously incorrect. 'The Racing Accident', *Hartlepool Northern Daily Mail* (30 March 1894), p. 3.
41 *Dublin Daily Nation* (20 June 1898), p. 2.
42 Diaries include Henry Hervey Molyneux (920 SEF/1), Charles Molyneux himself (920 SEF/2), Rose Molyneux (920 SEF/3), Helena Molyneux (920 SEF/4), and Frederick Molyneux (920 SEF/6), Liverpool Record Office.
43 Diary of Henry Hervey Molyneux, 920/SEF/1/28. A lack of candour is not the reason for omission of any details. Henry was happy to record a candid conversation with Osbert Molyneux (who succeeded

Men in the community 91

to the Earldom after his brother died) about his gambling debts. 920/SEF/1/26.

44 Yet his mental problems did not seem to change the young woman's feelings of disdain for the mad in general. She wrote about encountering a madwoman on her honeymoon in Paris. She writes that she 'couldn't help laughing at her all day & night ... Again laughed at the mad woman who seems to haunt us & shrieks at us everywhere we go.' Diary of Lady Helena Mary Molyneux, 920/SEF/4/1.

45 Diary of Rose Molyneux, 920/SEF/4/3.

46 J. Coxe, *Lunacy in Its Relation to the State: A Commentary on the Evidence Taken by the Committee of the House of Commons on Lunacy Law in the Session of 1877* (London, 1878), p. 37.

47 'Death of Lord Sefton', *South Wales Echo* (28 June 1897), p. 4.

48 Chancery proceedings were initiated by his mother and he did not object to the findings of his mind being unsound. NA, C211/63, 1897.

49 *London Daily News* (15 June 1898), p. 8. Not all papers were so circumspect in their coverage. For example: 'Lunatic Millionaire', *South Wales Echo* (15 June 1898), p. 2.

50 Diary of Lady Helena Mary Molyneux, 920/SEF/4/4.

51 'Obituary', *The Times* (3 December 1901), p. 6.

52 His uncle Frederick Molyneux, best known for his close connection to the royal family, was informed of his nephew's last illness by telegram. He left from London and found the family gathered around an unconscious Earl of Sefton. On 2 December he recorded that 'Poor Mull died about eight o'clock in the morning.' Diary of Frederick Molyneux, 920 SEF/6.

53 *Inverness Courier* (24 January 1856), p. 5.

54 *Morning Chronicle* (22 January 1857), p. 4.

55 One author noted that Meux's sister had no problem with the settlement of £18,000 he gave to her in March of that year, yet she would dispute his July 1857 codicil as seen below. J.C.B., 'Medico-Legal Trials and Inquisitions: Commission of Lunacy on Sir Henry Meux, Bart.', *Journal of Mental Science* 4 (1858), pp. 596–97.

56 'Sir Henry Meux's Insanity', *Devizes and Wiltshire Gazette* (24 June 1858), p. 3. This codicil was added to a will drafted in August 1856 after his marriage.

57 'The Commission of Lunacy on Sir Henry Meux', *Morning Chronicle* (11 June 1858), p. 6.

58 NA, C 211/32A/26, 1858.

59 'Sir Henry Meux's Insanity', *Devizes and Wiltshire Gazette* (24 June 1858), p. 3.

60 'Wills and Bequests', *The Times* (3 March 1883), p. 4.

61 *Fourth Annual Report of the Commissioners in Lunacy*, p. 10.
62 Shepherd and Wright, 'Madness, Suicide and the Victorian Asylum', p. 183.
63 W.R. Gowers, *Lunacy and Law: An Address on the Prevention of Insanity Delivered before the Medico-Psychological Association of Great Britain and Ireland* (London, 1903), p. 17.
64 In Scotland this system was on the whole a source of great pride and national distinction. J. Andrews, *'They're in the Trade ... of Lunacy/They "Cannot Interfere" – They Say': The Scottish Lunacy Commissioners and Lunacy Reform in Nineteenth-Century Scotland* (London, 1998); D. Hirst and P. Michael, 'Family, Community and the Lunatic in Mid-Nineteenth Century North Wales', in Bartlett and Wright (eds), *Outside the Walls of the Asylum*, pp. 66–85.
65 Renton, *The Law of and Practice in Lunacy*, p. 76.
66 *Fourteenth Report of the Commissioners in Lunacy* (London, 1860), p. 153.
67 P. Bartlett, 'The Asylum, the Workhouse, and the Voice of the Insane Poor in 19th-Century England', *International Journal of Law and Psychiatry* 21:4 (1998), pp. 421–32.
68 Great Britain Parliament, House of Commons. *Reports from Committees: Lunacy Law*, vol. 13 (London, 1877), p. 199.
69 The only reason Edmunds's movements are recorded is that his brother instituted proceedings in Chancery when George was transferred to private care. George did not object to his move, and he was found to be of unsound mind. NA, C211/35B/25, 1864.
70 Not only did Shaftesbury choose single care, but he also sent his son to a family in Lausanne. In private he was far more disparaging over care for the mentally ill in Britain. S. Wise, *Inconvenient People: Lunacy, Liberty and the Mad-Doctors in Victorian England* (Berkeley, 2013), p. 194.
71 E.G.T. Liddell, 'Gowers, Sir William Richard (1845–1915)', *Oxford Dictionary of National Biography*, 2004.
72 Gowers, *Lunacy and Law*, p. 4.
73 Gowers, *Lunacy and Law*, pp. 8–9.
74 A. Takabayashi, 'Surviving the Lunacy Act of 1890: English Psychiatrists and Professional Development during the Early Twentieth Century', *Medical History* 61:2 (2017), pp. 262–63.
75 'One of Them', *Mad Doctors* (London, 1890), p. 22.
76 Gowers, *Lunacy and Law*, p. 7.
77 'Unlawfully Harbouring a Lunatic', *Windsor and Eton Express* (15 March 1862), p. 2.
78 C. Dickens, *The Personal History of David Copperfield* (Boston, 1867), p. 110.

79 Dickens, *Personal History*, p. 115.
80 In 1851 there were fifty-seven Chancery lunatics with property of less than £100 per year. *Journal of Psychological Medicine and Mental Pathology* 4:16 (1851), p. 632.
81 Such advertisements offered residential care, massage, and other vague methods of treatment. For example: *Norfolk News* (27 October 1860), p. 1; 'Private Medical Advice', *Kendal Mercury* (10 September 1864), p. 2; *Essex Newsman* (12 September 1891), p. 4; *Morning Post* (2 November 1892), p. 1.
82 Such advertisements sometimes mirrored the language and tactics of patent medicines. This should not be surprising given the somewhat tenuous boundary between mainstream and quack medicines. L. Loeb, 'Doctors and Patent Medicines in Modern Britain: Professionalism and Consumerism', *Albion: A Quarterly Journal Concerned with British Studies* 33:3 (2001), pp. 407–8.
83 *Worcester Journal* (30 July 1859), p. 1.
84 'Lunatic in a Private House', *Nottingham Evening Post* (31 January 1903), p. 2. The severe £20 fine (or six weeks in prison) did not reflect a case of wrongful confinement, but rather a defiance of the 1890 Lunacy Act.
85 'Unlawfully Keeping Lunatics', *Portsmouth Evening News* (20 December 1879), p. 3; 'Unlawful Boarding of Lunatics', *Nottingham Evening Post* (6 September 1901), p. 2.
86 *Seventh Annual Report of the Commissioners in Lunacy*, pp. 30–32.
87 W. Edwards and B. Harraden, *Two Health-Seekers in Southern California* (Philadelphia, 1896), p. 130.
88 Travel was posed as a solution to madness in several works of fiction. For example: W. Collins, *Armadale* (New York, 1866), p. 17; J.S. Clouston, *The Lunatic at Large* (London, 1893), p. 9.
89 M. Frawley, *Invalidism and Identity in Nineteenth-Century Britain* (Chicago, 2004), pp. 83–94.
90 Collins, *Armadale*, p. 17.
91 C. Hoolihan, 'Health and Travel in Nineteenth-Century Rome', *Journal of the History of Medicine and Allied Sciences* 44 (1989), pp. 463–64.
92 W.R. Huggard and W.G. Lockett, *Davos as Health-Resort: A Handbook* (Davos, 1907), pp. 1, 200–202; D.C. Large, *The Grand Spas of Central Europe: A History of Intrigue, Politics, Art and Healing* (Lanham, 2015).
93 J. Adams, *Healing with Water: English Spas and the Water Cure, 1840–1960* (Manchester, 2015); H. Marland and J. Adams, 'Hydropathy at Home: The Water Cure and Domestic Healing in Mid-Nineteenth-Century Britain', *Bulletin of the History of Medicine* 83:3 (2009), pp. 499–529.

94 As Deborah Neill points out, the hydropathic spa of Ben Rhydding outside Leeds advertised a renewal of 'vital force' and removal of 'effete matter'. D. Neill, 'Merchants, Malaria and Manliness: A Patient's Experience of Tropical Disease', *Journal of Imperial and Commonwealth History* 46:2 (2018), p. 212.

95 For example: G.L. James, *Shall I Try Australia? Or, Health, Business, and Pleasure in New South Wales, Forming a Guide to the Australian Colonies for the Emigrant Settler and Business Man* (London, 1892); C. Nordhoff, *California for Health, Pleasure, and Residence: A Book for Travellers and Settlers* (New York, 1882); R.H. Otter, *Winters Abroad: Some Information Respecting Places Visited by the Author on Account of His Health: Intended for the Use of Invalids* (London, 1882); A.D. Walker, *Egypt as a Health Resort, with Medical and Other Hints for Travellers in Syria* (London, 1873); W.S. Wilson, *The Ocean as a Health Resort: A Practical Handbook of the Sea for the Use of Tourists and Health-Seekers* (London, 1881).

96 Thomas Carlyle, Charles Darwin, Aldous Huxley, G.H. Lewes, Alfred Tennyson, Herbert Spencer, George Meredith, and John Ruskin suffered some level of mental debility, depression, or hypochondria. B. Haley, *The Healthy Body and Victorian Culture* (Cambridge, 1978), pp. 13, 26, 28.

97 C. Sengoopta, '"One of the Best-Known Identity Crises in History?" John Stuart Mill's Mental Crisis and its Meanings', in R. Bivins and J. Pickstone (eds), *Medicine, Madness and Social History: Essays in Honour of Roy Porter* (Basingstoke, 2007), p. 174.

98 J. Tosh, 'Hegemonic Masculinity and the History of Gender', in S. Dudink, K. Hagemann, and J. Tosh (eds), *Masculinities in Politics and War: Gendering Modern History* (Manchester, 2004), p. 48.

99 Sengoopta, '"One of the Best-Known Identity Crises in History?"', pp. 175, 178.

100 J.R. Steward, 'Moral Economies and Commercial Imperatives: Food, Diets and Spas in Central Europe: 1800–1914', *Journal of Tourism History* 4:2 (2012), p. 183.

101 'A Lunacy Inquiry', *Daily News* (15 August 1891), p. 6.

102 'Lunacy Inquiry', *Sheffield Evening Telegraph* (15 August 1891), p. 3.

103 E. Jennings, *Curing the Colonizers: Hydrotherapy, Climatology, and French Colonial Spas* (Durham, 2006), p. 48.

104 Frawley, *Invalidism and Identity*, p. 115.

105 T.S. Dowse, *The Brain and the Nerves: Their Ailments and Their Exhaustion* (London, 1884), pp. 3, 76.

106 T.S. Dowse, *On Brain & Nerve Exhaustion: Neurasthenia, Its Nature and Curative Treatment* (London, 1887), pp. 56–58. The London

School of Hygiene and Tropical Medicine handbook recommended sea voyages for a number of ills. E. Hobhouse, et al. *Health Abroad: A Medical Handbook of Travel* (London, 1899), p. 93.

107 M. Honigsbaum, *A History of the Great Influenza Pandemics: Death, Panic and Hysteria, 1830–1920* (New York, 2013), p. 100.

108 Robert William Will defied his doctor's recommendation of asylum care and his friends set up travel with a retired army captain to France; he was certified and sent to an asylum after a suicide attempt. Manor House Asylum Case Notes, Male Patients, MS 6223, pp. 511–16.

109 Frawley, *Invalidism and Identity*, p. 127.

110 Manor House Asylum Case Notes, Male Patients, MS 6223, pp. 363–64.

111 Manor House Asylum Case Notes, Male Patients, MS 6223, pp. 363–64.

112 Manor House Asylum Case Notes, Male Patients, MS 6227, p. 32. John Whaley's name never appears in the Court of Chancery, and thus his family never sought to intervene to protect his assets. He therefore either recovered completely, or he returned to private care and travel.

113 As John Tosh notes, manhood was not something simply acquired at maturity in the nineteenth century; it needed to be constantly performed and reinforced in public. When a man could no longer fulfil this role in public, he was undermining his standing and reputation. Tosh, *Manliness and Masculinities*, p. 51.

114 A. McCarthy, 'Migration and Madness at Sea: The Nineteenth- and Early Twentieth-Century Voyage to New Zealand', *Social History of Medicine* 28:4 (2015), p. 707.

115 J.M. Moore, *New Zealand for the Emigrant, Invalid, and Tourist* (London, 1890), pp. 168, 218, 241.

116 J. Kain, 'The Ne'er-Do-Well: Representing the Dysfunctional Migrant Mind, New Zealand 1850–1910', *Studies in the Literary Imagination* 48:1 (2015), p. 86; J. Kain, *Insanity and Immigration Control in New Zealand and Australia, 1860–1930* (Basingstoke, 2019), pp. 3–4.

117 Hobhouse et al., *Health Abroad*, p. 178.

118 Frawley, *Invalidism and Identity*, pp. 76–77, 83–84.

119 'A Madman at Buckingham Palace', *Liverpool Mercury* (26 September 1865), p. 3.

120 'Terrible Murder by a Madman', *Edinburgh Evening News* (15 June 1874), p. 4.

121 'Terrible Murder by a Madman', *Dundee Courier* (16 June 1874), p. 3.

122 M.J. Wiener, *Men of Blood: Violence, Manliness, and Criminal Justice in Victorian England* (Cambridge, 2004), pp. 281–82.

123 In a strange scene in court, after the judge asked the witness if the young girl was afraid of her great-uncle, his daughter said no. The judge then had the little girl brought in to judge her reaction. She hugged Aitken and gave him a kiss immediately. 'Touching Scene in Court', *Bury and Norwich Post* (26 August 1873), p. 7.
124 'Central Criminal Court', *The Star* (26 August 1873), p. 2.
125 He had by that point lost his sight due to severe cataracts in both eyes. Letter from J. Lyons, 20 July 1876, Broadmoor, D/H14/D2/2/1/808/2. Berkshire Record Office.
126 Wiener, *Men of Blood*, p. 166.
127 Stories like that of Rosalind Hammond, confined and neglected by her husband and two maids in a bedroom for two years to cover up her doctor-husband's affair in the 1860s, were incredibly sensational. Another example was Harriet Richardson, a young woman on the boundaries of madness who was married against her family's wishes to a man who only wanted to secure her money; he confined her and starved her to death in 1877. Wise, *Inconvenient People*, pp. 205–7.
128 Pedlar, '*The Most Dreadful Visitation*', p. 162.
129 E. Yates, 'Mr. Wilkie Collins in Gloucester Place', in *Celebrities at Home, Third Series* (London, 1879), p. 150.
130 Over time the Commissioners grew more exasperated. Complaints about unregistered single lunatics were a a constant in the Commissioners' reports. In the autumn of 1896, they charged a woman in Hertfordshire with caring for two male lunatics for a fee without certification. In 1897 they noted that while the number of single lunatics was down, it was not due to more use of asylums but rather more people who continued to skirt the official rule. *Fifty-first Annual Report of the Commissioners in Lunacy* (London, 1897), pp. 42–43.
131 Sometimes reports came after the publication of Lunacy Commissioners' reports. 'Cruelty to Lunatics', *The Era* (1 October 1854), p. 15.
132 *Exmouth Journal* (29 August 1874), p. 7.
133 'Lunatics At Home', *British Medical Journal* (28 May 1870), p. 552.
134 *Eighth Annual Report of the Commissioners in Lunacy*, p. 36.
135 'Extraordinary Case of False Imprisonment', *North Wales Chronicle* (1 July 1853), p. 3.
136 'Carnarvonshire', *North Wales Chronicle* (29 July 1853), p. 2.
137 *Eighth Annual Report of the Commissioners in Lunacy*, p. 38. The North Wales Lunatic Asylum only opened in Denbigh in 1848, and thus would not have been available to the Roberts family when Evan was first ill. M.R. Olsen, 'The Founding of the Hospital for the Insane Poor, Denbigh', *Transactions of Denbigh Historical Society* 23 (1974), pp. 193–217.

138 K. Jones, 'Robert Gardiner Hill and the Non-Restraint Movement', *Canadian Journal of Psychiatry* 29:2 (1984), pp. 121–24; A. Suzuki, 'The Politics and Ideology of Non-Restraint: The Case of the Hanwell Asylum', *Medical History* 39:1 (1995), pp. 1–17.

139 Byrne's account of the case of Porter is used to highlight the need for the state to intervene on the part of private lunatics. He spared no detail in his sensational coverage. T.E.D. Byrne, *Lunacy and Law, Together with Hints on the Treatment of Idiots* (London, 1864), pp. 14–15.

140 *Eighteenth Annual Report of the Commissioners in Lunacy*, pp. 89–92.

141 Coverage was not limited to local or large dailies but was extensive across the nation. For example: *Cumberland and Westmorland Advertiser, and Penrith Literary Chronicle* (22 March 1864), p. 2; 'General News', *Dundee, Perth and Cupar Advertiser* (22 March 1864), p. 6; 'General News', *Herts Guardian* (22 March 1864), p. 2; 'The Cornwall Lunacy Case', *Newcastle Guardian and Tyne Mercury* (26 March 1864), p. 6.

142 'The Ill-Treatment of a Lunatic in Cornwall', *Morning Advertiser* (18 March 1864), p. 7.

143 'The Flushing Lunacy Case', *Leighton Buzzard Observer and Linslade Gazette* (29 March 1864), p. 3.

144 Byrne, *Lunacy and Law*, pp. 41, 12.

145 'The Doctor's Lunatic Brother', *Daily News* (17 August 1900), p. 3.

146 'The Doctor's Lunatic Brother', *Daily News* (1 September 1900), p. 3.

147 'The Doctor's Lunatic Brother', *Daily News* (5 September 1900), p. 7.

148 Tosh, *A Man's Place*, p. 145.

3

Personal shame: failures of morality and the will

> The youth who, in the vortex of pleasure, in the gleaming of the wine cup, in the whirl of gaiety, in the beastliness of lust, in the hallucinations of narcotics, in the excess of riot, and in the boisterousness of unclean mirth, drowns all that there is about him of purity, and principle, and honour, do I call him a 'man'?[1]

J.T. Davidson believed a man who followed his baser instincts and allowed himself to lose control was no longer a man. The associations of control and masculinity were wide and varied; there was a popular understanding that this loss of control could lead to madness. This was certainly the case in Anthony Trollope's novel *He Knew He Was Right*. It is unclear whether the main character, Louis Trevelyan, who becomes obsessed by the idea his wife has been unfaithful, is actually driven insane.[2] However, this was clearly Trollope's intent.[3] Trevelyan certainly loses control. His jealousy and suspicion drive him to the brink, and he alienates almost everyone around him. He tries to push away his anger and suspicion but fails in his attempts. Midway through the novel, a friend reaches out to him and beseeches him to make amends to his wife. In an appeal to put aside his anger his friend finally asks him: 'Can't you be man enough to remember that you are a man?'[4] His wife certainly believed her husband could not see reason. She argues that 'neither can the law, nor medicine, nor religion, restore to you that fine intellect which foolish suspicions have destroyed'.[5] Valerie Pedlar makes the point that madness is not feminized as such across Victorian fiction, but rather was characterized by a person out of control. Madness could be the result of a lack of masculinity, but it could also be driven by extreme machismo.[6] Men were held culpable for

Personal shame: failures of morality and the will

this loss of control, and their emasculated position was a source of shame to themselves and others.

A common response to the diagnosis of insanity was often anger (as discussed in chapter four) or a deep sense of shame. David Davidson, aware that he was demonstrating symptoms of a mental breakdown, was ashamed at his inability to stop his illness. In particular, when writing after his recovery, he frames his deep emotional turmoil as a failure of manhood:

> I was so blind, that I did not see it was utterly unmanly to give way like this, and that there was nothing whatever about my position that was unendurable or irremediable to anyone in a right state of mind, or possessed of a good spirit and proper determination.[7]

Davidson blames his breakdown on a lack of willpower and 'spirit'. His shame was compounded after he was treated and released from an asylum; his family wanted to pretend nothing had ever happened. He was angry at his family's decision to place him in an institution, and even more disappointed that they did not want him to publish his experiences 'both for the sake of their own feelings and, what hit me hardest, for the sake of my son's future'.[8] Davidson hoped to gain some agency over his experiences by writing about them; however, the shame was too much for his family.

Shame can be defined in a number of ways, but as Peter Stearns notes, it is a deeply self-conscious emotion at its core. It is a personal concern, but it is often reified by the fear of the judgement of others.[9] Having any kind of 'lunatic' in the family was often difficult to accept, even by those within the medical profession. Reginald Langdon Down spent his life caring for mentally ill children, but never disclosed that his own son was born as a 'Mongolian Idiot'. He cared for his son, but clearly wanted to keep his condition a secret.[10] The elaborate social expectations demanded in particular of the middle and upper classes were grounded in restraint and fear of being judged. A man who had no control was socially conditioned to feel shame. And self-conscious sufferers were well aware that theirs was an illness that cast a pall on their entire family.

Commentators outdid each other in outlining the disgrace and degradation that madness conferred (whether they believed it was justified or not). Even those fighting against stigma were often the first to highlight its existence. One physician prefaced his letter to the Earl of Shaftesbury, long-time head of the Lunacy Commission, with an acknowledgement of the horrors of lunacy. He described madness as:

> the heaviest of the Almighty's dispensations, – which involves in its course every conceivable calamity, loss of character, loss of friends, banishment from society, deprivation of fortune, to say nothing of physical pain, and even unreal torture, – is treated by modern society more as a crime than an affliction.[11]

While there were certainly empathetic reformers who wanted to combat the stigma of lunacy, they were a minority voice.

A diagnosis of lunacy was a humiliating and emasculating prospect partly because many believed it was avoidable. Without a clear explanation for lunacy, nor an ability to study it the way one could a diseased heart or broken limb, medical men often moralized their patients' disease. In 1849 John Barlow explicitly argued that the strongest men would never see the inside of an asylum unless they suffered a physical accident. No matter the mental turmoil or circumstances of life, Barlow believed the highly developed mind would keep its sanity. 'The wild whirl of passion which unsettles the brain of the ungoverned man, has no place in the mind of the Christian philosopher – fortune is lost or won with equanimity; for he has that self-sustaining power within which riches cannot give or take away.'[12] Such thinking helped shape the non-restraint movement, as the role of the doctor was transformed into that of motivator and moral sooth-sayer. The medical language of diagnostics continued to be permeated by moralistic language throughout the century. Arthur Gilbert explains this as part of a 'status anomaly' in the medical community, where doctors were asked to explain diseases that they had neither the training nor evidence to explain. Their answers, invariably, were to point to the moral failures of their patients as the cause of their illness, cloaked in medical language.[13] This philosophy never truly went away and led men to be ashamed of their mental breakdowns.

Madness, by its very nature, was characterized by a mind out of control. Morality was medicalized in the nineteenth century, and patients, families, and doctors often believed that mental disease was the result of a weak will or the inability to conquer a personal failing. While men might not have been able to control their hereditary

Personal shame: failures of morality and the will

predisposition, they were responsible for actions that could trigger insanity. The abuse of stimulants, and aberrant or excessive sexual practices were singled out as causes that people could and should control.[14] When men could not control their passions, such failures could trigger explicit feelings of shame and disappointment. This chapter will explore the value-laden landscape of diagnostic causation through the issues most related to personal shame: personal failure, sexual misconduct, and alcohol abuse. Men's shame was deeply linked to a judgement that they could not control themselves or their actions.

Shame and fear of breaking down

The shame of a mental breakdown was very real and dominated both cultural tropes of madness and men's personal experience. Certification as a lunatic led to a man losing control over his person, his family, his business, his wealth, and his property.[15] Given the patriarchal culture of the nineteenth century, the experience of being certified as a lunatic was even more disempowering for men than for women. Former heads of household were reduced to the legal status of children and could be placed in institutions or under enforced private care. One lawyer described the case of a man under a lunacy certificate as 'being consigned to a living death'.[16] Patients were often well aware of the stigma they would face should their institutionalization become public knowledge. One former Bethlem patient railed against those who might judge him: 'I do despise those who know I have been certified and judge ignorantly.'[17] The certificate held even more shame than treatment itself, as it signified a loss of independence. Lunacy Commissioners found a number of boarders at Holloway Sanitorium in the 1880s being held without certificates. Theirs were clear cases of lunacy, and while friends and relatives were happy for them to receive care, they did not want to formally acknowledge insanity with a lunacy certificate.[18] It was not the setting of the asylum that was a problem in such cases, it was rather the fact of certification.

Edgar Sheppard was well aware of the particular challenges that madness posed to the medical profession. In his inaugural lecture as chair at King's College in 1873, he acknowledged that diagnosing madness was distinct from diagnosing other diseases. To tell a man he had gout did not threaten his character or his family. Sheppard did not shy away from the potential disaster the diagnosis of madness could be both for the sufferer and his family. In particular, he highlighted the moral overtones of a lunacy diagnosis that were absent from most other somatic diseases.

> You could not frighten him more, or make him more indignant, if you said they were dishonest. It is almost to filch from him his good name, and stain him with a dye which is indelible. Insanity is a very serious issue. It involves in most cases the loss of personal liberty; it sets in motion the wheels of a costly and elaborate machinery.[19]

Any sufferer aware enough of his circumstances would be shamed by implications of a lunacy diagnosis, whether justified or not.

Even those sympathetic to the sufferings of lunatics and pushing for best treatment could not help but sometimes drift into moralizing. While acknowledging all patients were different, one observer believed that the root cause of insanity always traced to moral or spiritual causes.[20] Even the rise of theories of hereditary and biological determinism in the 1870s did not end the stigma and culpability of insanity. The blame for insanity was just spread throughout an entire family rather than an individual.[21] Biological determinism often blurred physical and moral pathologies and thus did little to allay stigma.

The association of shame and madness spread far beyond the medical community. The fear of oncoming madness was a powerful emotion, and popular novelists captured what the strain of expectations and self-doubt could do to the sensitive man.[22] Charles Reade published *It is Never Too Late to Mend* in 1856 as a way to highlight the abuses in the prison system. In doing so, he also wrote eloquently about the fear of madness. One of the many horrors of the Victorian prison he described was the use of solitary confinement to break even the toughest spirit. The hour-by-hour description of one man's tortuous experience in a dark and cold cell quickly descends into a battle against madness:

> Robinson was going mad. The blackness and solitude and silence and remorse and despair were more than his excitable nature could bear any longer ... He screamed, and cursed, and prayed, and dashed himself on the ground, and ran round the cell wounding his hands

and his face. Suddenly he turned deadly calm. He saw he was going mad – better die than so – 'I shall be a beast soon – I will die a man' – he tore down his collar – he had on cotton stockings, he took one off – he tied it in a loose knot round his naked throat – he took a firm hold with each hand ... A man to die in the prime of life for want of a little light and a word from a human creature to keep from madness.[23]

Robinson's fear that he was going mad is so terrifying and shameful that it pushes him to consider suicide as a more appealing alternative. In fearing he is becoming less than a man he does not fear becoming effeminate, but rather bestial in his madness.

Similar themes shape Wilkie Collins's *Heart and Science* published in 1882. The story introduces several characters who are haunted by the spectre of madness.[24] Its hero, Ovid Vere, pushes his constitution to the limit, and teeters on the edge of a breakdown. His 'morbidly-sensitive nerves were sadly shaken' and he is startled by the sound of a bell and horrified by the idea of killing a beetle.[25] Doctors warn him to leave London for his health, but he is enchanted by his young cousin and reluctant to leave. His struggle with his mental state is described by Collins as a struggle between emotion and manhood; his madness is presented as effeminizing. Vere sees his mental decline explicitly as a sense of weakness, and of failing strength. It is only by travelling to Canada, and sleeping in the open air, that Vere can restore his mind and health. Only manly courage staves off the incipient madness. On his return, with his aunt in an asylum and his beloved on the brink of madness and death, he is proud that he does not shed a tear and finds that 'Those once tremulous nerves had gathered steady strength, on the broad prairies and in the roving life'. Any unmanly sorrow was checked by 'the robust vitality that rioted in his blood' as grief struggled to find expression 'against the masterful health and strength that set moral weakness at defiance'.[26] A man who struggles to keep his mind through manly effort implies that a man who loses that struggle is less of a man. The language and metaphors of self-control strongly underscores the idea that to have a mental breakdown was to admit defeat.

While doctors and reformers tried to emphasize that to be sent to an asylum was a curative choice no different from any other hospital, it is clear that many patients and family members understood institutionalization as shameful. Working-class autobiographer Sam

Shaw grew up in a family whose patriarch slowly lost control of his health and his family's well-being. His father first lost his sight, then lost his employment, and finally lost his mind. He was sent to an asylum around 1891 and the family was broken apart. Looking back years later, Shaw felt little sympathy for his father, simply seeing him as a failure, unable to keep himself and his family together. His need for institutionalization was proof of his failure as a man and a father.[27] Shaw blamed his father for his descent into madness.

Shame is a marker of community values; when members of a society did not tailor their feelings and their actions to the norms and expectations of the broader community by staying out of the workhouse or the madhouse, they were shamed by others, or embodied their own sense of shame.[28] The experience of enforced institutionalization was more degrading if it was paired with an economic degradation. One asylum inmate defined himself as a rate-payer who had donated to various charities, and he was appalled to find himself eventually sorted through the workhouse system.[29] There are glimpses even in the terse admission records that some men had internalized such a sense of failure. William Tamlin was a plumber who suffered from melancholia. Notes reveal he told doctors that he worried he was 'not a perfect man'.[30] While patients were consistently advised to seek out medical help as soon as possible, the shame of admitting you needed help often compounded men's struggles. Much of a family's social status was tied up with men's economic labour, and any failure to live up to expectations tended to be interpreted as a failure of a man's character.[31] Poverty and business failure had even greater stigma attached to them in an era that increasingly prioritized self-sufficiency; the shame involved in business failure ran deep.[32] The need for men's earning power led to a particular problem for men dependent on a regular pay cheque who might have identified early signs of mental distress. Commercial and professional men could not afford private care and would not admit themselves to a pauper asylum.[33] While some families did make the financial sacrifice and put their male breadwinners in private asylums, it was not possible for all families, nor was it possible for many more in the long term.[34]

Men who had the means and resources to live independently could delay any intervention. The case of a Mr A, recorded in the Lunacy Commissioners' annual report, outlines how shame could prevent men from seeking help, and independent resources could lead to men avoiding any interference. Mr A was a British army officer and when his regiment disbanded in 1857 he took up lodgings in a European hotel. He was a man of considerable means whose only living relative was an aunt who lived in London. He settled into his hotel, bought a number of horses, and maintained the habits of a gentleman. He visited his aunt and a few sporting acquaintances for a few years but increasingly began to retreat into his rooms in the hotel. As of 1863 he allowed no one but the hotel manager and his property manager to visit, and stopped responding to his aunt even when she invited him to her wedding. She tried to visit him yearly at his hotel but was refused entry. By 1868 his business manager had stopped visiting and then it was the hotel manager alone who had any access. It is not clear who alerted the Lunacy Commissioners to the Englishman's state, but one of their medical members went to visit.[35] They found Mr A locked away in two rooms that were stacked floor to ceiling with furniture and garbage. He was filthy, unkempt, and dressed in rags with his feet covered in cloth. The bedroom was filled with pots and vessels filled with excrement. Aged only thirty-five, he was confined to a horsehair sofa, and was unable to walk as he suffered severe rheumatism.

While ashamed of his current conditions, Mr A was adamant he would oppose any proceedings in lunacy that would rob him of his autonomy. In fact, he believed his shame about his situation proved his sanity. The medical inspector, however, perceived the case differently. 'His gentlemanly demeanour contrasted throughout my interview most painfully with his disgraceful condition. The strongest proof, and I might almost say, the only proof, of his insanity was his own explanation of what he saw.'[36] Mr A explained away his matted beard, his filth, and his surroundings as the result of being trapped in the hotel with no one to help him leave. He expressed a wish to leave but said he could find no help to do so. He was deeply ashamed to have anyone see his surroundings but had refused any help from his friends or relative. The shame was a natural reaction, but his inability to act was proof of madness.

Mr A eventually agreed to see an old family doctor who worked at a county asylum and he was temporarily removed there. He was bathed and groomed, and his legs were found to be permanently crippled. In trying to explain how he had allowed himself to fall into such a state, the patient explained to the doctor that 'he felt himself for some time different from other young men; that he felt he was looked upon by the people as a lunatic; that he gave way to his feelings with the result I now saw before me'.[37] Mr A improved rapidly at the asylum and his Lunacy Commission was postponed several times until proceedings were stayed and the Lords Justices declared him sane and in full management of his property.[38] In this case, shame at a deteriorating condition and fear of being institutionalized drove a man into seclusion and squalor.

Asylum patients were often wracked with guilt and shame about real and imagined faults. William George Boyle was a busy man, and by the time he was forty he was an MP, Lieutenant-Colonel in the Coldstream Guards, and Justice of the Peace.[39] In 1870 he began to display symptoms of paranoia, worsening to hallucinations and finally suicidal behaviour. That same year he was admitted as a private patient to the Manor House Asylum. While the casebooks note some hopeful signs in the first months of his admission, these trends were never sustained. By all accounts he seemed a sensible, hard-working, honourable man throughout his life. But doctors worried he 'worked his brain to a very freak [sic] extent'.[40] He was overwhelmed by fears that he had brought unspeakable shame to his family. While the doctors noted there was no truth to this fear, and that it was a symptom of his delusional mania, his fear of disappointing his family and letting down his military comrades helped drive Boyle out of his senses. Sometimes men were not ashamed of their mental distress, but their shame was in fact a symptom of their insanity. Boyle would live the rest of his life, thirty-eight years, in the asylum with little improvement.[41]

Whether motivated by fear of bestial madness or effeminate indolence, men felt the social stigmas of madness and doctors had very little success shifting such opinion among their patients, the general public, or even their own ranks. The fact that most families would want to keep lunatic relatives secret was an oft-repeated sentiment.[42] One report noted that 'the natural desire' to conceal lunacy was a reason that census statistics on idiots and imbeciles were not reliable.[43] James Coxe, a Scottish physician, emphasized the general public's distaste for acknowledging lunacy in their own families. He noted that there was a powerful motive to keep such illnesses private, despite the fact that lunacy was a disease like any other. But unlike most disorders, 'the interest and prospects of families are far more seriously affected by an imputation of lunacy, than by any bodily disorder'.[44] Examples from this section show how deeply internalized shame could be among patients who retained a sense of self-awareness.

Intemperate madness

Medical experts believed any number of factors could predispose a person to lunacy, ranging from social and institutional circumstances to individual lifestyle choices.[45] In attempting to identify the preventable causes of madness, one author in the *Westminster Review* identified alcohol, tobacco, drugs, overwork, and lack of sleep as primary causes.[46] While the intent of such warnings might have been to spare readers the ravages of mental disease, they also implied that those who did suffer had allowed themselves to become ill.[47] Those seen as most at fault for their own breakdowns were often those whose cause of insanity was listed as the opaque term 'intemperance'. This prejudice never fully dissipated, as men who drank were often held up as complicit in their own mental breakdowns.[48] Many patients and families hoped to trace mental illness to a physical injury, which held the least stigma. When men's actions could be blamed for their madness, their shame was magnified.

The link between drunkenness and insanity was longstanding. Seneca's maxim that to be drunk was a form of self-inflicted madness would have been well known to physicians educated in the classics.[49] From the moment that the Commissioners in Lunacy began taking national surveys of the causes of mental breakdown, it was clear that alcohol was listed as the predisposing cause more often than any other reason apart from 'unknown'. This problem was particularly acute for men, as statistics from the 1890s demonstrate (Figure 3.1).

It is difficult to overestimate how frequently the Victorians blamed insanity on drink.[50] While alcohol was a daily part of most men's lives, doctors increasingly worried that it was not a harmless pleasure. Henry Maudsley, mental specialist of the last decades of the nineteenth century, believed that alcohol took a toll on everybody, and was a vice to be avoided.[51] Alcohol acted like a 'pawnbroker or the usurer, it is a present help at the cost of a frightful interest'.[52] Temperance

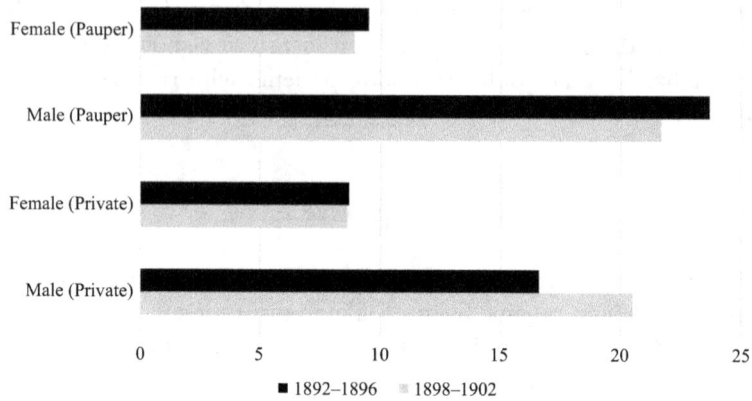

Figure 3.1 Intemperance in drink as formal cause of insanity (Yearly average number of instances in which each cause was assigned during the five years)

advocates consistently warned against the serious danger of alcohol to the nervous system.[53] Alcohol abuse was framed as a failure of willpower, and alcohol itself a substance that could destroy the will.[54]

Drinking crossed class, regional, and religious boundaries, but by the nineteenth century there was a renewed focus on problematic or excessive drinking. While the temperance movement(s) varied over the course of the century, from radical teetotallers pushing for government intervention to moderate temperance advocates arguing for personal responsibility, there was a general disapproval of drunkenness.[55] To be drunk in the nineteenth century became proof of a problem: either an anti-social vice, a medical illness, or a side-effect of crushing poverty. Scholars note that while men were the gender most likely to be defined as 'habitual drunkards', there was an intense social panic about women.[56] Most scholarship has focused on Victorian women and drinking; women were often pointed out as suffering the most from the excesses of alcohol.[57] However, for men drunkenness was increasingly seen as a lack of manly self-control leading to the madhouse.

Temperance novelists used every trick of sensation to highlight the dangers of alcohol.[58] While there are a number of such sources centring on women, there were a number of both visual and textual narratives of the patriarch's descent into oblivion. G. Cruikshank's series of etchings dubbed 'The Bottle' outlines a family tragedy that begins when a man introduces alcohol into the home. A strong father becomes a wreck of a man over the series of eight plates. He murders his wife in a fit of drunken madness, and ends up in the asylum, destroying himself and his family.[59]

Perhaps the most powerful exploration of this theme is in the work of popular novelists who portrayed tormented wives helpless in the face of their husbands' drinking. Such tales extended beyond temperance literature to general tales of sensation. One of the most iconic of such characters is Arthur Huntingdon, the dissipate aristocrat in *The Tenant of Wildfell Hall* who destroys himself and almost destroys his family with his intemperate life. He is oblivious to his own failings and feels no shame or grief at his actions. In contrast, Lord Lowborough avoids such a fate, seemingly because of his sense of shame. Huntingdon mocks his friend's conscience, and laments that 'in his sober moments, he so bothered his friends with his remorse and his terrors and woes, that they were obliged, in self-defence, to get him to drown his sorrows in wine'. His friends would push Lowborough to drink to excess, but the next day he would 'lament his own unutterable wickedness and degradation'.[60] He gains his happy ending eventually through force of will, with a solid, loving, and sensible wife who helps him stay on the right path. In this instance, shame is the only thing keeping a man from ruin.

Novelists explored popular understandings of the complex balance between drinkers' rights and the damage they could do to society. Wilkie Collins's novel *Man and Wife* details several unhappy and dysfunctional marriages. Hester Dethridge is a housekeeper with a dark history: she killed her husband. She explains how she was driven to murder after her husband became a violent alcoholic who ran through her fortune. She sought out help from the police and a lawyer but could find no relief. Hester could not understand why her husband could not be classified as a madman and sent to an asylum:

> Mad people, as I understand it, are people who have lost control over their own minds. Sometimes this leads them to entertaining delusions; and sometimes it leads them to committing actions hurtful to others or to themselves. My husband has lost all control over his own craving for strong drink. He requires to be kept from liquor, as

other madmen require to be kept from attempting their own lives, or the lives of those about them. It's a frenzy beyond his own control, with *him* – just as it's a frenzy beyond their own control, with *them*. There are Asylums for mad people, all over the country, at the public disposal, on certain conditions. If I fulfil those conditions, will the law deliver me from the misery of being married to a madman, whose madness is drink?[61]

The lawyer simply answers that no – neither he nor the state could help her. Her husband's lack of control led to his wife taking desperate measures.

Coulson Kernahan, a popular novelist in the 1890s, wrote a fictional confessional that traced how a writer destroyed his life through an inability to stop drinking. The narrator turns to whiskey to deal with his writing workload. A social and occasional drinker quickly descends into an addict and a wreck of a man.[62] His narrative highlights the dangers of the idea that liquor fuelled artistic output and postulates that alcohol ultimately leads to the destruction of creativity.[63] The fictional author of the memoir is ashamed of his choices, and this is presented as the appropriate response to such a failure. In another short story, a young woman's early and reckless marriage to a hard-drinking man turns into a nightmare after he breaks and begins raving. The doctor has to tell the young woman that 'he is out of his mind, in fact – the inevitable result of the life he has led. I am terribly sorry for you, but it was bound to end so.'[64] The selfish husband's lack of control has cost him his mind and left his wife doomed as the living widow of a madman. Fiction was a powerful tool to highlight the particular dangers of drinking.

The links between insanity and alcohol were most marked in the diagnosis of *delirium tremens*. It was classified as a form of temporary insanity that did not meet the threshold for certification as a lunatic; however, it did require specialized medical care.[65] Doctors could not understand why some heavy drinkers suffered while others did not; they agreed, however, that *delirium tremens* mimicked the conditions of madness, at least in the short term, and could lead to long-term insanity. Dr Alexander Peddie believed that it was a disease that particularly affected men and spared even the most inveterate female gin drinkers.[66] *Delirium tremens* was the clearest example of alcohol directly leading to insanity.

Personal shame: failures of morality and the will   111

The illness was a potentially dangerous one both for the sufferer and those around them. A marine deployed during the Zulu wars, C. Fleming, went on a four-day drinking venture while on leave. He returned to his ship bruised and cut, but ready enough to return to work with his shipmates. That evening, the ship's surgeon noticed signs of 'incipient delirium tremens'. His symptoms worsened as he began hearing voices and developing paranoia. Fearing he was going to be executed, he grabbed a bayonet and chased his fellow shipmates. He was ill for twenty days before he was stable enough to be sent to hospital.[67] Military authorities treated alcohol abuse seriously and they understood that *delirium tremens* could be a serious threat to the health and well-being of their troops.[68]

Asylum authorities were also aware that a temporary case of *delirium tremens* could often lead to sustained madness. Thomas Whitlaw Barclay was a carriage driver who suffered numerous attacks of *delirium tremens* due to his alcohol abuse. He was finally admitted to Glasgow Royal Lunatic Asylum 1895 after he became suicidal and obsessed with death. On admission it was noted that 'He makes up the bedclothes to represent dead bodies and seems to think he is performing his duties at funerals.'[69] John Taffenden was a publican admitted to Bethlem by his brother-in-law. He was then suffering from mania, but the root cause of the disease was listed as *delirium tremens*.[70] Doctors understood that hard drinking or withdrawal from such could trigger an attack of *delirium tremens* and potential longer-term madness.

The outlines of *delirium tremens* were well known, and fictional characters suffering the ailment were typically presented as powerful and out of control. In *Caged*, the heroine of the story can see the severity of her driver's drinking problems so well she deduces he cannot go long without a drop. After she throws away his flask (he is trying to kidnap her) he admits that 'I shall have the horrors if I have to do the next six miles without a drink … I shall be dancing, whooping mad in five minutes if I don't get a fresh bottle … I can feel 'em coming on now; there's a green snake with magenta eyes just over your head.'[71] Without even naming the illness, the reader is expected to recognize the symptoms of *delirium tremens* in the driver.

Alcohol was singled out as a particular trigger for madness, and the overindulgence of alcohol manifested as a form of madness itself. While there were growing voices in the medical community that saw addiction to alcohol as a kind of disease, for most people it was simply understood as a problem of willpower. A man whose madness was linked to alcohol was represented as complicit in his own breakdown and was conditioned to feel shame about his illness. Women should abstain from alcohol altogether, but a man should be able to drink in a controlled and restrained manner. Moral causes of insanity were always linked most explicitly to a lack of control and could be characterized as unmanly vices rather than medical conditions.

Pathologized desire and sexuality

Sexual excess was accepted to varying degrees by doctors and moralists as a potential cause of mental breakdown.[72] In listing the top causes for insanity, sexual issues – or, more particularly, sexual vice – consistently made the list for most medical authorities.[73] It was thus at the forefront of doctors' minds when diagnosing and assessing their patients. Sexual standards and maintaining codes of respectable behaviour hinged on a foundation of shame.[74] Value judgements could weave into diagnoses just as easily as they could into a sermon. Sexual desires had to be controlled and channelled into healthy expressions or else they threatened relationships and feelings.[75] Sexual behaviours were pathologized to varying degrees that sometimes depended on symptoms, but more often than not were shaped by class and gender. For men of the middle and upper classes, the desire for respectability and reputation necessitated a tremendous amount of self-control and restraint on issues of sexuality. Working-class men were assumed by medical authorities to be less able to control their base desires, but the anxieties and strictures of Victorian sexual mores shaped all men's and women's lives to varying degrees.

There is no evidence that men were ever institutionalized simply for their excessive sexual activities (and little evidence women were). Sexual intemperance was listed as a formal cause of insanity in only a very small number of patients (Figure 3.2). Beyond the statistics, however, there is ample evidence that some men actively struggled with their desires to an almost pathological extent. To doctors, sexual delusions or unrestrained sexual acts were part of a larger

Personal shame: failures of morality and the will 113

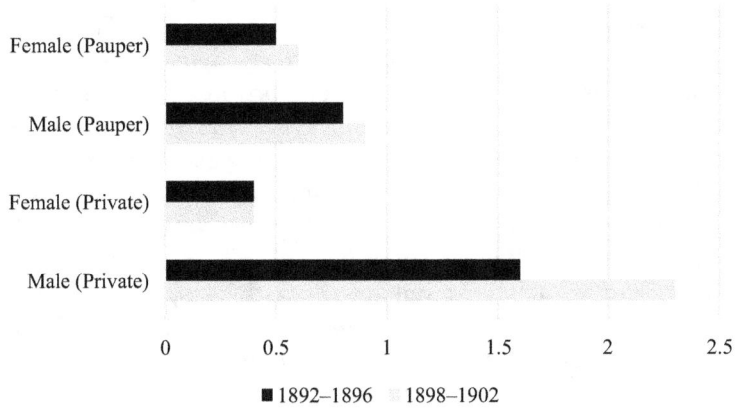

Figure 3.2 Sexual intemperance as formal cause of insanity (Yearly average number of instances in which each cause was assigned during the five years)

cluster of symptoms or triggers pointing to a mind out of control. This medical context traces networks of shame, and how doctors balanced their own prejudices against the overall health of their patients. Patients revealed their own, internalized beliefs about normative and abnormal sexual behaviours that sometimes aligned with their doctors', and sometimes did not. When looking at people charged with sexual insanity and doctors writing about sexual perversion, it is rare to find a balanced view.

There was a tacit agreement that men were sexual creatures, subject to sexual urges that they frequently indulged. However, not all doctors or commentators accepted that men were unable to control these sexual desires. Doctors helped give medical justification to restraint. Lionel Beale, physician to King's College Hospital, argued that the sexual organs were unique in the body as they did not need to be used, and should be controlled by the mind.[76] Sexual desire was masculine, but the inability to control those urges was emasculating.[77] Social purity advocates challenged those who believed men were sexual creatures by nature who had to indulge their passions; to promote such a belief according to one reformer was 'to degrade manhood'.[78]

Shame cloaked most frank conversations about sexuality and could make diagnosing sexual insanity more difficult. Those who could not control their urges were often condemned, but should they seek release in dark alleyways and in private spaces theirs were seen as moral and not mental failings. A series of detailed cases from Manor House Asylum demonstrate that when these urges were coupled with socially unacceptable actions, or when men confessed to sins they had not committed, that is when doctors diagnosed a problem. Reginald Wynne Simpson was full of perverse sexual fantasies and would burst out into 'beastly' language.[79] George Bernard's delusions took on a sexual tone, though there was no mention of sexual perversity.[80] Doctors were concerned when patients' own shame turned into obsession or was coupled with delusions. Alfred Yeames was a fifty-seven-year-old unmarried merchant who was convinced he had serious sexual troubles. In this case he believed he was impotent, although the doctors' notes seem to imply this was a delusion rather than reality.[81] They also noted his was a serious case and did not trivialize the man's fears. The anxieties could be just as problematic as the behaviour.

Casebooks are a frustrating resource at times – one often has to guess at cause and effect, and marvel at why some patients are released and others are not. Why are some patients seen as incurable while others have good prospects? Why do doctors seem to find some patients instantly unlikeable? The case of Rev. Arthur Henry Delmé Radcliffe, admitted to Manor House Asylum in 1890 at the age of forty, illuminates the difficulties in unpacking medical judgements. A married man of good health with five children, he was an upstanding rector in the Church of England. His admission notes are quite positive in tone, and they simply acknowledge he suffered syphilis when an undergraduate at Cambridge, was treated and recovered. These admission notes, while brief, are illuminative of first impressions, and Radcliffe received none of the negative or suspicious remarks that sometimes dog these cryptic entries. The causes of his insanity were listed as overwork that led to a breakdown of his stomach and bladder and vague 'sexual troubles'. Yet the case notes go out of their way to note that the man was of general temperate habits and had led a 'blameless life'.[82]

Once admitted to the asylum, Radcliffe had numerous delusions, some of money and fame and miracles, but also clearly sexual

Personal shame: failures of morality and the will 115

delusions. At one point, doctors noted that his 'considerable sexual excitement' was exacerbated by visits from his wife so they had to monitor them closely; his excitement could quickly turn to violence.[83] A few of Radcliffe's drawings, preserved within the casebook, highlight his confused thinking. Many deal with bombs and guns, and there is a recurrent theme of women and suffragettes as the source of degeneration (Figures 3.3 and 3.4). The doctors worried that the presence of his wife excited him so much sexually that he might turn violent. While most of the commentary is vague as to what his sexual delusions were, it does mention he once said his bed was 'full of young ladies' that were sent to him by God. Despite this, the medical staff demonstrated great patience with him, and never showed signs of annoyance or revulsion.[84] (And the doctors

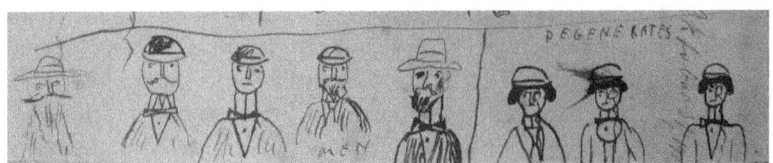

Figure 3.3 Drawing of 'Men' and 'Degenerates' in case notes of Rev. Arthur Henry Delmé Radcliffe

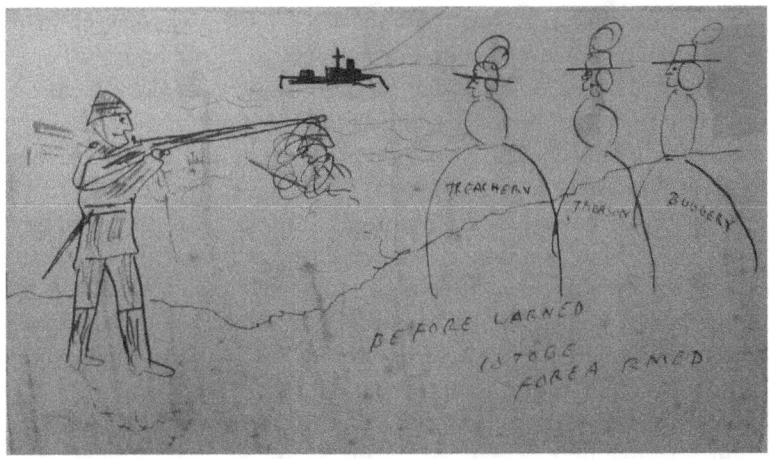

Figure 3.4 Drawing of 'Before Warned is to be Forearmed' in case notes of Rev. Arthur Henry Delmé Radcliffe

at Manor House clearly made it known when they did not like a patient, or found their behaviour disgusting.) Because of the other contexts of his life – a clergyman, family man, a man who worked hard – whatever his past peccadillos as an undergraduate might have been, they did not influence doctors' judgement of his present condition. His fantasies and desires were seen as strictly a product of his mental illness, and not an actual reflection of his true character or inner desires.

Many sexual delusions at their core centred around shame. Herman Edmund de Pury entered Manor House Asylum in 1907 a married man with three children. In recounting his own case history, he noted that he had been excited and tempted before his marriage, but, in his own words, never 'went wrong'.[85] Yet even these temptations preyed on him, as he was convinced that he had committed a horrible crime (a common delusion). For at least two men at Manor House the idea they had participated in a heinous sexual act or acts was the root of their melancholy.[86] For others, fear they had contracted a venereal disease was the keystone of their illness.[87] Doctors did not always accept their patients' narratives as fact and were sceptical that such behaviours ever took place. This does not mean they simply ignored or made light of patients' beliefs, however.

There are cases where doctors did understand their patient's sexual behaviour as proof of moral weakness and the cause of disease. Marmaduke Simpson was admitted to Manor House Asylum in 1881 at the age of twenty-one. He had suffered from lung problems as a child, he had been spoiled, and given an irregular education. It is clear from the outset that this young man was not liked by the staff. His constant theatre attendance, lack of exercise, and inattention at church marked him as an indolent young man. Dr Tuke's first impression of him was that he suffered from exhaustion and sexual indulgence.[88] Simpson himself admitted he had indulged in 'venereal excess' since the age of fifteen. He confessed that he seduced his mother's housemaid and her sisters. Doctors were so unimpressed with his character, and so disdainful of his manliness, that they came to doubt whether these sexual dalliances were even real. His confessions were reconstructed as delusions because of his perceived failures to live up to gendered norms.

Doctors engaged in moral judgements of men's sexual behaviour, marking out actions and feelings they believed were responsible for mental illness. It is difficult to unpack why some patients were marked as sexual deviants while others were not. Sometimes symptoms appeared on the surface, at other times they had to be secreted out. But oftentimes it was patients themselves who were plagued by shame of their sexual past. And doctors' role could be to mitigate their patients' guilt if it hampered their recovery.

Masturbation

Victorians' obsession with masturbation is so well known it verges on the caricature. Exploitative works of quack doctors and moralizing lectures of clergymen and educators warned of the horrors of masturbation into the twentieth century. As Lesley Hall notes, 'in a climate of sexual ignorance, guilt, and fear, the quacks were able to build a profitable edifice on the site of masturbation, giving shape to inchoate male anxieties'.[89] James Barker's *A Secret Book for Men* was typical of the genre, warning of the dangers of carnal sin and trumpeting his own miracle cure. In quoting a number of doctors he attempts to solidify his claim that masturbators 'find their way into lunatic asylums and similar institutions, through their becoming stark mad, or lapsing into such a confirmed state of imbecility that they are unfitted for decent society'.[90] Others offered less dramatic, but equally clear, warnings that masturbation could be a sure path to the asylum.[91] While most doctors offered tempered warnings, those on the boundaries or outside official medical circles were less circumspect.

Masturbation had long been censured as a moral sin and physical waste; medical opinion in the nineteenth century reached a consensus that seminal excitement and emissions were generally problematic for the healthy male body. Mainstream medical thinking promoted an idea that essentially 'pathologiz[ed] normal male sexuality itself'.[92] Whether it was the older theory of seminal loss or newer theories about nerve power, such beliefs affirmed that any time sperm left the body a man damaged his physical and mental health. The spermatorrhoea panic was spurred by medical thinkers but enthusiastically pursued by men of the middle classes. Any man who suffered from involuntary seminal discharge (wet dreams, premature ejaculation, and so on) could be caught up in this panic. Men often self-identified their own sexual disfunctions. Many men believed that their sexual shame was visible for all the world to see as it destroyed their physical and mental health.[93] To cure themselves, men sought out painful and sometimes damaging treatments.[94]

In the nineteenth century, masturbation was often listed as a cause of madness – not just by social purity campaigners, but also by asylum officials.[95] As early as 1845, at the elite Brislington House Asylum, doctors listed ten patients with 'self-pollution' identified as the cause of their insanity. This was the highest of all of the so-called physical causes.[96] Statistics from other sampled asylums put the number of admissions due to masturbation at anywhere from 2 to 3 per cent. This was felt to be underreported, as 'the extensive mental mischief' caused by the practice must be much higher, one doctor reckoned.[97]. In his study of the Bethnal House Asylum, Robert Peel Ritchie believed that out of 1,345 patients admitted between 1845 and 1861, 8.84 per cent of male patients were suffering from madness caused by 'vicious indulgences'.[98] Official Lunacy Commission reports in the last decades of the century registered small numbers of sexual self-abuse as the official cause of insanity (Figure 3.5). It was always significantly higher among men than women, and in private asylums versus pauper institutions. However, this only records the final ascertained cause of the medical officers, and neglects suspicions about a cause, or masturbation as a symptom. Beyond this, hard numbers only tell us part of the story. The anti-masturbation panic is important to unpack precisely because it reveals doctors' and patients' personal values about sexuality and the mind more broadly.

The fact that asylum doctors paid so much attention to masturbation should not be surprising. Those who worked in asylums frequently witnessed patients masturbating, often without shame.[99] Those who believed it dangerous could go to extremes to curb the practice. Alexander Elder spent time at Glasgow Royal and Baldovan asylums and he was variously described as being an epileptic or imbecile. His longstanding insanity made him helpless to survive on his own and he had been living as a pauper. Doctors noted that he was addicted to masturbation, and at some point he had pins placed through the foreskin of his penis to prevent the practice. Doctors noted that the treatment seemed to have decreased his epileptic attacks and his bodily health improved. When the pins loosened,

Personal shame: failures of morality and the will 119

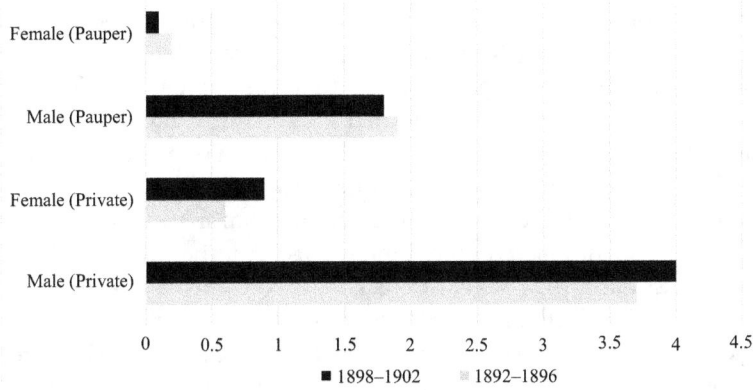

Figure 3.5 Self-abuse as formal cause of insanity (Yearly average number of instances in which each cause was assigned during the five years)

he began masturbating again. They had to remove the pins when they began ulcerating the skin, but doctors worried that now he was even more devoted to the practice even in public, and would kick and bite anyone who tried to stop him.[100] The hopelessness of Elder's case was linked to the persistence of his masturbation.

In one of Henry Maudsley's early publications, he wrote that while self-abuse was often listed as a cause of insanity, it was more likely that it was a symptom of an underlying disease.[101] For a materialist like Maudsley, masturbation was problematic because it proved an example of a physical act that damaged the nerves and therefore the brain. He interpreted masturbation as an essentially anti-social act, and believed that uncontrolled passion and selfishness was the gateway to criminality and madness for both current and future generations.[102] It is no surprise that practitioners might make such causal connections.[103] While some doctors distanced themselves from the theory that masturbation paved the road to the asylum, it lingered into the twentieth century.[104]

Less reputable specialists encouraged men to fear their masturbatory habits and nocturnal emissions. Published case histories characterized the masturbator as not only a lunatic but also as sexless or effeminate. Patients often fed the narrative as well, as it was common practice for doctors to quote case histories of patients who admitted they believed masturbation caused their insanity.[105] One twenty-two-year-old philosophy student sought help from a doctor with early symptoms of a nervous disorder. When describing his sexually explicit dreams, the doctor noted that the student's voice was 'whimpering and unsteady' and that his tone was 'fawning'. In the case of a landed young gentleman, the 'last scion of an ancient noble line', he was described as looking like a decrepit old man at twenty-four years of age. He confessed to indulging in masturbation from a young age, and now suffered impotence. Another man confessed to onanism and then sexual excess that led to his wrecked frame; the doctor described him 'staggering into my consulting room' broken and diseased.[106] In all such cases the doctor compares the emasculated patients with their cured selves, who are typically stronger, fitter, and most often prove their new manly vigour through successful marriage and procreation.

Masturbation was not simply a symptom, but a catch-all explanation for moral judgements that many people used to justify a dislike of a person or their lifestyle.[107] Doctors and patients alike understood sexual symptoms as unmanly. In his anonymous description of life inside a London asylum for the poor, one author related his own experiences along with fellow patients'. He judges the patients based on their symptoms and the cause of their illness. One patient he described as having 'a nasty habit in the bedroom, which soon reached the doctor's ears, and we were not sorry when he was removed to another asylum'.[108] The author alternatively described this patient as 'proud, vain, arrogant, and a bully' whom no one liked or respected. He was described as effeminate, duplicitous, and an exhibitionist.[109] The man's masturbation was highlighted as definitive proof that he was beyond hope.

Masturbation was listed as the cause of insanity in several cases at Manor House Asylum.[110] The main course of treatment for masturbation involved rigorously watching patients, in particular at night, and the use of bromides. Such treatments had mixed results. Charles William Pardoe suffered delusions that the doctors believed were caused by masturbation. Admitted to Manor House at the age of thirty-four, he had suffered two previous attacks, the first at the age of twenty-one. With a good family history and no obvious cause, doctors strongly suspected masturbation, though Pardoe was too confused in thought to confirm or deny. Doctors may have assumed this cause as he was anxious, tried to flee from people, and repeated that he was dirty and not fit to be in company.[111] Pardoe had clearly internalized a deep sense of shame and the doctors extrapolated the most likely cause for such a reaction.

In other cases masturbation was 'proven' as a cause of illness. Reginald Balfour was diagnosed at sixteen with hysteria triggered by masturbation. He quickly recovered but a dozen years later overwork spurred another attack, according to doctors. Institutionalized in 1903, he varied between periods of mania and despondency, and for several weeks was violent. While masturbation was not initially listed as a cause for this breakdown, he later revealed he had been masturbating in secret. Balfour was identified as a man susceptible to insanity caused by sexual excitement; his track record showed masturbation was dangerous to him in ways it might not be to other men.[112] Such cases highlight why just counting the cases where masturbation was listed as an official cause of insanity downplays its significance in medical treatment; Balfour's first incarceration listed masturbation as a cause while his second did not.

These assessments cannot be dismissed as moralized reactions to a normal sexual behaviour; while the idea that masturbation could cause insanity seems laughable today, patients and doctors internalized these fears. Morgan William O'Donovan was admitted to Manor House Asylum at the age of nineteen with delusions and melancholy. The cause of his disease was listed as masturbation. But the doctors quickly became more disturbed by his delusions than his masturbation. O'Donovan was convinced he had committed extreme sexual sins. He was horrified by his own self-diagnosed spermatorrhoea that he believed was caused by masturbation. A measure of how he had internalized some of the most dire religious warnings of the sin of onanism is that he insisted that his sin needed to be paid for with blood. He wanted to cut off his left hand and tear out his eyes, and at least once was found with a knife in his hand. His doctors were more concerned to lessen the shame of his actions than to heap their own blame on the young man. He was discharged as cured within a few months of admission – in this case doctors provided a sympathetic audience and comforted him that his masturbation was not the end of the world.[113]

Doctors specializing in lunacy had to walk a fine line between acknowledging masturbation as a potential cause of mental breakdown and being lumped in with charlatans peddling miracle cures. One specialist on neurasthenia and hysteria believed that masturbation could lead to mental breakdowns, but not in a clear-cut manner. It was in fact patients' shame over their past behaviour and fear of being revealed as a childhood masturbator that created a 'constant wearing influence on the central nervous system'.[114] Even at the height of the masturbation panic in the 1880s, there was a widespread recognition across the medical profession that the warnings over masturbation could cause as much damage as the practice itself.[115] And as social purity campaigners increased their fear-mongering over masturbatory insanity after 1885, the majority of medical practitioners began to downplay its influence.[116]

Evidence of masturbatory panic is easy to find among doctors and more particularly in patient populations. Men were conditioned to feel shame about their masturbatory habits and told that the secret vice would eventually be made visible through physical or mental ailment. To have sexual urges and anxieties was normal, but a man was supposed to be able to control and overcome such urges. The belief that a man should have full control over his body was proclaimed by doctors and religious figures from boyhood. Diane Mason points out that such propaganda both demonized and provided a roadmap to sexual vices.[117] When a man was told or believed that his lunacy was the result of masturbation, shame was the socially proscribed emotion. His failure to embody self-control had led to an emasculating madness. Yet sometimes that shame became so pathologized that doctors had to counteract that self-loathing lest it do more damage than the original 'sin'.

Homosexuality

While doctors debated the significance of masturbation as a cause and/or a symptom, perhaps the most serious sexual perversion from a social point of view was homosexuality. Unlike other forms of deviance or intemperance, however, homosexual acts were regulated by law.[118] Medical debates over whether same-sex desire was inborn or acquired were overshadowed by the very real fact that its sexual expression was punishable by law. Just as the born criminal might not have been able to stop his descent into crime, so too the 'uranian' might not be able to resist acting on his desires, according to experts at the time. Doctors were split on whether such offenders should be sent to an asylum or to prison. Same-sex longings existed among layers of shame crafted by religious, moralistic, and legal strictures. For medical experts who encountered men's same-sex desire, it was categorized as a pathological sexuality to be suppressed or 'cured'.

The epicentre of medical thinking on same-sex desire was clearly on the continent, and there were few British sexologists exploring pathbreaking research in the field. Some scholars have argued there was less public debate on the topic than on other forms of aberrant sexuality.[119] While the leading thinkers were undoubtedly German, this does not mean British physicians were ignorant of continental developments.[120] Early British alienists discussed homosexual acts along with other aberrant forms of sexuality such as masturbation or excessive fornication. An article published in *Brain* clearly outlined same-sex desire as a form of perverted sexual feeling and included a number of continental case studies.[121] Ivan Crozier notes that British readers were introduced to cutting edge sexological writings about homosexuality, and British doctors reviewed such work in their scholarly publications.[122] There was also a popular understanding about same-sex acts between men, and men could hardly feign ignorance about the practice.[123]

Doctors, sociologists, and lawmakers saw same-sex desire as a source of deep shame and perversion that could and should have been controlled. A doctor working at an asylum in Perth explained 'The common sot destroys his mental functions by his inveterate habit, which might well have been kept in check at the beginning of his vicious career.'[124] Dr Rumler believed that some people were born with the desires through congenital defect, but also stated that 'they may be developed if the persons concerned are greatly weakened by onanism or immoderate sexual pleasures, and are entirely deadened to natural sexual intercourse'.[125] As such, the sufferer was to blame for his unnatural desires and should feel shame; same-sex desire was essentially framed as a failure of self-control and thus a failure of masculinity.

Medical case studies clearly reveal how men internalized their shame about same-sex desire. One young man was sent to Dr George Savage by a religious advisor when he was suicidal. The cause of his distress was that 'he felt so ashamed of his unnatural state that he wished he were dead ... He says the sight of a fine man causes him to have an erection, and if he is forced to be in his society he has an emission.'[126] This unnamed man was deemed perfectly normal in his senses and reasoning powers, but unable to change his sexual desires. This patient's deeply internalized shame led to dangerous, self-destructive behaviours. Mainstream physicians offered few solutions to such desires beyond general admonitions of hygiene and improved physical health. In the fourth edition of his work on hypnotism, C. Lloyd Tuckey offered some hope to 'cure' homosexual desire; however, he admitted it was very hard work and required absolute commitment from the patient and careful oversight by the doctor.[127] Dr Albert von Schrenck-Notzing was well known for an intensive treatment to cure sexual inverts. With heavy use of hypnosis, he attempted to remap sexual desires, and was not adverse to using the brothel as a training zone.[128] While not all doctors went to such extremes, the idea that a man could 'cure' his same-sex feelings through control and training was widely believed.

Some doctors did not believe such cases were appropriate for treatment by medical men, but rather the church or the justice system. Others, however, saw homosexual acts as an early symptom of larger mental derangement. There was no unified consensus on whether same-sex desire was congenital, acquired, or a symptom of a more generalized mental illness.[129] In one case study from Richmond Asylum in Dublin, same-sex desire appeared as a symptom, rather than the root issue. J.D. was a twenty-one-year-old man admitted to the asylum with serious melancholia. Before his illness he enjoyed good mental health and had no history of masturbation or same-sex desires. In fact, he was perhaps too sexually active with women in the two months leading up to his admission. But in the asylum, he began to display sexual symptoms: namely masturbation and sexual attraction to men. After a month in the asylum, as his melancholia began to wane, he fell in love with a fellow patient. He would stare at the man 'ecstatically, following him about' and admitted quite freely his love was sexual. But as J.D. continued to recover, such expressions ended and the feelings receded. According to his physician, 'the condition of perverted sexual feeling was merely an episode in the melancholic attack'.[130] Doctors in this case believed J.D. had a temporary attack of homosexual feelings as one of the symptoms of his lunacy.

Personal shame: failures of morality and the will 125

Havelock Ellis's text *Sexual Inversion* was first published in German and then translated into English in 1897. His descriptions of homosexuality are empathetic, and aside from his horror at the idea of sexual inverts reproducing, he generally proposed they be left in peace.[131] He clearly wanted to dismantle the religio-moral stranglehold on sexual behaviours and instead focus on the strictly scientific.[132] Patients, however, often demonstrated deeply inscribed feelings of shame and disgust. A forty-one-year-old man wrote to Havelock Ellis asking about possible treatments for his longstanding sexual attractions to men. He was adamant that he had never acted on his desires but he was hoping for a way to reduce his struggle. 'The shame of this has made life a hell, and the horror of this abnormality, since I came to know it as such, has been an enemy to my religious faith.'[133] Ellis clearly found this case worthy of inclusion to suit his larger perspective on same-sex desires.[134] The anonymous writer understood his homosexual urges as a temptation he had to resist.

While it is difficult to tease out ordinary men's experiences with same-sex desires, there are enough well-known figures who wrote of their experiences that one can glean some sense of their struggles. The shame over homosexuality could be instilled at an early age. E.F. Benson describes a terrible scene at his school, Temple Grove, when two boys were publicly shamed in front of the entire school. The headmaster claimed they brought '"utter ruin and disgrace" on themselves and had broken their parents' hearts'. They were immediately expelled as 'their presence was filthy and contaminating'.[135] Benson cautioned that the strength of the feelings of young boys could be dangerous as 'this strong beat of affection may easily explode into fragments of mere sensuality, be dissipated in mere "smut" and from being a banner in the clean wind be trampled into mud'.[136] Benson's solution was self-control.

While some scholars have questioned Benson's sexuality, he was adamant in his own writings that his attraction to other boys at school was non-sexual.[137] Benson believed most young men kept their childhood friendships pure but understood how it stirred strong emotions. Benson was resolute that such attractions were innocent, and not sensual.[138] His brother Arthur struggled with his own sexual feelings in his private diary, desperate to separate his sentimental, intellectual fascination and desire for young men from any actual action. 'I should not want to give anything, only take a little ripple of emotion – how hideous to talk so!'[139] Even the idea of flirtation with men filled Arthur Benson with horror.

Reformers tried to push for a view of same-sex longings that defied medicalization or shame. John Addington Symonds explicitly rejected the idea that the 'uranian' was diseased or degenerate.[140] Even Symonds took a long time to reach this level of acceptance; when he was a young man, he had a strong sexual attraction to men and was terrified of masturbation. He was so concerned about his involuntary emissions that he allowed a doctor to cauterize him through the urethra. This procedure did little to stem his emissions or his attraction to men.[141] In his later autobiography Symonds was still struggling to reconcile his same-sex desires with his masculine self-identity; he turned to the Greeks as a potential way to solve the seeming contradiction.[142] He did know that his society had not yet figured out what to do with those plagued by such feelings. 'But the Urning is neither criminal nor insane. He is only less fortunate than you are, through an accident of birth, which is at present obscure to our imperfect science of sexual determination.'[143] Symonds was a minority voice arguing for sympathy and compassion.

The extraordinary case of Sir George Grant Suttie is a thoroughly documented story of a man who could or would not stop propositioning men.[144] While shame could reach pathological levels, a complete lack of shame of homosexual desires could be equally pathologized. Suttie was declared a lunatic and kept under certificates for almost his entire life. In his early years, he clearly exhibited multiple mental symptoms such as rage, random outbursts, and mental distraction. When his fits of violence passed, his only remaining symptoms were being somewhat childish and unable to abide by Victorian strictures on sexual conduct. At this stage doctors were doubtful he would meet the standard for a new certification.[145] However, his complete lack of restraint around men struck his doctors as justifying his constant supervision, for fear he would otherwise land in prison.

Suttie's first mental disease was at the age of twenty-three, and within four years he had tried travel, the Crichton Royal Asylum, and finally admission as a private patient under an urgency order to Manor House Asylum.[146] Admission papers at Manor House state that he had a hereditary predisposition to insanity, and that he had demonstrated sexualized symptoms from a young age.[147] As a child he had a violent temper and a habit of masturbation so intense his hands were restrained at night at the age of ten. More troubling, they noted that he developed sexual habits at Eton and later at Oxford, where he met 'the most evil persons who fostered and encouraged him in unnatural propensities'. Suttie had been blackmailed and removed from Oxford. He had openly spoken of being in love with men and sending them presents. Doctors in Scotland recommended he be put under restraint immediately.[148] His doctor wrote, 'He is absolutely untrustworthy and I do not consider him fit to be at large, as no stranger of his own sex can be said to be safe from him & he requires constant watching.'[149]

Suttie transgressed both gender and class expectations. He flirted with male servants, and made several explicit propositions to other men, all while under certificates. At one point the doctor notes, he 'seems to attach himself to strange men if he has any opportunity'. He did try to conceal his activities from the doctors at times, but he never stopped. At one point he was showing good progress, and case notes explicitly praised his more masculine behaviour. 'He was more manly in many ways.' And yet soon it was evident that nothing had changed. Letters were intercepted that the doctor characterized as 'vicious correspondence' just when he seemed to be improving.[150]

Case notes reveal the doctors' frustrations. One can also detect that had Suttie been able simply to pretend more convincingly, and stop making covert advances, they would have been happy to let him go. In some ways it was as much about his lack of control as his sexual desires. It was the inability to fake social proprieties that truly doomed Suttie to confinement. He was eventually transferred to private care, where he continued to live his very long life in seclusion. Signs of improvement were always matched by setbacks.[151] Letters preserved in his file record that he continued to write to young working-class men, and he displayed 'cunning' trying to send them unnoticed.[152] Evidence in these intercepted letters indicates some men might have returned his affections. Suttie wrote to a man named Donald in 1908 thanking him for his note and gift of heather. Suttie wrote with obvious sexual desire and no sense of shame:

> I wish I had you here to give you some kisses and get you on my knee again; and I should like to see you in bed with me without any clothes on. Tell me if you would like this when you write. Don't shew this to <u>anyone</u>.
> With love xxxxxxx[153]

It is impossible to know how many other letters like this were written. Suttie was not institutionalized because of his love for men, but once he was declared a lunatic it is clear this was a main reason to keep him under restraint. By refusing to succumb to the medico-moral narratives of normative sexuality, Suttie lived free of shame, but paid a heavy price.

Some men sought out medical or religious treatment for their same-sex desires in the hope of avoiding prison. An Australian doctor submitted a case history to the *Journal of Mental Science* in 1891, detailing the life of such an English patient. The young man had a troubled family, and a head injury as a child. It was this latter injury that marked a significant change in the boy according to his mother. He masturbated frequently and preferred the company of male children only. When a young man, he began 'indecent habits towards boys, but denies sodomy'. He was unable to form any healthy attachment to women and was ashamed of his desires towards young men. When he heard the police were inquiring about his habits, he obtained poison, but before killing himself went to a London physician with his story. He was admitted to Murray's asylum as a voluntary patient. His doctor clearly found little to recommend in his patient, describing his expression as 'effeminate', his manner 'nauseous and unmanly'.[154]

A detective from London arrived at the asylum and removed the patient to stand trial for indecent practices. His solicitor asked for a review of the case to try to help his client; this inspired the doctor to ponder the correct treatment for the young man. The solicitor advised the young man to plead guilty with extenuating circumstances, rather than pleading actual insanity. The judge asked the question of what should be done with the man; if he could not be detained as a lunatic, he was sure to end up back in the court soon enough having committed the exact same sexual offence. But the law had only a limited sentencing power, so he was given one year's hard labour.[155] Clearly some members of the legal system saw the 'uranian' in similar ways to the inebriate; men who could not control their desires, and, while not insane, could not live in society.

Suttie's longstanding, unrepentant, and persistent same-sex advances made him a difficult patient. For much of his life his family made the decision to keep him under medical supervision for fear he would end up in prison. Doctors viewed homosexual desires in a similar way as other sexual vices, and yet it was the only symptom that could lead to prison if pursued. Thus, while there was some medical compassion and understanding, it is no surprise that most medical authorities saw same-sex desire as a pathological behaviour that needed to be removed. Most patients and doctors agreed that these were sick and sinful desires that needed to be suppressed.

Conclusion

In writing about sexual inversion, Havelock Ellis warned doctors in general not to judge their patient's symptoms or their lifestyle; their job was to treat and not to condemn. 'The physician who feels nothing but disgust at the sight of disease is unlikely to bring either succor to his patients or instruction to his pupils.'[156] Yet neither patients, their families, nor doctors could completely divorce their personal feelings from their assessment of behaviour. In a Darwinian age where most believed that not only genetic diseases but also moral temperaments and failings could be passed down, there were real-world consequences to moral failings. As Daniel Noble's influential 1853 psychological textbook explained, a number of factors could lead to insanity. Along with grief, alcohol, and insomnia, he lists a number of more value-laden causes, including alcohol, sexual excess, syphilis, and 'the moral conduct of the parents' that could then be passed along to their children.[157] In an era with rising asylum rates and lowering hopes of cure, the spectre of insanity loomed large, and men were shamed should they succumb to a preventable cause. Men were held more accountable for their inability to control their base desires because self-regulation was central to the masculine ideal. The men in this chapter largely accepted the opprobrium of society and blamed themselves for their mental breakdowns. Yet not all men accepted such judgements so readily, and some refused to accept there was anything wrong with them or their behaviour or mental state.

Notes

1 J.T. Davidson, *Wanted, a Man! Manly Talks* (London, 1893), p. 22.
2 The exact state of Louis Trevelyan's mind has been much debated among literary scholars. Goodman, 'Madness in Marriage'; C. Wiesenthal,

Figuring Madness in Nineteenth-Century Fiction (Houndmills, 1997), pp. 63–96.
3   D.D. Oberhelman, 'Trollope's Insanity Defense: Narrative Alienation in *He Knew He Was Right*', *Studies in English Literature, 1500–1900* 35:4 (1995), p. 802.
4   While Trevelyan is sometimes ashamed of his behaviour, he cannot control his suspicions and wild thoughts, and is eventually broken by them. A. Trollope, *He Knew He Was Right*, vol. 1 (Leipzig, 1869), p. 184.
5   Trollope, *He Knew He Was Right*, vol. 1, p. 337.
6   Pedlar, *'The Most Dreadful Visitation'*, pp. 132, 160.
7   Davidson, *Remembrances of a Religio-maniac: An Autobiography* (Stratford-on-Avon, 1912), p. 40.
8   Davidson, *Remembrances of a Religio-maniac*, pp. 288, 3.
9   P. Stearns, *Shame: A Brief History* (Champaign, 2017), pp. 15, 73.
10 Cohen, *Family Secrets*, pp. 88–89; O. Ward, 'John Langdon Down: The Man and the Message', *Down Syndrome Research and Practice* 6:1 (1999), pp. 19–24.
11 E.J. Seymour, *A Letter to the Right Honourable The Earl of Shaftesbury on the Laws Which Regulate Private Lunatic Asylums* (London, 1859), p. 6.
12 J. Barlow, *On Man's Power over Himself to Prevent or Control Insanity* (London, 1849), p. 40.
13 A.N. Gilbert, 'Masturbation and Insanity: Henry Maudsley and the Ideology of Sexual Repression', *Albion: A Quarterly Journal Concerned with British Studies* 12:3 (1980), p. 269.
14 There was consistent belief in the medical community that there were numerous preventable causes of insanity that simply demanded self-control. For example: J.M. Clarke, *Hysteria and Neurasthenia* (London, 1905), pp. 183–84; W.W. Moseley, *Twelve Chapters on Nervous or Mind Complaints* (London, 1860), pp. 67–80.
15 A. Scull, *Hysteria: The Disturbing History* (Oxford, 2011), p. 97.
16 'The Inquiry in Lunacy', *Morning Post* (8 April 1884), p. 7.
17 Quoted in Chaney, '"No 'Sane' Person Would Have Any Idea"', p. 18.
18 *Forty-third Annual Report of the Commissioners in Lunacy*, p. 101.
19 E. Sheppard, *Lectures on Madness in Its Medical, Legal, and Social Aspects* (London, 1873), p. 25.
20 W. Williamson, *Thoughts on Insanity and Its Causes and on the Management of the Insane. To which are Appended Observations on the Report for 1850, of the Lunatic Asylum of the North and East Ridings of Yorkshire* (London, 1851), p. 4.

21 A. Wynter, *The Borderlands of Insanity* (London: Henry Renshaw, 1877), pp. 62, 287.
22 Male lunatics were popular figures in imaginative writings throughout the century. Goodman, 'Mad Men'; Pedlar, *'The Most Dreadful Visitation'*, p. 15.
23 C. Reade, *It is Never Too Late to Mend: A Matter of Fact Romance* (London, 1911), p. 170.
24 The story follows the machinations of a vivisectionist doctor obsessed with the human brain and an evil aunt trying to disinherit her young niece by driving her mad. In the end the scheming aunt loses her mind and is sent to a private asylum.
25 W. Collins, *Heart and Science: A Story of the Present Time*, vol. 1 (London, 1883), pp. 111–13.
26 Collins, *Heart and Science*, vol. 3, p. 230.
27 Doolittle, 'Fatherhood and Family Shame', p. 94.
28 D. Nash and A. Kilday, *Cultures of Shame: Exploring Crime and Morality in Britain 1600–1900* (London, 2010), pp. 17–18.
29 Anon., *Fastened-Fellow: A Man's Adventure* (London, 1878), pp. 4–6, 12.
30 William Lang Tamlin, Bethlem, ARA 37, 1896.
31 Oppenheim, *'Shattered Nerves'*, pp. 150–51.
32 Stearns, *Shame*, p. 83.
33 This was a common refrain of doctors and the general public in the popular press. For example: A Physician [pseud.], 'Lunatic Asylums and the Lunacy Laws', *The Times* (19 August 1858), pp. 8–9; *The Times* (17 February 1870), p. 9; *The Times* (10 June 1880), p. 9.
34 MacKenzie, *Psychiatry for the Rich*, p. 114.
35 Lunacy Commissioners' reports tended to anonymize names and identities except in the case of criminal acts.
36 *Twenty-fifth Annual Report of the Commissioners in Lunacy* pp. 80–86.
37 *Twenty-fifth Annual Report of the Commissioners in Lunacy*, p. 85.
38 *Twenty-fifth Annual Report of the Commissioners in Lunacy*, pp. 88–91.
39 *Colburn's United Service Magazine*, vol. 2 (1870), p. 300.
40 Manor House Asylum Case Notes, Male Patients, MS 5725, p. 2.
41 Manor House Asylum Case Notes, Male Patients, MS 5725, pp. 2, 38, 59, 75; Manor House Asylum Case Notes, Male Patients, MS 6223, pp. 57, 326, 631; Manor House Asylum Case Notes, Male Patients, MS 6224, pp. 3–4.
42 In one sensation novel, a grandfather reveals that there is a terrible family secret that will doom his beloved granddaughter and bring ruin to her and the rest of her family if she ever married. She assumes it

to be madness, as do other characters in the novel. M.A. Fleming, *A Wife's Tragedy* (New York, 1881).

43 *Report of a Special Committee of the Charity Organisation Society on the Education and Care of Idiots, Imbeciles, and Harmless Lunatics, Etc.* (London, 1877), p. 6.

44 Coxe, *Lunacy in Its Relation to the State*, p. 36.

45 For example, a man may not be able to control being born into an overcrowded city but it was a choice to be a money-obsessed miser. Both were risk factors for insanity according to Maudsley. H. Maudsley, *Physiology and Pathology of the Mind* (London, 1867), pp. 204–5.

46 'Mental Deterioration: Some of its Avoidable Causes', *Westminster Review* (July 1888), pp. 64–81.

47 Like John Barlow, who blames mania on men's 'ungoverned passions'. Barlow, *On Man's Power over Himself*, p. 88.

48 The identification of alcoholic insanity as a failure of moral willpower survived into the twentieth century. J.R.G. Digges, *The Cure of Inebriety: Alcoholism, the Drink and the Tobacco Habit* (London, 1904), p. 14.

49 A. Vleugels, *Narratives of Drunkenness: Belgium, 1830–1914* (New York, 2015).

50 Peter McCandless cites one temperance preacher who believed that 75–90 per cent of Britain's insane population got that way because of alcohol. P. McCandless, '"Curses of Civilization": Insanity and Drunkenness in Victorian Britain', *British Journal of Addiction* 79:4 (1984), p. 49.

51 As co-editor of the *Journal of Mental Science* for fourteen years and President of the Medico-Psychological Association, Henry Maudsley was one of the most influential and successful practitioners of the age. He did not believe that lunacy was increasing, but rather that more people were being identified and treated. E.F. Torrey and J. Miller, *The Invisible Plague: The Rise of Mental Illness From 1750 to the Present* (New Brunswick, 2007), pp. 79–80.

52 H. Maudsley, *Responsibility in Mental Disease* (New York, 1874), pp. 285–86.

53 There were two recognized diagnoses particularly related to alcohol: dipsomania (a chronic desire to drink to excess) and *delirium tremens* (acute reaction to hard drinking or withdrawal of alcohol). J.W. Bradshaw, *Use and Abuse of Stimulants: On Dipsomania and Its Results, Etc.* 2nd ed. (London, 1867), pp. 6–9; G.R. Wilson, *Drunkenness* (London, 1897), p. vii.

54 M. Valverde, '"Slavery from Within": The Invention of Alcoholism and the Question of Free Will', *Social History* 22:3 (1997), pp. 251–68.

Personal shame: failures of morality and the will 133

55 Despite the consistent messaging of restraint, there is little evidence that rates of alcohol consumption changed. L.L. Shiman, *Crusade against Drink in Victorian England* (London, 1988), pp. 240, 244.
56 Between 1870 and 1895, 75 per cent of those labelled habitual drunkards were men. B. Morrison, 'Controlling the "Hopeless": Re-visioning the History of the Female Inebriate Institutions c. 1870–1920', in H. Johnston (ed.), *Punishment and Control in Historical Perspectives* (Houndmills, 2008), p. 138.
57 T. Hands, 'Sobering Up the Magdalenes' Drunken Sisters: The Institutional Treatment of "Female Drunken Pests" in Scotland, 1900–15', *Social History of Alcohol and Drugs* 27:1 (2013), pp. 62–81; G. Hunt, C. Mellor, and J. Turner, 'Wretched, Hatless and Miserably Clad: Women and the Inebriate Reformatories from 1900–1913', *British Journal of Sociology* 40:2 (1989), pp. 244–70; C. Soares, 'The Path to Reform? Problematic Treatments and Patient Experience in Nineteenth-Century Female Inebriate Institutions', *Cultural & Social History* 12:3 (2015), pp. 411–29; J. Wallis, 'A Home or a Gaol? Scandal, Secrecy, and the St James's Inebriate Home for Women', *Social History of Medicine* 31:4 (2018), pp. 774–95.
58 S. Zieger, *The Mediated Mind: Affect, Ephemera and Consumerism in the Nineteenth Century* (New York, 2018), pp. 48–49.
59 G. Cruikshank, *The Bottle* (London, 1847). It also inspired a short novel of the same name. K. Makras, '"The Poison that Upsets my Reason": Men, Madness and Drunkenness in the Victorian Period', in Knowles and Trowbridge (eds), *Insanity and the Lunatic Asylum*, p. 144.
60 A. Brontë, *The Tenant of Wildfell Hall* (London, 1854), pp. 148, 346.
61 W. Collins, *Man and Wife*, vol. 3 (Leipzig, 1870), pp. 220–22.
62 J.C. Kernahan, *A Literary Gent: A Study in Vanity and Dipsomania* (London, 1897), pp. 23, 29, 37. Dipsomania was not always characterized as a form of madness, although it was subject of much debate. McCandless, '"Curses of Civilization"', pp. 49–58.
63 The connection between alcohol and creativity long pre-dated the Victorian period and continued into the twentieth century. O. Laing, *The Trip to Echo Spring: On Writers and Drinking* (New York, 2014).
64 G. Rayne, 'London's Little Love Stories XX. – the Barfier', *Vanity Fair* (26 July 1911), p. 118.
65 Doctors continued to debate the best forms of treatment, however, along with the issue of whether *delirium tremens* was the result of the withdrawal of alcohol by a long-time abuser or the result of long-term, extreme abuse. See, for example, the evolving debate in *The Lancet*. G.W. Balfour, 'Clinical Lecture on the Treatment of Delirium Tremens',

The Lancet (1 February 1879), pp. 146–48; 'Record of a Night with the Charge of a Delirium Tremens Patient', *The Lancet* (27 November 1880), pp. 872–73; 'A Case of Delirium Tremens following Sea-Sickness, and Occurring in an Opium-Eater', *The Lancet* (2 February 1888), p. 218; 'Sunstroke or Delirium Tremens', *The Lancet* (24 September 1898), p. 823; 'Certain Clinical and Etiological Aspects of Delirium Tremens', *The Lancet* (15 July 1899), p. 169; 'The Management of Delirium Tremens', *The Lancet* (14 March 1906), p. 779.

66 A. Peddie, *On the Pathology of Delirium Tremens, and Its Treatment, Without Stimulants or Opiates* (Edinburgh, 1854), p. 6.

67 Henry Frederick Norbury, Journal of Her Majesty's Flag Ship Corvette (1 January 1879–25 October 1879), NA, ADM 101/156/1, p. 10.

68 For example, the 14th Brigade kept a list of their deceased soldiers; *delirium tremens* was a frequently listed cause of death. Registry of Deceased Soldiers, 14th Brigade (1859–1877), NA, WO 69/596/626.

69 While he was discharged within a month, he was readmitted within a year. House surgeon's notes for physician: Male, Records of Glasgow Royal Lunatic Asylum, HB 15/5/130, 1895.

70 Admission Register, Bethlem, ARA 24, 15/05/1861.

71 F.E. Grainger, *Caged! The Romance of a Lunatic Asylum* (London, 1900), p. 91.

72 Robert Ritchie, physician at Bethnal House Asylum, believed many of his peers failed to recognize or write about masturbation as a cause of young men's insanity. 'Let us not ignore so powerful a cause of mental disease merely because it is a nameless vice, and one we blush even to allude to.' R.P. Ritchie, *An Inquiry into a Frequent Cause of Insanity in Young Men* (London, 1861), pp. 6, 7.

73 J.C. Bucknill and D.H. Tuke, *A Manual of Psychological Medicine, Containing the Lunacy Laws*, 4th edn (London, 1879), p. 91.

74 Stearns, *Shame*, p. 72.

75 S. Seidman, 'The Power of Desire and the Danger of Pleasure: Victorian Sexuality Reconsidered', *Journal of Social History* 24:1 (1990), p. 49.

76 In fact he argues that it is one of the defining differences between man and animal – that our sexual urges are completely under our own mental control. L.S. Beale, *Our Morality and The Moral Question: Chiefly from the Medical Side* (London, 1887), p. 43.

77 L.A. Hall, 'Forbidden by God, Despised by Men: Masturbation, Medical Warnings, Moral Panic, and Manhood in Great Britain, 1850–1950', *Journal of the History of Sexuality* 2:3 (1992), p. 375.

78 In this pamphlet, the author identifies prostitution as the greatest social evil, and lambasts the double standard that shuns promiscuous

Personal shame: failures of morality and the will 135

women but accepts such men. J.A. Rawlings, *The Greatest Evil of Our Time: An Address to Men* (London, 1891), p. 28.
79 Manor House Asylum Case Notes, Male Patients, MS 6223, p. 425.
80 Manor House Asylum Case Notes, Male Patients, MS 5725, pp. 146, 147, 153, 233; MS 6223, p. 64; MS 6224, pp. 33, 34, 51, 52, 69, 70.
81 Manor House Asylum Case Notes, Male Patients, MS 6227, p. 143.
82 Manor House Asylum Case Notes, Male Patients, MS 6222, pp. 277–78.
83 Manor House Asylum Case Notes, Male Patients, MS 6222, p. 281.
84 Manor House Asylum Case Notes, Male Patients, MS 6223, pp. 279, 281, 282.
85 Manor House Asylum Case Notes, Male Patients, MS 6224, p. 63.
86 Henry Witherby (admitted in 1885) and Robert William Will (admitted 1900). Manor House Asylum Case Notes, Male Patients, MS 6222, p. 51; MS 6223, p. 512.
87 Manor House Asylum Case Notes, Male Patients, MS 5725, p. 7.
88 Manor House Asylum Case Notes, Male Patients, MS 5725, p. 410.
89 Hall, 'Forbidden by God, Despised by Men', p. 369.
90 Barker was a self-proclaimed Professor of Phrenology and a registered dentist working in Brighton. J.A. Barker, *A Secret Book for Men: Containing Necessary Personal and Confidential Light, Instruction, Information, Counsel, and Advice for the Physical, Mental, Moral & Spiritual Weal of Boys, Youths, and Men* (Brighton, c. 1888), p. 10.
91 Sheppard, *Lectures on Madness*, pp. 21–22.
92 R. Darby, 'Pathologizing Male Sexuality: Lallemand, Spermatorrhea, and the Rise of Circumcision', *Journal of the History of Medicine and Allied Sciences* 60:3 (2005), pp. 285, 314.
93 Stephens, 'Pathologizing Leaky Male Bodies', pp. 428–29.
94 Treatments for spermatorrhoea were invasive and punitive, and the many volunteers speaks to a deep level of shame and desperation. Stephens, 'Pathologizing Leaky Male Bodies', pp. 427–29.
95 Similar ideas were dominant in France and Germany. C.K. Codell, 'Infantile Hysteria and Infantile Sexuality in Late Nineteenth-Century German-Language Medical Literature', *Medical History* 27:2 (1983), pp. 186–96; Hewitt, *Institutionalizing Gender*, p. 23.
96 *Fourth Annual Report of the Commissioners in Lunacy*, p. 23.
97 In this case the York Asylum at 2.5 and the Northampton State Lunatic Hospital at 3 per cent among male admissions. Bucknill and Tuke, *A Manual of Psychological Medicine*, p. 98.
98 Ritchie, *An Inquiry into a Frequent Cause of Insanity*, pp. 8–9.
99 Gilbert, 'Masturbation and Insanity', p. 273.

100 House surgeon's notes for physician: Male, Records of Glasgow Royal Lunatic Asylum, HB 13/5/61, 1876–1893.
101 H. Maudsley, 'On Some of the Causes of Insanity', *Journal of Mental Science* 12 (January 1867), p. 489. He later even more explicitly distanced himself from the idea that masturbation could cause insanity. L.A. Hall, '"It was Affecting the Medical Profession": The History of Masturbatory Insanity Revisited', *Pedagogia Historica* 39:6 (2003), p. 697.
102 Gilbert, 'Masturbation and Insanity', pp. 270–71, 277.
103 Others believed that masturbation was a symptom of a larger mental illness. For example, one observer at Claybury Asylum noted that epileptics often became masturbators over the course of their disease. T.E.K. Stansfield, 'Notes on Insanity with Case Notes from Claybury Asylum', 8 March 1896, MS 6806.
104 A. Hunt, 'The Great Masturbation Panic and the Discourses of Moral Regulation in Nineteenth- and Early Twentieth-Century Britain', *Journal of the History of Sexuality* 8:4 (1998), p. 576.
105 Hall, '"It was Affecting the Medical Profession"', p. 690.
106 Rumler, *The Causes, Nature, and Cure of Neurasthenia in General, and of Nervous Disorders of the Generative System in Particular.* 15th edn (Geneva, 1901), pp. 244–76.
107 T.D. Savill, *Clinical Lectures on Neurasthenia* (London, 1899), pp. 23–24.
108 Anon., *Fastened-Fellow*, p. 31.
109 Anon., *Fastened-Fellow*, p. 30.
110 There are also clearly cases where some level of masturbation was detected but it was tied to larger problems of sexual perversion and delusions. On one of Henry E. Bessemer's certificates the doctor notes that the patient related a confused story about friends who mesmerized him and forced him to masturbate. Manor House Asylum Case Notes, Male Patients, MS 6223, p. 596. In the case of James Wild Stranham, his insanity was sparked by a love affair gone wrong, but doctors worried about a cluster of sexual symptoms including excitement, seminal emissions, and masturbation. Manor House Asylum Case Notes, Male Patients, MS 6223, p. 112.
111 Manor House Asylum Case Notes, Male Patients, MS 5725, pp. 464–65, 468.
112 Manor House Asylum Case Notes, Male Patients, MS 6223, p. 625.
113 Manor House Asylum Case Notes, Male Patients, MS 5725, p. 354.
114 Clarke, *Hysteria and Neurasthenia*, pp. 243–44.
115 Hall, 'Forbidden by God, Despised by Men', p. 376.

116 Hunt, 'The Great Masturbation Panic', p. 593. There were, of course, medical holdouts like Dr Henry Morris, who still warned young people that masturbation would age them prematurely. J. Stengers and A. Van Neck, *Masturbation: The History of a Great Terror*, trans. K.A. Hoffmann (New York, 2001), p. 138.

117 D. Mason, *Secret Vice: Masturbation in Victorian Fiction and Medical Culture* (Manchester, 2013), pp. 13–14, 18–19.

118 In 1533 buggery was made a crime under civil law, though it was equally named a vice and a sin. The penalty was death. This was the foundation of homosexual convictions up to 1885. It was not until 1861 in England and Wales and 1889 in Scotland that the death penalty was formally removed for sodomy. Section 11 of the Criminal Law Amendment Act expanded the criminalization of sexual acts to include any homosexual acts committed in public or private. Finally, the 1898 Vagrancy Act included punishments for any homosexual soliciting. J. Weeks, *Coming Out: Homosexual Politics in Britain from the Nineteenth Century to the Present* (London, 1977), pp. 12–15.

119 H.G. Cocks, 'Making the Sodomite Speak: Voices of the Accused in English Sodomy Trials, c. 1800–98', *Gender & History* 18:1 (2006), p. 87.

120 J. Weeks, *Sexuality and its Discontents: Meanings, Myths, & Modern Sexualities* (London, 1985), pp. 67–68.

121 J. Kreug, 'Perverted Sexual Instincts', *Brain* 4:3 (1881), p. 368.

122 I. Crozier, 'Nineteenth-Century Psychiatric Writing about Homosexuality before Havelock Ellis: The Missing Story', *Journal of the History of Medicine and Allied Sciences* 63:1 (2008), pp. 75–77, 93–101.

123 C. Upchurch, 'Full-Text Databases and Historical Research: Cautionary Results from a Ten-Year Study', *Journal of Social History* 46:1 (2012), pp. 89–105, 99–100.

124 Urquhart, 'Case of Sexual Perversion', *Journal of Mental Science* 37:156 (1891), p. 94.

125 Rumler, *Causes, Nature, and Cure of Neurasthenia*, p. 201.

126 G.H. Savage, 'Case of Sexual Perversion in a Man', *Journal of Mental Science* 30:131 (1884), p. 390.

127 Crozier, 'Nineteenth-Century Psychiatric Writing', p. 92.

128 Ellis was horrified by such ideas, as such a course of action would imply adding vice and perversion to a patient already troubled by aberrant sexual desires. H. Ellis, *Sexual Inversion* (Philadelphia, 1901), pp. 195–96.

129 Crozier, 'Nineteenth-Century Psychiatric Writing', pp. 83, 91.

130 W.C. Sullivan, 'Notes on a Case of Acute Insanity with Sexual Perversion', *Journal of Mental Science* 39:165 (1893), pp. 225–26.
131 The fact that John Addington Symonds was a collaborator on the work undoubtedly helped set a more humane tone.
132 J. Dixon, 'Havelock Ellis and John Addington Symonds, Sexual Inversion (1897)', *Victorian Review* 35:1 (2009), p. 74.
133 Ellis, *Sexual Inversion*, p. 199.
134 I. Crozier, 'Pillow Talk: Credibility, Trust and the Sexological Case History', *History of Science* 46:4 (2008), p. 381.
135 E.F. Benson, *Our Family Affairs, 1867–1896* (New York, c. 1921), pp. 88–89.
136 Benson, *Our Family Affairs*, p. 151.
137 B. Masters, *The Life of E.F. Benson* (London, 1991).
138 Benson, *Our Family Affairs*, p. 155.
139 Quoted in S. Goldhill, *A Very Queer Family Indeed: Sex, Religion and the Bensons in Victorian Britain* (Chicago, 2016), p. 139.
140 J.A. Symonds, *A Problem in Modern Ethics: Being an Inquiry Into the Phenomenon of Sexual Inversion* (London, 1896), p. 99.
141 It was only when he later began having sex with male partners that his earlier sexual symptoms disappeared. Darby, 'Pathologizing Male Sexuality', p. 305.
142 O.S. Buckton, *Secret Selves: Confession and Same Sex Desire in Victorian Autobiography* (Chapel Hill, 1998), pp. 94, 5.
143 Symonds, *A Problem in Modern Ethics*, p. 100.
144 His name was variously spelled as 'Suttie' or 'Suttee' across various records.
145 In 1945, at the age of seventy-four, doctors conferred on his case and believed that living under certification as a lunatic did him no harm, and that should he be left alone the 'consequences might be disastrous for himself and others'. Unsigned letter, 31 July 1945. Sir George G. Suttie, NA, MH 85/29/5127.
146 Walter Forsyth Chevers, Certificate of Medical Practitioner on Sir George G. Suttie. Single Patients, NA, MH 85/29.
147 In this case his deceased father's family was noted as having a history of intemperance and his mother, who signed the admission orders, had suffered epileptic attacks for years.
148 Manor House Asylum Case Notes, Male Patients, MS 6223, p. 281.
149 Walter Forsyth Chevers, Certificate of Medical Practitioner on Sir George G. Suttie. Single Patients, NA, MH 85/29.
150 Manor House Asylum Case Notes, Male Patients, MS 6223, p. 450.
151 He would occasionally express regret at his actions to his doctor. George Suttie to Dr. Needham, 15 January 1904, NA, MH 85/29.

152 G. Wickenham to Lunacy Commissioners, 7 February 1907, NA, MH 85/29.
153 George Suttie to 'Donald', 20 August 1908, NA, MH 85/29.
154 Urquhart, 'Case of Sexual Perversion', p. 94.
155 Urquhart, 'Case of Sexual Perversion', p. 95.
156 Ellis, *Sexual Inversion*, p. 216.
157 Noble, *Elements of Psychological Medicine*, pp. 231–51.

4

Madmen out of the attic: reputation, rage, and liberty

> Those who had true love for their relatives did not take steps to proclaim to the world that a father was a hard living man, or to bring to light all the various private particulars of his life.[1]

The author of the statement above was critiquing families who publicized their loved ones' mental trials through contentious lunacy proceedings. The author, and many like him, believed that discretion, if not outright secrecy, was the best way to protect both personal and family reputations when it came to the question of madness. The process of certification did not always allow such discretion, however. Despite the challenges of social stigma and pressures of friends and family to hide or downplay men's madness, the most sensational public lunacy scandals tended to emerge. And in some cases, men branded with the label of lunatic chose to make their stories public. In such cases, men believed that the risk of publicity was worth the benefit of restoring their reputation or gaining their freedom. The men who fought against the label of madness knew very well what was at stake in being formally labelled as madmen; they were fighting to protect or restore their identities.

There were a number of ways to be declared a lunatic, depending on circumstances outlined in chapter one. In all of these scenarios, a man was formally declared incapable of managing himself and/or his property. Even for a man who seemingly did not challenge his diagnosis, the fact of his certification and detainment could be galling.[2] And those who believed they had been coerced, tricked, or were the victim of a conspiracy felt the sting all the more. They lost control of themselves, of their families, of their wealth and property, and, essentially, they lost the right to do as they pleased.

Treatment without consent was common practice throughout the nineteenth century, and most believed the mad needed to be cared for by medical experts. And yet, from the 1860s onwards, there was a growing counter-movement about the need to get greater consent from patients.[3] As ideas of individual rights and freedoms became the intrinsic defining characteristics of manhood in the West, the position of being labelled mad was increasingly degrading.[4] Not only was a man's masculinity at risk, but so too was his full personhood; the gender norms at the time dictated that a man should fight the diagnosis of insanity.

These struggles against the label of madness were fought in very personal and very public ways. The main antagonists included family members, doctors, and the courts in what often became publicized battles of will. Supposed lunatics frequently showed great capacity and creativity in defending their actions and rationalizing seemingly irrational activity. Some were victorious in their struggles while others found themselves confined, if not entirely silenced. Organizations devoted themselves to publicly fighting for the rights of the wrongfully certified. While the first half of this book has focused on private stories, and those who sought to keep their experiences of lunacy quiet, this chapter shifts to explore very public debates about madmen.

Those who publicized their fight against a diagnosis faced significant scepticism. Some commentators pathologized the desire to seek out publicity for what they clearly saw as a shameful blight. In summing up Lord Chelmsford's speech in Parliament, a journalist noted that to limit public exposure in the certification process was impossible because lunatics by their nature craved a spectacle:

> It was a peculiarity of insane persons to have a very exalted idea of their own importance, and he had no doubt many of them would prefer the notoriety of a trial before a Superior Judge to the secrecy of a quiet and unpretending inquiry before a Master in Lunacy.[5]

Like a self-fulfilling prophecy, the fact of seeking out justice was seen as proof of one's madness. And yet the best way to prove one was undeniably not mad was to win the decision in the court of public opinion. When a person was recognized as having been unjustly detained or certified as a lunatic, the public was incredibly sympathetic to the sufferer.

It is impossible with medical hindsight to separate those who were truly suffering mental illness from those whose eccentricities simply confounded or outraged their relatives.[6] That is not the purpose of this chapter. What studying the voices of those who challenged their status as mad can provide is a nuanced understanding of public and private understandings of what it meant to be labelled a 'madman' in Victorian Britain. It is important to look at men's lives and experiences as patients in connection with discourse from doctors, lawyers, family members, and the general public.[7] Mental illness was deeply imbued with meaning for the sufferers, and touched on their identities as husbands, fathers, property-holders, and citizens.[8]

Seeking out the voices of the 'mad' has often been a politicized endeavour, in particular when issues of power, social class, and gender collide.[9] In this instance, wealth and class have the most direct influence on sources and storytelling. Records of the county asylum were geared to demonstrating insanity, rather than recording people protesting their incarceration.[10] The general public did not see the wrongful incarceration of pauper lunatics as a real problem as they were a financial burden on the state; there was no financial motive to certify them.[11] However, this should not discount the fact that individuals who were incarcerated at county asylums were in fact or believed themselves to be sane; it simply reflects the lack of larger public outrage and limited resources to publicize their discontent. And while many of these struggles are lost, there are a variety of sources that can tell their stories. Sometimes men turned to acts of civil disobedience or crime in order to draw attention to their cases. Court records outline many instances of poor men publicly fighting against the label of madness, rejecting witness and legal testimony that they were insane, even if it might have aided in their defence.

Men of the middle and upper classes had both the best opportunity to publicly protest their incarceration and were also believed to be most vulnerable to wrongful incarceration because of the financial incentive. Private asylums were dependent on the high fees of paying patients. Men of education and means could reach out to the public directly through published memoirs and politicized tracts or challenge their diagnosis through the Court of Chancery. Educated and wealthy men were aware of the system and their rights within it, and they knew how to get their voices heard. Certification as a lunatic touched on broader issues of personal liberty and men's power within their family and society.

This chapter explores how men challenged the label of madness through the various methods at their disposal. Men took on their own families, doctors, the courts, and the government at various stages. Several groups organized to fight on behalf of those who believed they were wrongfully incarcerated as lunatics, while other men fought on their own. This chapter begins with the formal organizations that were founded on behalf of supposed lunatics. These advocacy groups worked to amplify individual stories and fight for collective change. It ends with a series of well-publicized case studies exploring how and why different men challenged their diagnoses. Men's chief justification for telling their stories can be grouped into three main motivations: an attempt to reassert their patriarchal control, an attempt to regain their freedom, or a desire to restore their reputation.

Creating a public scandal: organized protest

While some vented their outrage alone, others formed groups to fight for their own and others' interests. Victorian advocacy groups such as the Alleged Lunatics' Friend Society and the Lunacy Law Reform Association (LLRA) specifically campaigned for people who felt they had been unlawfully certified as mad.[12] They shone a bright and not always welcome light on abuses, both rumoured and verified, in the public and private madhouse trade. The most prominent members of these groups often had first-hand experience of the madhouse system and were motivated both to free people from wrongful incarceration and to highlight cases where family members deprived their relatives' of liberty for selfish or self-serving reasons. These activist groups raised the profile of wrongful incarceration cases and helped individuals find public redress.

The Alleged Lunatics' Friend Society was founded in 1845 out of a group of like-minded men who had either experienced wrongful confinement or believed the issue to be a serious concern. Its driving force was John Perceval, who became an outspoken activist after being committed to a private madhouse in 1830.[13] He published his story in 1838 and went on to become the honorary secretary of the ALFS from the 1840s through to the 1860s.[14] This group was male only, and took up cases at a rate of twenty-two men to five women; however, they expressly stated that both sexes could be vulnerable to scheming relatives and unscrupulous doctors.[15]

Captain Childe was in a protracted battle with his father over the state of his mental health for fifteen years before he found help from the ALFS.[16] The Society went so far as to send their own legal counsel to support Childe when his case came before the courts in 1854. Lawyers for the plaintiff objected to the presence of such counsel, claiming in opening statements that the group could be an 'officious and injudicious' influence on the proceedings. Counsel for the prosecution specifically highlighted that it was the influence of this group that rendered public a matter that should have been kept private. The defence used such claims to argue that the prosecution was biased and relying on prejudice to win their case. The group justified their presence as necessary because the case had both personal and national significance.[17]

With or without the Society's involvement, the case was likely to garner widespread attention as it dealt with the highest members of British society. Captain Childe was by all accounts an excessively handsome man. Even Lord Shaftesbury, who interviewed Childe in 1852, agreed that while the man was decidedly unsound, he would have been 'an ornament to any society, if he could keep himself under control'.[18] Childe's father believed that his son had been slowly declining in mental health for years before he intervened in 1839. Childe's behaviour was so shocking that military authorities warned his father that were the young man not confined, they would remove him to the military hospital at Chatham.[19] Childe was placed under Dr Monro's care at St John's Wood after doctors confirmed that he was no longer safe to be at large. He was then transferred to Hayes Park Asylum in 1851, when his condition worsened.[20] The young man's central problem, according to his family and the medical evidence, was rooted in a perverse egotism and sense of grandeur; he developed a fixed delusion that the Queen was in love with him. He claimed that the Queen had made advances to him and that they had some form of secret understanding. Dr William Conolly of Hayes Park believed that his patient had no self-control, and that if at large the Queen and anyone involved in his incarceration might be at risk.[21] Given that the Queen had survived several assassination attempts by this point, it was not a threat many would have taken lightly.

And yet his defence claimed that everyone was overreacting and that this rather vain young man had simply allowed his bravado to run away with him. Appearing on the stand, Childe explained that he believed in the past the Queen's manner towards him had been marked. The letters he wrote to her were the mistakes and vanities of youth, and the fact he wrote countless later letters in a cypher was simply a diversion to occupy his mind while under confinement.[22] His counsel emphasized that while their client had been mistaken about the Queen, to be incorrect was not the same as harbouring a delusion.[23] They also stressed that any strange behaviour or lingering beliefs their client possessed were due to his twelve years of wrongful treatment as a lunatic, and that the surest cure was to release him immediately.[24] Childe made a positive impression in the court; however, his previous actions could not be ignored. As a journalist for the *Berkshire Chronicle* noted, while 'his demeanour was such as to produce a feeling in his favour, the circumstances were such as evidently to impress the jury with the reality of the alteration of his intellect'.[25]

While he impressed many with his bearing in the court, Childe's dogged insistence on explaining and justifying his past conduct rather than absolutely denouncing it lent credence to the idea that his rationality was suspect. Asked about his previously stated belief that the Queen's marriage was a sham, he admitted it was not a fixed opinion, but explained it was a rational supposition based on her conduct. This remained hard to reconcile with reality. Childe's outrage at his detention failed to sway members of the jury or members of the press that his actions had proved him anything but unsound.[26] Midway through the trial, the ALFS excused itself from the case, leaving Childe without an advocate to communicate to the public or the media.[27] To imply the Queen was sexually interested in his person was so far outside the class and gendered rules of Victorian society it is no surprise that it was seen as a form of madness.

While confirmed cases of wrongful confinement were rare, there were a few celebrated instances of sane men and women spending time in the madhouse.[28] Edward Fletcher used both the ALFS and novelist Charles Reade to prove his was one such case. Fletcher's uncles claimed the young man had led a reckless life, and that he was dissolving in an alcoholic haze of madness.[29] However, there was more to the story. The young man countered that his uncles wanted him confined for purely mercenary ends. Charles Reade took up the young man's cause after Fletcher escaped from a private asylum where his uncles had sent him. He took the young man to his own independent medical men for examination and was convinced Fletcher's uncles were trying to deprive him of his freedom to benefit from his estate. Reade kept the case in the public eye by writing to the newspapers as the trial was delayed time and again. For Reade, and by extension Fletcher, the young man's life was in limbo until his day in court. As a suspected madman he was denied 'his footing in society, his means of earning bread, and his place among mankind. For a lunatic is a beast in the law's eye, and society's; and an alleged lunatic is a lunatic until a jury pronounces him sane.'[30]

With the help of Reade and the ALFS, Fletcher's case finally came before the Queen's Bench. In this case, however, it seemed the parties agreed to a compromise rather than extend public scrutiny. It was Reade and the Society who felt the most outrage, whereas Fletcher was more willing to come to a private understanding. Fletcher and his family settled on the second day of the trial. Fletcher dropped any charges of improper motives in his detainment, and his uncles agreed to pay the young man an annual £100 annuity. The young man received financial compensation and a unanimous verdict that he was of sound mind.[31] Fletcher's vindication in his freedom to live his life as he pleased was enough to satisfy his outrage.

It was not, however, enough for Charles Reade. If stories like Fletcher's read as if they were taken from the plot of a sensation novel many were, in fact, indistinguishable from works of popular fiction at the time. Charles Reade was inspired by Fletcher's case when he wrote his epic novel *Hard Cash*, first serialized in 1863. One of the main plots of Reade's story follows the tale of Alfred Hardie, a young man who is tricked and confined to a lunatic asylum by his own father. The book is merciless in its portrayal of what Reade clearly viewed as a corrupt system. Two doctors brought in to consult on Alfred's case quickly decided a normal boy in love was suffering from erotic monomania.[32] Specific echoes of Fletcher's case made their way into the story as Alfred is locked in an asylum by a scheming, money-seeking father. Mr Speers, one of the certifying medical men in the novel, tells Alfred he seems in good mental shape apart from his 'little delusion' over monies owed.³³ Just like in Fletcher's case, the money owed is no delusion; but once labelled mad and placed in an asylum, it is hard to prove otherwise. The text spends much time in various madhouses demonstrating the variety of treatment methods and variances of misdiagnosis, corruption, and ignorance. While the book is a rollicking example of sensation fiction, Reade consciously wrote the book as a serious piece of social advocacy.³⁴

Reade was at pains to demonstrate that his was a work of fiction grounded in very real facts; in the preface to the first London edition Reade emphasized the accuracy of his depiction of madhouses in particular.³⁵ In 1863 he printed a circular asking for stories of unlawful confinement to prove 'this great question did not begin with me in the pages of a novel'.³⁶ Reade was well aware of contemporary critiques of sensation fiction, and of the use of madness as a lazy plot device.³⁷ Reade took to the newspapers to defend himself against the accusation that his work slandered the good name of lunacy doctors without basis in fact.³⁸ He reminded readers of his previous experience actively intervening in Fletcher's case, and that this was just the beginning of a period of intense research on both the certification and the madhouse system. He claimed that his work was not a flight of fancy but rather a realistic portrayal of the state of lunacy laws whereby 'any English man or woman may without much difficulty be incarcerated in a private lunatic asylum when not deprived of reason'.³⁹

Sensation novelists helped keep the issue of wrongful confinement in the public consciousness when formal associations waned. In one story, a young man's father uses the asylum to force him to marry a wealthy industrialist's daughter instead of his true love.⁴⁰ The constant stream of potential wrongful confinement cases in novels and the press helped undermine lunacy 'experts'.⁴¹ Indeed, one of *The Lancet*'s frequent critiques of private lunatic asylums deemed them 'incessantly in conflict with the rights of individual liberty, and as degrading to the members of a learned profession'.⁴² The shadow of wrongful confinement was never entirely absent from public discourse, and each scandalous individual case found a ready audience.

There was hardly a period when the Lunacy Commission was in existence (1845–1913) that there were not calls to change the policies and practice of certification in Britain.[43] Slight variations to the law, and even more numerous failed reform attempts, kept the issue cycling through the public consciousness. As new Lunacy Bills wound their ways through committees and the Houses of Parliament, and as individual cases seemed to test these laws, the topic was easy fodder for an active press.[44] Two major lunacy panics led to the House of Commons appointing select committees in 1858–59 and 1876–77 to investigate potential abuses in the system.[45] And despite findings that there was no widespread problem, fears persisted. Even when the 1890 Lunacy Act introduced new provisions to protect both private and pauper lunatics, the *British Medical Journal* complained that the provisions provided only the smokescreen of reform and few actual benefits.[46]

After the ALFS faded from view, another major advocacy group formed in the 1870s to take up the cause. Louisa Lowe formed the Lunacy Law Reform Association in 1873 to extend her personal campaign against lunacy laws.[47] The new group had a far more balanced gender makeup, and its most impassioned advocates were often women. The prominence of Lowe and the excellent work by historians of women could leave some observers with the impression that the LLRA's central mission was rescuing women from madhouses. It is undeniable that women had a particularly vulnerable legal status due to the combination of lunacy laws and married women's lack of property rights for much of the century.[48] However, the group was dedicated to seeking out abuses in the lunacy infrastructure of Great Britain as a whole, with a focus on the plight of wrongfully confined men *and* women.[49]

At one public meeting of the Association in 1875, Dr Pearce related two cases of patriarchs conspiring with doctors to lock up troublesome young men. In the first instance he claimed that a father locked his son in an asylum as a result of a serious family quarrel. In another, a father institutionalized his daughter's new bridegroom in an asylum because he disapproved of the match. The meeting was full of anecdotal examples of the asylum being used as the ultimate weapon in family squabbles.[50] Inside and outside of the adversarial courtroom, advocates could tell their stories without question and be assured a ready audience and widespread coverage in the media.[51] Such groups were a perennial frustration to the lunacy experts who believed they were little more than an outlet for the delusional and the disgruntled.[52] Yet, as Louisa Lowe was keen to stress, advocates spoke out not to seek publicity, but rather out of a belief that secrecy would be more damaging than truth.[53] In fact advocacy groups, lawyers, doctors, and the press all fought about the meaning of the same high-profile cases in very public ways.

Louisa Lowe highlighted many specific cases in her lengthy published critiques of private madhouses. Perhaps one of the strangest was that of Reverend H.J. Dodwell, who was sentenced as a criminal lunatic.[54] Dodwell's troubles began when he lost his job as Chaplain to Brighton Industrial schools. He felt his dismissal was unfair and was frustrated by his inability to get a hearing. Unable to find work, he appealed to the Court of Chancery who declared it out of their jurisdiction.[55] Dodwell believed the only way to get attention and satisfaction was through an act of civil disobedience. He wrote a letter to a friend explaining that after 'five and a third year's of incessant struggling I have come to the most unwelcome conclusion that I can gain a hearing, not a grand thing for any man in any country, only by breaking the law'.[56] He returned to court in March of 1878 and fired a pistol at the Master of the Rolls.

At the subsequent criminal trial for assault Dodwell insisted on representing himself. Court records confirmed he waited for the Master of the Rolls and fired one shot at him from twelve feet away. The intended victim first introduced a question as to the defendant's sanity, stating he believed the defendant had delusional thoughts and believed in a conspiracy against him. When directly asked if he thought the defendant was sound, the Master of the Rolls stated that 'the prisoner's act was that of an insane person'.[57] The jury found that Dodwell did not intend to kill or seriously injure his victim, and thus he was not guilty of the more serious charge of attempted murder. In the case of common assault, the jury found him not guilty on the ground of insanity.[58]

While the affronted Reverend never published memoirs, his voice did make it into the public domain.[59] Some of his Latin verse was read into evidence during the trial. One poem imagined the scheming thoughts of his intended victim, the Master of the Rolls, and the compliance of the press:

> Oh, Press, enable me to deceive, enable me to appear just and upright, throw the darkness of night over my sins, and a cloud over my frauds; and let not the shouting boys and hoarse girls vend their wares in Fleet Street or the Strand, lest the Queen, as she runs through the evening papers, may read the unjust judgment, and the well-founded

complaints of the oppressed suppliant, and the words of Her Majesty despised; and lest the Lady, who rules over Asia, as an avenger may demand satisfaction both for outraged shame and broken faith. May you suppress with me all rights, divine and human.[60]

Dodwell believed that if only the press and, more specifically, the Queen knew of his plight, they would surely intervene. During his trial he delivered a lengthy closing statement detailing his grievances. He was quite successful in attracting supporters and public interest to his case.

After he was sent to Broadmoor, his specific grievances shifted from his employment failures to his detention as a lunatic.[61] His status as a lunatic inherently negated any justifiable complaint against his former employer; thus fighting for his sanity became his most pressing concern. Dodwell found sympathizers not only among the advocacy community, but also some unlikely allies in the medical community. Drs Forbes Winslow and Winn both went to Broadmoor on the insistence of his friends to interview Rev. Dodwell, and with the sanction of the Home Secretary. After several visits with him at the asylum, the doctors concluded that Dodwell was perfectly sane. His supporters did not deny that the Reverend had an overdeveloped sense of grievance; however, they argued that this was hardly the threshold for madness. Both doctors felt this case set a dangerous precedent.[62] In the words of Forbes Winslow, 'Mr. Dodwell is a gentleman and a scholar, acutely conscious of his wrongs, thoroughly truthful' and should not be found unsound.[63]

The influence of Dodwell's case stretched beyond the popular and medical press to Parliament. After Winn and Forbes Winslow went public with their findings, the Home Secretary sent new medical experts to examine the Reverend at Broadmoor. They found that Dodwell very much belonged there. However, this did little to end the debate; MP Thomas Burt asked that copies of their reports be made available to the House. While this was denied on privacy grounds, the government was firm that not only was Dodwell of unsound mind, but also that releasing him would be dangerous to the public.[64] The next year another MP in the House asked if the Lunacy Commissioners had anything to say about Dodwell in their annual report; they did not.[65]

Despite widespread coverage in the press and the intervention of two prominent doctors on Dodwell's behalf, he remained in

Broadmoor until his death.[66] The superintendent of Broadmoor was convinced that Dodwell likely inherited a tendency to madness and that he had fallen victim to 'morbid introspection'.[67] In some ways his case highlights the struggles of the LLRA. If their goal was to release those unlawfully confined and radically transform the lunacy certification system, theirs was an absolute failure. However, as Nicholas Hervey points out, as an advocacy group they were remarkably successful in keeping these issues constantly in the public eye.[68] Louisa Lowe mentioned Dodwell in her *Bastilles of England* as an example of a man still unlawfully confined in 1883.[69] Public attention rarely waned as a succession of royal commissions, inquiries, and shifting legislation tried to address abuses within the lunacy system, as all the while the state vastly increased the number of people under care. Despite the fact that the government and most experts agreed that cases of wrongful confinement were extraordinarily rare, patient advocacy groups gave individuals a voice and a platform to express their anger and frustration in a system that deemed them mad.

Men's challenge of their diagnosis did not always lead to the result for which they were hoping. In terms of cases of wrongful confinement where people gained their freedom or a retroactive assertion that they had never been mad, such vindications were rare. And different constituencies could take diverse lessons from the same case. Dodwell's case sparked outrage among his supporters; however, in 1880 his case was also used as an example in a legal text as an unambiguous case of a criminal lunatic. The author acknowledged that 'like all real lunatics, he strongly denied that he was insane', but reaffirmed that the public interest was best served by having such an unstable individual confined.[70] Within ten years of his committal, Dodwell committed another act of violence at Broadmoor, just as the government and his medical team insisted he would.[71] To his supporters, of course, such an action simply proved that years of unjust confinement had finally broken the man.

Lunacy Commissioners did periodic checks to investigate the issue of wrongful confinement but consistently found that it was not a problem. However, organizations such as the ALFS and the LLRA were very effective in convincing the general public that there was a problem and they kept pressure on the government to change legislation. Such organizations gave support to individuals fighting for their freedom and gave a sense of community to those who believed they were wrongfully confined. High-profile cases helped undermine doctors' authority and expertise in the ability to conclusively draw a line between sanity and insanity.

Patriarchal authority: Laurence Ruck and indignation against control

In a system that advocated the denial of liberty as the first step in treatment, it should come as no surprise that the issue of wrongful confinement was a perennial topic. As *The Lancet* noted, 'Every now and then, when more absorbing topics fail, the discovery is made that the jealously-prized and arrogantly-boasted liberty of the British citizen may be successfully assailed under cover of the Lunacy Laws.'[72] The case they were referring to here was that of Laurence Ruck, a Welsh country gentleman sent to a private asylum. Mary Ann Ruck was able to send her husband away against his wishes without consulting him or his family. While most agreed that Ruck's behaviour was unacceptable, popular opinion was deeply divided on whether or not she had acted appropriately. Was her husband actually mad, or was his behaviour the result of alcoholic excess? Mrs Ruck's decision was not made in haste, but when undertaken it had fundamental and immediate effects: Ruck's rights as head of household were instantly stripped. A common critique of wrongful confinement is that it subverted patriarchal authority. Ruck was furious with his wife and demanded both his freedom and vengeance on all who had a hand in his confinement.

Ruck's friends noticed troubling signs of instability in 1856. At one social gathering he randomly kicked his friend, ran outside, and performed an unnamed 'indecency'.[73] He locked up his mistress in a room for a day and a half, threatening to shoot her if she left, and charging her with killing their two illegitimate children.[74] His behaviour culminated in a fervent belief that his wife was a prostitute.[75] His wife, terrified at his conduct and concerned for her safety, signed an order along with a doctor and family friend to send her husband as a private patient to Moorcroft House, where he was treated for ten months.

Ruck improved at Moorcroft, but obstinately denied any implication that his behaviour had been anything but an excess of alcohol. Laurence Ruck demanded his day in court and thrust his private struggles into the public sphere rather than try for any private solution. He asked his wife to petition the Court of Chancery to settle the status of his lunacy once and for all. Chancery's role was not to determine whether or not Mr Ruck had ever been mad, but rather to investigate if at the time of the trial he was still unsound and incapable of managing himself and his affairs. After collecting affidavits from ten people over the course of three weeks, Ruck was granted an Inquisition by jury. For five days jurors heard evidence.[76] The trial gained national attention, forming the heart of a trio of unlawful confinement controversies in 1858.[77] Ruck's trial was subject to enormous press coverage, highlighting competing ideas of the limits of self-control.

No one challenged the narrative of Laurence Ruck's actions, nor did anyone try to defend them. What was up for debate was the cause of these actions: was it madness or was it drink?[78] Mrs Ruck and her supporters believed it was more than alcohol, and in particular focused on his delusion that his wife was a prostitute. To be cuckolded by one's wife could be justification for the deprivation of her property, her children, and her reputation in the 1850s. And yet to besmirch a woman's reputation without cause was the sign of a cad, and perhaps even a madman, and later in the century would carry serious repercussions.[79] Thus a key element in the trial centred on the conduct of Mary Ann Ruck. Mary Ann Ruck testified to a happy marriage with six children that had only recently broken down. Her husband would drive around the country or take long purposeless walks at night. He began to be suspicious of his wife's actions, charging her with flirting with men in carriages, and, finally, in her words he accused her of 'general prostitution'.[80] Lawyers on both sides agreed that the charges against Mrs Ruck were absolutely untrue, and the trial established Mary Ann Ruck's sterling reputation.[81]

From the point of view of the medical witnesses for the prosecution, Ruck was still deluded on the specific topic of his wife's fidelity, and until that delusion was truly gone, he was not sane. The famed Dr John Conolly centred his decision that the man was still mad on the fact he remained angry with his wife and showed no remorse for his suspicions.[82] Conolly understood that it would be hard for the jury to see madness in a man who seemed so calm and rational in the courtroom:

> Mr. Ruck is a man one cannot see without liking, and I am sorry to have to express my opinion of his malady in his presence. I should think it the most cruel thing in the world to have him taken out of the asylum, because he entertains insane delusions of the most extravagant kind, and I have not the smallest shadow of a doubt that those delusions might lead him to very dangerous lengths.[83]

Had he simply been an inebriate, his anger towards his wife would have quickly dissipated; had he been mad and recovered, he would have acknowledged his suspicions were delusions. Dr Forbes Winslow testified that while Ruck had largely recovered, he might still harbour some delusions, and warned that cases such as his were prone to relapse.[84]

Mr Ruck's conduct in court helped his defence as it was so greatly at odds with descriptions of his past actions. His deportment in the courtroom was generally praised, contrasting the 'modest, rational, and unassuming' man with the shocking evidence of Ruck's previous actions.[85] His answers on the stand only confirmed the impression of a man in control of his emotions. Speaking in his own defence, Ruck acknowledged that his behaviour had been appalling, but that it was not madness but an excessive amount of alcohol that was the root cause.[86] He admitted that he became convinced of his wife's infidelity when he was 'in an agitated state of mind from drink'. He insisted if he had only been allowed to investigate his suspicions, that he would have been satisfied with the results and it would have calmed his mind.[87] As head of his household, he thought any and every suspicion he might have had, even if inspired by drink, was worthy of inquiry. The more he was challenged in this belief, the angrier and more frustrated he became. Doctors brought in to defend his sanity agreed his was a case of drunken mania and any delusions were strictly caused by alcohol and by his misdiagnosis and treatment in an institution. They all agreed that the proper course of treatment should have been a hospital, not an asylum.[88]

A senior surgeon at St Bartholomew's and Bethlehem, a witness for the defence, found the man sane. And yet even he could not assert it was absolutely safe to discharge him, and worried he would return to his previous drinking habits.

Had some difficulty in saying whether he ought to be altogether discharged – a difficulty arising out of the present state of the law, which only recognized sane men and insane, whereas there are infinite gradations between the two.[89]

However, there was no place in the English justice system for such murky definitions. In the criminal courts a defendant either possessed *mens rea* or they did not; in the Court of Chancery, a defendant was either of sound mind or not. There was no room for partial insanity.

One member of the jury understood that the sticking point revolved around Ruck's attitude to his wife; he asked Ruck on the stand if he could guarantee he no longer harboured suspicions against his wife. While Ruck answered in the affirmative, he related a very different version of his marriage from any other witnesses. He testified that he had always been unhappy with his wife as she had refused intercourse with him.[90] From the certifying doctors' point of view, this simply confirmed that Ruck still harboured continuing delusions about his wife as all other witnesses confirmed it had been a happy marriage. However, the jury found in Ruck's favour, he was declared sound at the time of the trial, and the spectators cheered.[91]

The timing of the trial in 1858, at the height of a lunacy panic, influenced how many interpreted the verdict. One reporter for the *Saturday Review* concluded the jury's decision in Mr Ruck's favour was not about whether or not the man was ever mad. Instead, it was an opportunity to put private lunatic asylums as an institution on trial. 'There is a war against these institutions – they are capable of abuse, and they are abused.'[92] And Ruck's next steps seemed to confirm that impression. He was not content simply to have his rights over himself and his property reaffirmed; he wanted his diagnosis of madness completely overturned, and those responsible punished.

He launched a suit against the proprietor of the asylum where he was sent and the doctor who certified him. His family supported him, believing the family's reputation had been sullied through his confinement. In particular, one point of the trial focused on the actual medical certificate signed by Mrs Ruck. Under causes for disease, it listed intemperance (which no one disputed) and also hereditary causes. Mrs Ruck admitted the family doctor and co-signer of the order filled it out, and she simply signed without looking.[93] The Ruck family did not agree that they had a hereditary taint of madness.

Competing issues of reputation and privacy were key to this case. As one former Lunacy Commissioner stated, the problem was that Mrs Ruck, in seeking to spare the publicity of her husband's illness, usurped her husband's authority and that of his family:

> A gentleman of irregular habits, and addicted to indulgence in wine, being alone in the country, occupied himself largely in drinking. By degrees his mind became obscured with insane ideas of the infidelity of his wife; and when she found every word, and even action, became polluted by this morbid idea, she placed him in a lunatic asylum of the best kind without conferring with his sisters, his brother, or his mother.[94]

Ruck believed this second trial was the only way he could restore his family honour. In this case, his efforts paid off and he was found to have never been properly certified and he was granted £500 in damages.[95]

The Lancet in 1858 acknowledged that the grievance that best exemplified the era was that of the supposed lunatic, unjustly detained. While the author acknowledged that most asylums were run properly, 'there is nothing which can offer an assurance to us, or to anyone, that the most flagrant injustice is not commonly perpetrated in the incarceration of persons, accused of insanity by interested relatives, upon certificates too easily granted'.[96] While most doctors involved in treating lunatics vigorously challenged the validity of such claims, the fear of unlawful confinement persisted throughout the century.[97] To many this was an abstract anxiety, no greater or lesser than other social issues of the day. However, for those directly involved, their outrage knew no bounds. Whether it was denying events that supposedly took place, or explaining that delusions were anything but, many men took to the courts, to the media, and to advocacy groups to rail against the system.

Challenging the doctors: Charles Merivale and rewriting case history

Outraged men often sought to publicize their experiences due to a personal desire for justice without thought to potential publicity. Other men explicitly sought a public hearing of their grievances out of a more calculated desire to protect or restore their reputations. Patients and doctors alike were well aware of the stigma of insanity, and that certification 'disqualif[ied] the sufferer for social life and, at least temporarily, degrad[ed] him from the ranks of humanity'.[98] While some men likely sought privacy and secrecy as the best way to protect their reputation, others needed to counter stories already circulating in the press or in gossip circles. The most straightforward way to restore one's reputation was to claim misdiagnosis. Symptoms that might have seemed to indicate madness were simply something else. Delusions caused by fever were not classified as madness and could be treated in the home without any need for certification.[99] Madness fuelled by alcohol could be dismissed as a temporary condition, not meeting the threshold of true insanity. Most doctors (both legitimate and less so) agreed that hysteria, nerve prostration, neurasthenia, and general nervous disorders were separate ailments from true insanity.[100] As doctors were often loath to fix a hard line dividing madness from other nervous disorders, patients could easily gain sympathy by claiming such a misdiagnosis.

Victorian men of science of various types were bound to defining and upholding acceptable 'canons of behaviour'.[101] Perhaps there was no type of doctor more invested in the project than those defining lunacy, and no patient more apt to challenge those definitions than the supposed lunatic. The case of Herman Charles Merivale, a famed dramatist and author, provides unique insight into the differing perspectives of doctors and patients outside the charged atmosphere of a Chancery or criminal court. Official asylum records present a very clear picture of a mentally troubled man. Doctors were clear in their diagnoses and believed Merivale could only be aided by asylum care. Merivale challenged his doctors in the asylum, and later took control of his narrative as he rewrote his history of institutionalization in a memoir. He blamed doctors of various types for exacerbating his illness instead of curing him. Turning the tables on the doctors, he questioned their professional reputations and their knowledge. Such public criticisms placed doctors' own gentlemanly status in question, marking a pattern seen across the sciences where professionals often had to defend their status as professional gentlemen.[102]

Merivale was first institutionalized in Manor House Asylum at the age of twenty-nine for twelve months. Two years later witnesses claimed he attempted suicide. He was then admitted to the even more exclusive Ticehurst Asylum. His appearance at admission was described as 'wild', he was suffering delusions, and had attempted to drown himself in deep water.[103] He was often confused, and in his early months doctors believed he suffered epileptiform seizures. A long-time friend visited him after a few months of care and still found he suffered the delusion he was under the influence of an 'evil one'. [104] He improved and was discharged as relieved after seven months.[105] Doctors were well aware that Merivale was not happy with either his diagnosis or treatment as he sent them a detailed letter a month after his release that was transcribed into the casebook. It was copied without comment, although someone had highlighted the section where Merivale admits to being 'tempted to commit the foolish act at Southampton'. For the medical staff at Ticehurst, his admission of a suicide attempt was the only relevant fact at hand, and proved his incarceration was justified.[106]

Merivale's letter shows a clear displeasure with his incarceration and treatment at Ticehurst. After suffering what he believed was simply 'a long nervous disorder' that reached a climax of 'hypochondriacal despondency' he was sent to an asylum against his will. He stated it was not a true suicide attempt, but rather an act of childish bravado when he jumped into the water. Among a number of complaints he had about his care, Merivale singled out Dr Newington's careless indifference as particularly cruel. He felt belittled and ignored, put under care of an attendant he already distrusted.[107] A few years later Merivale published a memoir about his experiences of asylum care where he more fully explained his frustrations. While admitting he had struggled from some form of mental exhaustion, he would not admit to madness and insisted there had been no need to deprive him of his liberty in an asylum.[108] He again pointed to 'religious hypochondria' which he believed was more like nervousness than madness.[109] The term 'hypochondria' was used widely in the later nineteenth century as a broad category to cover many physiological and emotional disorders.[110] Merivale concluded that he suffered only from a failure of the spirit, and not true madness. 'I deny distinctly, deliberately, categorically, that I have ever been insane; and I say that the fancies of delirium or hypochondria are as clearly to be distinguished from those of madness as midday from midnight.'[111]

Merivale re-diagnosed himself with something he felt more suitable and palatable to his sensibilities.

Charges of wrongful confinement were grounded in competing authorities. Men were not fighting abstract concepts or diagnoses, but the capacity of the doctors who signed their certificates and the government that created the laws. And while men under asylum care felt they needed to restore their personal reputations, the burgeoning psychiatric community was just as keen to assert their own professional standing. Doctors' expertise was challenged in the courts, by governments, and within families. Merivale named lunacy doctors as the lowest form of medicine; he believed 'the lunacy trade (with marked and fine exceptions, of course) [was open] to the doctor who is no good for any other "specialty", and knows he is not'.[112] To Merivale, Dr Henry Maudsley was clearly one of the exceptions. At some point he must have sought out Maudsley for a second opinion, as Merivale wrote that he redefined his hysterical seizures not as epilepsy but as a form of hysterical weakness.[113]

Merivale attempted to place his illness in a different category from insanity, and to claim the separation between madness and sanity was the difference between night and day. However, few experts in lunacy agreed. The definition of madness was not accessible to all, but rather a variegated spectrum that required specialized knowledge to discern.[114] Lunacy doctors' expertise was rooted in the fact it required specialized knowledge to diagnose. And while Merivale dismissed the seriousness of his symptoms, to the psychiatric and legal community delusions of any sort were the surest sign of madness, and a suicide attempt incontrovertible proof.[115] Merivale might have appeared lucid to some (and to himself), but his doctors clearly saw a dangerous madness.

Merivale published his memoir less than five years after his time in asylums following a marriage and a return to writing. Merivale clearly understood differences between acceptable and unacceptable versions of mental distress. Neurasthenia, neurosis, 'religious hypochondria', or an extreme physical weakness that clouded his brain were acceptable diagnoses to him. However, his diagnosis of insanity and placement in an asylum were gossiped about by his friends and acquaintances, and Merivale believed it had damaged his professional reputation.[116] Merivale transformed his diagnosis from one that implied he was a helpless wastrel to a form of overwork consistent with a man of genius. Merivale understood how the curse of inheritable madness lingered.[117]

According to Merivale's narrative, his wrongful certification was a philistine reaction to the artistic, the cultured, or the genius. This would have resonated with a late nineteenth-century audience who accepted the link between madness and genius. The hangover of phrenology, Lamarkian ideas of heredity, and cerebral localization theory combined to create the idea that genius could lead to madness.[118] One author writing in the 1870s noted that men of creative gifts were often lumped in with madmen simply because they were misunderstood. 'Frequently we see a man of brilliant gifts, of dazzling wit, infinite culture, and fascinating manners, which are able to promulgate even a new faith, but he is considered mad because he sees too far, penetrates too deep, and tells us too much truth, which we dislike.'[119] By its very nature genius lived on the boundaries of madness. By claiming this definition Merivale not only challenged his diagnosis, but he also reaffirmed his genius.

Men like Merivale challenged not only their diagnosis, but also the very foundations of the system of certification. They refused to accept the expertise of lunacy doctors, and instead asserted their own ability to know and understand their bodies and minds. This tension is an example of a competition among different kinds of privileged white men for an authoritative masculinity.[120] Rising expectations of the professional ideal made both doctors and middle-class patients ever more likely to be defensive of their reputations.[121] Merivale was aware that a diagnosis of insanity undermined his professional standing as an author. His insistence of a diagnosis of 'religious hypochondria', and his right to choose his illness and a doctor who would back him up, challenged the creditability of lunacy specialists. Doctors defended their diagnoses against critique to preserve their own authority.

Freedom: William Windham's quest to do as he pleased

Sometimes what a man accused of lunacy fought for was simply the ability to be left alone to pursue his own desires. The most famous, lengthy, and costly Chancery lunacy trial centred on a young man that no one argued should be put in an asylum, nor even certified as mad.[122] While doctors might have charged the courts with being too inflexible in their binary view of madness and sanity, Windham's situation proved a test case for the idea of a more limited intervention for a slightly mad individual. Even before the trial began it was the focus of national attention.[123] The press quickly recognized this trial might set a new standard for the boundaries of madness, and that extremes of folly and eccentricity might now come under the purview of the Commissioners of Lunacy.[124] It also became a media sensation, and thus a wonderful opportunity to see how ideas of madness were aired in public discourse.[125] The Windham trial centred on a struggle between opposing visions of a gentleman's duty in society. Windham's family was concerned about the family's reputation and his obligation to future generations. Windham believed that in order to be a man, he needed to assert his personal autonomy above any obligations to his class or his status.

William Windham was from an old Norfolk family. He came of age, married a courtesan, and began running through the family fortune. His behaviour, even by the standards of the day, went beyond merely eccentric, rakish, or unconventional. Over the holiday season of 1861–1862, a jury of twenty-four men and Masters in Lunacy oversaw an Inquiry at the Court of Exchequer in Westminster before bursting crowds to decide whether that behaviour reached the threshold of madness. No less than fifteen of William Windham's relations petitioned the court to have the young man declared incapable of looking after his affairs.[126] The trial ended after thirty-four days on 28 January, at a cost £20,000.

Windham's agency in his fight for independence was one of the central issues the court was asked to tackle. The prosecution claimed that Windham was not acting on his own will, but in fact was being manipulated by his wife and her paramour into conflict with his family.[127] His family did not think he was quite insane to the point he needed to be institutionalized, but they did think he was not responsible to make major life decisions. In essence, they asked the courts for an extended minority status whereby William Windham would be a permanent legal dependant, his marriage would be annulled, and his family would take control of his estates.[128] Whether coerced or compelled, Windham clearly expressed a desire to fight against any restrictions on his behaviour. He was active in his defence, attending the trial regularly and seeking out a strong legal and medical team to support his claims. While this was not a case of wrongful incarceration, and there was no threat of an asylum, his defence counsel characterized his family's proposed restrictions on Windham as an 'icy corpse-like grasp of legal incapacity and legal restraint'.[129] Windham was not fighting for his freedom from incarceration, but his freedom to exercise his manly prerogative to establish his own family.

Windham's marriage to a well-known courtesan is what spurred his uncle, General Windham, to start proceedings in Chancery. Windham was hardly the first aristocrat to marry a courtesan, and no one argued that this in and of itself was proof of madness. However, Agnes Willoughby seemed to have had no affection for her husband before or after the marriage.[130] In a separate proceeding, one of Windham's lawyers was actually condemned for drawing up a wedding contract between the two knowing full well Windham was not yet of age and that the match was clearly unsuitable. While there was no charge proven against the lawyer, the judge was scathing in his judgment, stating the lawyer acted recklessly as he

> knew all throughout that Mrs. Windham never displays the slightest affection for her intended husband, yet he is content to see this infatuated young man about to marry a woman of worthless character, who feels an absolute repugnancy for him, without taking any step to protect him.[131]

But it was for a jury to decide if the young man needed such formal protection.

It was not the fact of Mrs Windham's past that most troubled the doctors, but rather the fact that she continued to seemingly have relationships with other men, and that Windham was aware of the fact. This included, perhaps, on the eve of her wedding to Windham. Windham was living with his wife's paramour (or pimp), a Mr Roberts, at the time of the trial, which greatly disturbed the medical witnesses for the prosecution. Forbes Winslow was shocked by Windham's nonchalance:

> When he told me that Roberts was a good fellow he giggled and laughed, and when he referred to the *sobriquet* under which Roberts was generally known [Bawdy House Roberts] he laughed loudly, as if he thought it a good joke. There was a peculiarity about his expression and his laugh. I attach no importance, however, to his mode of

laughing, though I thought it rather strange his laughing at all upon the subject.[132]

Windham found the idea that his wife was cuckolding him with his supposed friend unimportant at best, and funny at worst. Forbes Winslow found such a lack of moral outrage deeply disturbing.

Windham's case touched on one of the main bugbears of Victorian lunacy: moral insanity. This was a category of insanity first formulated by James Cowles Prichard in the 1830s to explain the moral degeneracy of his age. It was not accepted by the legal profession and was a contested idea even within the medical community.[133] David Skae's outlining of moral insanity came down to an inability to master self-control. Born with an inherent weakness, such boys grew to be 'credulous and silly' men.[134] The year of Windham's trial, John Charles Bucknill's classic *Manual of Psychological Medicine* gave cautious support to the idea of moral insanity, but would not commit to pointing out when moral failing turned into moral insanity, deferring that he was 'neither the legislator nor the administrator of the law'.[135] The concept was popular with social purity campaigners and those trying to understand the connections between morality and rationality.[136]

In his writings, Forbes Winslow was a staunch defender of the idea, and outlined the concept of people who had mental capacity but were 'moral idiots'.[137] These people did not suffer delusions or hallucinations but were subject to their impulses. Called as a witness in the Windham trial, he described the young man's diagnosis as 'a paralysis of the moral sense'.[138] While Windham's case would seem ripe fodder for the proponents of moral insanity, the term had a toxic reputation in the courtroom.[139] Dr Mayo, a witness for the prosecution, was keen to distance himself from the idea of moral insanity in Windham's trial, even though in essence it was what his relations believed was at fault. Mayo pointed out that in cases of gradual mental decline, it was often moral imbecility that came before the dissolution of rational decision-making.[140]

Lawyers for the family tried to establish that from an early age Windham had been unlike other children, and that his failures had only intensified with age. They claimed he had always been mentally weak, so much so that his father consulted a specialist when the boy was only six.[141] His uncle, the Marquis of Bristol, testified that around the age of seven young Windham came to visit with his mother and she carried a little whip to keep him in control at luncheon.[142] Another uncle testified that the boy, when told he could not have any tart, seized a carving knife and threatened his mother with it.[143] Many witnesses acknowledged the young man had some sort of cleft palate, although his uncle was adamant it did not explain or justify the man's strange, 'foolish' expression when he laughed.[144] A surgeon long familiar with the family and involved with lunacy for over twenty years testified not only to the lack of discipline in the Windham household, but also to a potential predisposition to madness as his father was 'hot-tempered' and his mother 'excitable'.[145] The petitioners sought to portray a young man with a hereditary taint of insanity whose mental degeneration only accelerated as he grew up.

While the young man was twenty-one at the time of the trial, witnesses focused on the fact that he acted in many ways like a child, in particular through his extremes of passion and his inability to control his emotions.[146] Witnesses testified that not only was Windham often reduced to tears, but also that when he cried he did so like a baby. He was generally accepted as being uncouth, and his gluttony and slavering at the mouth while eating obviously disgusted many observers.[147] There was evidence he was consistently disruptive in his public behaviour. His love of trains bordered on the obsessive, and his habit of acting as a railway guard on multiple occasions was seen as potentially dangerous.[148] The accusation that he had actually once driven the engine was presented as reckless and irresponsible.[149] His general behaviour in society was beyond the pale; he screeched and danced around at formal events, and his approach to ladies was so odd it frightened them. Such behaviour might have made Windham an unpopular dinner guest, but the jury was asked to decide if such behaviour meant he was unable to manage his affairs.

Some of the most damning evidence came from the Llewellyns, Windham's landlords since he came of age. Mrs Llewellyn testified that the young man was subject to rages, that he swore, that he yelled out of the windows, that he only washed when told and was 'insensible to the calls of nature'.[150] Her husband confirmed her testimony and added that Windham was reckless with money and constantly told lies.[151] Their portrait of a completely unhinged young man, however, did not stand up under cross-examination. The defence characterized the landlords themselves as disreputable characters, and implied the pair had been bribed for their testimony and acted as spies to Windham's uncle (charges they vehemently denied).[152]

The Llewellyns' evidence was the most extreme example of what the petitioners believed was Windham's inability to understand his position as a gentleman. In his family's estimation, his boorish behaviour was not a choice, but rather a compulsion. He was most comfortable in the presence of servants and working-class people and had been known to help with their tasks and socialize with them. When a young man, his father even had a suit of livery made up for him.[153] For many Victorians, this cross-class behaviour was certainly strange; the doctors framed it as pathological. Boyhood eccentricity became a fixed preference as he grew to manhood. The petitioners connected the idea that a man who failed his social and gendered obligations so thoroughly was not completely in control of himself.

Some journalists were convinced that Windham was a man who needed to be controlled. As the *Gloucester Journal* noted:

> The facts already given in evidence tend to prove the mental incapacity of the unfortunate young man, who was unable to acquire knowledge, had an extraordinary fondness for low company, much affected washing dishes, and stoking &c., on railways, was excessively dirty, violent, and impulsive, and had contracted habits of the worst character.[154]

Press outlets sympathetic to General Windham and the family in general accepted the narrative that a simple-minded young man had been caught in the grip of unsavoury characters who were trying to drain his personal fortune.

However, this was largely the minority opinion. Most of the press coverage was in fact far more sympathetic to young Windham. Instead of a tale of a simpleton being manipulated by an unscrupulous wife, such accounts held that General Windham was simply worried his spendthrift nephew would squander the family inheritance. Windham's supporters did not defend his behaviour but they did feel it did not meet the threshold of necessitating a permanent custodianship. The *Cheltenham Chronicle* dismissed all of Windham's unsavoury behaviour as simply 'a variety of harum-scarum boyish pranks'.[155] According to this narrative, all the prosecution had proven was that Windham was not an ideal man. Moreover, the worst incidents of a man's life did not necessarily equal madness. And what the prosecution represented as moral insanity, many other witnesses dismissed as simply youthful enthusiasm or bad judgement. The defence provided a wealth of witnesses from fellow militiamen to fishmongers to railway men to testify to the soundness of Windham's mind, if not the soundness of his character.[156] His marriage had been regrettable and, as his lawyers summarized, it was 'improper and distasteful to society' but not proof of madness.[157]

The defence was able to capitalize on the unpopularity of the concept of moral insanity in the English courtroom.[158] Dr Seymour explicitly stated that moral insanity did not exist. 'If a young nobleman were to choose to act as a sweep, and carry a soot-bag in the streets, I should not therefore consider him of unsound mind.'[159] Defence witnesses were just as willing to testify and explain behaviour that seemed inexcusable in the eyes of the prosecution. His slow learning as a child was due to high spirits, and his poor behaviour when being led around Britain and Europe by a series of tutors and companions was simply a young man straining under the yoke of being confined like a child.[160]

The public (at least in the courtroom) seemed to agree that to restrict a man who was simply on the road to ruin was 'cruel, most unjust, and most unjustifiable'.[161] Windham was declared sound, and able to manage himself and his affairs. The jury decided he was a disreputable man, but he was a man capable of making his own decisions.[162] The court agreed with the defence counsel and medical men who 'found in deliberate vice, debauchery, and excess of every kind, adequate explanation for Mr. Windham's shameless indifference to personal honour, and utter disregard for the esteem and respect of his fellow creatures'.[163] *The Times* assured that the decision was just, and were also confident that Windham would likely pursue 'a career of folly, prodigality, and vice, will decline through a stage of brutal dissipation and unpitied beggary, and will die neglected and forgotten'.[164]

The crippling costs of the Inquisition might have ruined Windham even if he had been a shrewd and cautious man.[165] He was neither of these things, and what his relatives had worried of soon came to pass; his life rapidly unravelled and he was soon virtually bankrupt. He was reduced to living off a weekly allowance of one pound from his uncle, General Windham. He died in February 1866 at the age of twenty-five.[166] William Windham's name came to be a shorthand term for scandal, debauchery, and disgrace.[167] But in the end, he had won his right to that reputation.

William Windham was happy to sacrifice a great deal for the sake of his unfettered freedom. He either did not care what the general public thought of him, or thought it was more important they thought him sane than thought him good. Counsel representing the interests of Windham's mother, Lady Sophia, best encapsulated what was most at stake for Windham in the trial. In directing the jurors in their duty,

> He hoped they would pause long before they fixed upon Mr. Windham the stain of insanity – before they took from him on the very threshold of manhood that which made manhood a thing to be prized – the sense of personal freedom and personal independence.[168]

Windham was fighting for the ability to live his life unfettered by the tenets of respectable society as represented by his uncle and the rest of the family. Windham's public supporters did not think he was a good man, but that as a man he had a right to his autonomy and personal choice as inherent to his identity.

Getting back to work: George Gilbert Scott and competing reputations

Many lunacy disputes centred on competing notions of reputation, and what was in the best interest of a person versus that of the family at large. George Gilbert Scott prioritized his public professional reputation over his family's desire to maintain family honour and morality. In choosing to protect his paid, productive work as an architect, Scott was adhering to Victorian respect for a professional work ethic and identity that was becoming omnipresent in the period. In doing so, however, he was willing to sacrifice the other pillar of manhood: the home.[169] Scott believed proof of his ability to continue working while destroying his family through erratic and uncharacteristic behaviour was enough to establish his sanity. The Chancery Court had to decide if this rejection of the balance of work and home was the action of a heartless rake or a maniac.

Scott was a prominent, well-respected architect who married in 1872 and seemed to get along with his family. According to his wife's testimony, they lived happily for almost ten years until he had a period of very strange behaviour lasting almost six months. She attributed the cause to overwork and mental strain in his effort to complete a book he was writing.[170] He seemed to recover and no additional action was taken by either his wife or the wider family. However, this was only a brief return to normalcy before a much more dramatic change in his habits and attitude less than a year later. On a visit to his brother's house in Wimbledon in the autumn of 1883, he seemed to have a breakdown, once brandishing a knife. He wandered about the fields for several nights consumed with thoughts of conspiracy and villainy. The family immediately consulted a doctor, and later convinced Scott to travel to meet with another. Both doctors signed the requisite certificates, and he was placed in Bethlehem hospital.[171] This decision was in keeping with much medical orthodoxy at the time that prioritized quick treatment as the only hope of recovery. However, to his defence counsel it was cruel treatment at the hands of supposed friends. 'They had made haste to shut him up in a madhouse instead of waiting to see what might be done by private restraint and influence.'[172] His fame drew more than usual media attention to the case when it reached Chancery.[173]

The case for the prosecution emphasized Scott's good character in trying to emphasize the insanity of his later acts. Mr Webster, a witness for the family, described Scott before recent events as 'a highly intellectual man and a perfect gentleman'.[174] According to this interpretation, it was only his madness that excused his actions and protected Scott's character. In closing arguments, the prosecution stated: 'If he were not mad no language could be too strong wherewith to describe the grossness of his conduct.'[175] To his family, his sudden change of character could only be explained by an attack of madness, echoing his previous, milder breakdown. What else could explain the complete change in the character of a man from upstanding architect and family man to a suspicious louche? Would a sane gentleman bring his French mistress into his home and introduce her to his children? His family were united and acted quickly to protect their brother's, and their own, reputation.

Given the choice between being labelled a cad and being labelled a madman, however, Scott chose the former. The case for the respondent told a very different tale, one that in many ways presented Scott in a much more unflattering light. His defence claimed this was no sudden attack of madness, but in fact a slow descent into heavy drinking. According to Scott, excessive drinking had actually caused all of his subsequent 'mad' acts. A doctor's testimony for the respondent recalled his meeting with Scott, who admitted that in 1880 he had begun drinking brandy for the first time in aid of his writing. In stating that he believed Scott was capable of managing himself and his affairs, the doctor did so while acknowledging the man was now leading an 'irregular' life.[176]

Scott's history leading up to the Chancery trial demonstrated his resistance to having his professional reputation sacrificed for the sake of his personal reputation. He was not content to sit in Bethlehem but rather escaped and travelled to Rouen. He drifted back to England after his certificates expired, and in the autumn he was arrested and charged with threatening a servant. Instead of facing criminal trial, he was removed to a private lunatic asylum near Maidstone. He escaped again in December 1883.[177] He remained free, though under family surveillance, until the Chancery lunacy case in April 1884. Throughout his ordeals, he remained in contact with his major architectural client, the Duke of Norfolk, about the building of a new church. In fact, his letters to the Duke were submitted to the court to demonstrate the man's 'shrewdness and common sense'.[178] Scott's defence was that his business acumen, and his ability to continue working, were the best proof of his sanity.

In his summation, Justice Denman was quite explicit about the problems of the case and disagreed with Scott's defence on principle. He explained to the jury that the definition of being capable of managing himself and his affairs could not simply be proven by the fact that a man kept his business going. He explained that a man's affairs included his life beyond simply his career and included managing his wife, his children, and his home. Denman also recognized that simply because a man was fond of drink, and ignored its harmful effects, this did not necessarily make him mad. However, in a case where a man suddenly transformed, it did not exclude it. 'If a man, through drink, or through excessive erotic passion, or through overwork, or anything else, becomes of unsound mind – it does not matter how he became so – it is none the less unsoundness of mind.'[179] Scott's behaviour had radically altered whether under the active influence of alcohol or not.

Scott was not present when the jury decided on his case, claiming to be too ill with a cold to be there for a final interview.[180] He seemed to take a rather light-hearted or at least fatalistic approach to the case, sending a series of sarcastic poems about the legal system to a friend during the trial. Whether fearing the outcome of the trial, or simply preferring the company of his French mistress in Rouen, he was out of the country when the jury unanimously found him to be of unsound mind. Scott wrote from Rouen to a friend and remarked that his position was 'droll ... I am thus insane in the Kingdom of England and sane in the Republic of France. What a difference the Channel makes.'[181] When he returned to England in 1885 he found he was still considered mad in England and was confined in St Andrew's hospital for a short time. He was back in hospital in 1888, and finally from 1891–1892 before his death in 1897.[182] Scott failed to secure vindication of either his professional or personal reputation.

While a diagnosis of madness certainly conveyed a certain stigma, Scott's was not the only example where the disgrace of madness might have been preferable to the alternative.[183] Men like Scott adhered to the belief that a professional reputation was the only one that mattered; and proof of the ability to continue to work was the best evidence against madness. To his friends, family, and the judge at his trial, Scott's sudden changes of behaviour in his private life proved he was not in control of his mind no matter what architectural work he could complete. His distraught wife saw an asylum as the only hope for her husband, and the only way to rehabilitate his reputation.

Conclusion

Men fighting against wrongful incarceration, a Chancery decision, or even the imputation of madness realized they had much at stake. While men critiqued the medical and legal system in ways similar to their female counterparts, their stories recognized they had much more to lose. Primarily this was because, as the privileged sex, men simply had more power and position to lose in the first place. But in addition, wrongful certification and incarceration proved a threat to their gendered identity in ways it did not for women. To be declared an irrational subject was to be unmanned. Thus, when men fought to express their outrage, to restore their reputations, or to regain their independence, they were also fighting to restore elements of their manhood.

Notes

1. 'The Lunacy Inquiry', *Daily News* (16 February 1891), p. 7.
2. C. MacKenzie, 'Social Factors in the Admission, Discharge, and Continuing Stay of Patients at Ticehurst Asylum, 1845–1917', in W.F. Bynum, R. Porter, and M. Shepherd (eds), *The Anatomy of Madness*, vol. 2, p. 147.
3. Fennell, *Treatment Without Consent*, pp. 4, 9.
4. H. Fabrega Jr, 'The Culture and History of Psychiatric Stigma in Early Modern and Modern Western Societies: A Review of Recent Literature', *Comprehensive Psychiatry* 32:2 (1991), p. 111.
5. 'Parliamentary Intelligence', *The Times* (12 March 1862), p. 5.
6. Bynum and Neve described the pitfalls of this approach in an early article. W.F. Bynum and M. Neve, 'Hamlet on the Couch: Hamlet Is a Kind of Touchstone by Which to Measure Changing Opinion – Psychiatric and Otherwise – about Madness', *American Scientist* 74:4 (1986), pp. 390–96.
7. As Alan Beveridge ably demonstrates, one can neither discount the narratives of asylum patients as meaningless nor accept them fully as the voice of the unfairly persecuted. Such accounts could be telling a person's truth and still demonstrate mental illness. A. Beveridge, '*Britain's Siberia*: Mary Coutts's Account of the Asylum System', *Journal of the Royal College of the Physicians of Edinburgh* 35:2 (2005), p. 180.
8. R. Porter, 'The Patient's View: Doing Medical History from Below', *Theory and Society* 14:2 (1985), p. 193.
9. R. Huertas, 'Another History for Another Psychiatry: The Patient's View', *Culture & History Digital Journal* 2:1 (2013), pp. 3–4.
10. Bartlett, *The Poor Law of Lunacy*, pp. 158–61. However, case studies of more robust patient histories indicate that poor patients did protest to asylum authorities and their families about their incarceration. For example: Beveridge, 'Voices of the Mad', pp. 902–4; Smith, '"Your Very Thankful Inmate"', pp. 243–44.

11 Wise, *Inconvenient People*, p. xvii.
12 Such groups built on critiques of wrongful confinement stretching back to the eighteenth century. N. Hervey, 'Advocacy or Folly: The Alleged Lunatics' Friend Society, 1845–1863', *Medical History* 30:3 (1986), p. 246.
13 A. Scull, *Madness in Civilization: A Cultural History of Insanity, from the Bible to Freud, from the Madhouse to Modern Medicine* (Princeton, 2015), pp. 239–40; D. Trotter, 'A Media Theory Approach to Representations of "Nervous Illness" in the Long Nineteenth Century', *Journal of Victorian Culture* 24:2 (2019), pp. 146–58.
14 J.T. Perceval, *A Narrative of the Treatment Experienced by a Gentleman, during a State of Mental Derangement; Designed to Explain the Causes and the Nature of Insanity, Etc.* (London, 1838).
15 Wise, *Inconvenient People*, p. 92.
16 He is referred to both as 'Child' and 'Childe' in various publications. 'Commission of Lunacy on Captain Child: Extraordinary Case', *Daily News* (18 July 1854), p. 9.
17 'Commission in Lunacy on Captain Childe', *Morning Chronicle* (22 July 1854), p. 3.
18 'Commission of Lunacy on Capt. Child', *Daily News* (19 July 1854), p. 7.
19 'Commission in Lunacy on Captain Childe, Late of the 12th Lancers', *Reynolds's Newspaper* (23 July 1854), p. 4.
20 'Commission of Lunacy on Captain Child', *Daily News* (18 July 1854), p. 9.
21 'The Commission of Lunacy on Captain Childe', *Daily News* (21 July 1854), p. 7.
22 'Commission in Lunacy on Captain Childe, Late of the 12th Lancers', *Reynolds's Newspaper* (23 July 1854), p. 13.
23 'Commission of Lunacy', *The Examiner* (22 July 1854), p. 464.
24 'Commission of Lunacy on Captain Childe', *Sunday Times* (23 July 1854), p. 8.
25 'Extraordinary Delusions', *Berkshire Chronicle* (22 July 1854), p. 6.
26 'Commission in Lunacy on Captain Childe, Late of the 12th Lancers', *Morning Post* (22 July 1854), p. 4.
27 'Commission of Lunacy', *The Examiner* (22 July 1854), p. 464.
28 Scull, 'The Social History of Psychiatry in the Victorian Era', in *Madhouses, Mad-Doctors, and Madmen*, p. 25.
29 'At the Court of Queen's Bench', *Illustrated London News* (16 July 1859), p. 69.
30 C. Reade, 'Our Dark Places. No. IV', in *Readiana* (New York, 1887), p. 67.

31 'At the Court of Queen's Bench', *Illustrated London News* (16 July 1859), p. 69.
32 C. Reade, *Hard Cash* (Leipzig, 1864), pp. 477–80.
33 Reade, *Hard Cash*, p. 595.
34 Pedlar, *'The Most Dreadful Visitation'*, pp. 87–90.
35 Reade, *Hard Cash*, pp. v–vi.
36 C. Reade, *'The Complete Writings of Charles Reade*, vol. 7 (London, 1895).
37 'Madness in Novels', *The Spectator* (3 February 1866), pp. 134–35.
38 J.S. Bushnan, letter to the editor, *Daily News*, 23 October 1863, p. 6; 'The Author of "Very Hard Cash"' [C. Reade], letter to the editor, 28 October 1863, p. 2, in *The Complete Writings of Charles Reade*, vol. 7, pp. 615–16.
39 C. Reade, 'Correspondence Elicited by the First Edition of "Hard Cash"', in *The Complete Writings of Charles Reade*, vol. 7, p. 621.
40 J.S. Borlase, 'The Lass o' Gowrie; or, a Husband for an Hour', *Dundee Courier* (6 December 1881), p. 7.
41 P. McCandless, 'Liberty and Lunacy: The Victorians and Wrongful Confinement', *Journal of Social History* 11:3 (1978), p. 374.
42 *The Lancet*, 74:1870 (1859), p. 14.
43 Fennell, *Treatment Without Consent*, p. 6.
44 For example: 'The Acomb Lunatic Asylum', *The Times* (30 July 1858), p. 12; 'The New Lunacy Bill', *Journal of Mental Science* 8 (1862/1863), pp. 152–58; 'Report of the Lunacy Commissioners', *Saturday Review* (12 August 1871), pp. 208–9; 'The Reform of The Lunacy Laws', *The Times* (29 August 1885), p. 10; 'Lunacy Law', *Chepstow Weekly Advertiser* (15 March 1890), p. 2; 'Lunacy Law', *Exeter and Plymouth Gazette* (20 December 1912), p. 6.
45 McCandless, 'Liberty and Lunacy', p. 366.
46 'The Working of the New Lunacy Act', *British Medical Journal* 2:1542 (1890), pp. 156–57.
47 Lowe had a long and, despite outside appearances and six children, a deeply unhappy marriage. Her developing beliefs in spiritualism led her to leave her husband, who then had her confined to a private asylum. She was unsuccessful winning recourse in the courts; however, she did draw positive attention to her case. H. Nicholson, 'Introduction to the Writings of Louisa Lowe', in R. Porter, H. Nicholson, and B. Bennett (eds), *Women, Madness, and Spiritualism: Georgina Weldon and Louisa Lowe* (London, 2016), pp. 140–43.
48 Nicholson, 'Introduction to the Writings of Louisa Lowe', p. 139.
49 M.J. Clark, 'Does a Certificate of Lunacy Affect a Patient's Ethical Status? Psychiatric Paternalism and its Critics in Victorian England', in

A. Wear, J. Geyer-Kordesch, and R. French (eds), *Doctors and Ethics: The Earlier Historical Settings of Professional Ethics* (Amsterdam, 1993), p. 283. The group later splintered over fears of Louisa Lowe's association with spiritualism to form the Lunacy Law Amendment Society in 1876.

50 'Lunacy Law Reform Association', *Daily News* (21 May 1875), p. 3.
51 Such meetings were reported on with regularity across the nation. For example: 'Lunacy Law Reform', *Glasgow Herald* (19 March 1874), p. 7; 'Lunacy Law Reform', *Yorkshire Post and Leeds Intelligencer* (21 May 1875), p. 3; 'Illegal Detention of Lunatics', *Merthyr Telegraph, and General Advertiser for the Iron Districts of South Wales* (16 June 1876), p. 3; 'Lunacy Law Reform', *Leicester Chronicle and the Leicestershire Mercury* (17 November 1877), p. 2; 'The Action for Detention in a Lunatic Asylum', *London Evening Standard* (7 November 1879), p. 2.
52 L.S. Forbes Winslow, letter to the editor, *Daily News* (31 May 1875), p. 2.
53 L. Lowe, letter to the editor, *Daily News* (9 June 1875), p. 2.
54 L. Lowe, *The Bastilles of England: Or, the Lunacy Laws at Work* (London, 1883), pp. 35–39.
55 Lowe, *The Bastilles of England*, p. 38. Lowe's account, however, overlooks the fact that this was the second school to have dismissed Rev. Dodwell, and in fact he appeared before Sir George Jessel three times for three separate incidents where Dodwell tried to get the law to intervene on his behalf.
56 Henry John Dodwell, 11 March 1878, t18780311-365, OBP.
57 Henry John Dodwell, 11 March 1878, t18780311-365, OBP.
58 Henry John Dodwell, 11 March 1878, t18780311-365, OBP.
59 He did write up his case, however, while at Broadmoor in 1899. It was never published, but clearly demonstrated he believed his to be a case worthy of attention. Cited in J. Shepherd, 'Victorian Madmen: Broadmoor, Masculinity and the Experiences of the Criminally Insane, 1863–1900' (PhD Dissertation, Queen Mary University of London, 2013), p. 277.
60 These were verses written in Latin addressed to Justice Denman and seized by the Governor of Newgate. Henry John Dodwell, 11 March 1878, t18780311-365, OBP.
61 The two were interconnected; by declaring him a lunatic, the courts had therefore also undermined the validity of his initial complaints.
62 *London Medical Press and Circular* (26 June 1878), p. 533.
63 L.S. Forbes Winslow, letter to the editor, *British Medical Journal* (17 August 1878), p. 271. Forbes Winslow was a committed activist for

the cause, also writing to *The Times* that he would put up any amount of money or resources to guarantee the man's safety if authorities would 'rescue a sane man from being incarcerated in a living tomb'. L.S. Forbes Winslow, letter to the editor, *The Times* (2 July 1878), p. 11.
64 HC Deb. 30 July 1878, vol. 242, c643.
65 HC Deb. 13 March 1879, vol. 244, c821.
66 Forbes Winslow was adamant that it was confinement that led to Dodwell's madness, and that all of his actions up to and including firing at the Master of the Rolls were the actions of a sane man. L.F. Winslow, *Recollections of Forty Years* (London, 1910), pp. 116–26.
67 The medical inspector of convict prisons agreed and found that Dodwell was unable to obey the law if it impeded what he believed to be his own sense of justice. Shepherd, 'Victorian Madmen', pp. 263–65.
68 Hervey, 'Advocacy or Folly', p. 246.
69 Lowe lamented that in the case of Rev. Dodwell, 'medical men see as a rule what they are sent and paid to see'. Lowe, *The Bastilles of England*, p. 39.
70 A.S. Taylor, *A Manual of Medical Jurisprudence* (Philadelphia, 1880), p. 808.
71 Dodwell attacked a medical superintendent with a heavy stone, seriously injuring the man. According to the authorities, the crime demonstrated premeditation and intent, highlighting that while the man might have experienced lucid intervals, his proper place was in an asylum. 'The Defence of Insanity in Criminal Cases', *Law Journal* (18 October 1884), p. 610.
72 *The Lancet* 72:1827 (1858), p. 259.
73 Mr C.F. Thruston was no more specific than to say that Ruck committed 'an act of indecency'. This was the first indication he had that the man was mad.. 'Commission in Lunacy', *The Times* (24 August 1858), p. 10.
74 This woman, Mary Jones, as later revealed in the trial, started staying over at the family home when Mrs Ruck was absent. At first this did not cause much suspicion among the servants as she was a relative of Mrs. Ruck. 'Commission of Lunacy', *Daily News* (24 August 1858), p. 6.
75 He did not keep his suspicions as to his wife's conduct secret; he wrote to his children's governess about his wife's supposed infidelity. 'Commission of Lunacy on Mr. Ruck', *Morning Post* (25 August 1858), p. 2.
76 NA, C211/32/57, Chancery: Commissions and Inquisitions of Lunacy, 1857–59.

77 The cases of Mr Ruck, Mr Leech, and Mrs Turner all centred on the issue of confinement in private asylums. Each highlighted problems in medical testimony; however, none was a clear-cut case of sane people being illegally detained. Rather, they concerned questions of mental capacity and technicalities of confinement. Hervey, 'Advocacy or Folly', pp. 261–62.

78 The difference is key as it entailed radically different treatment. While medical and social reformers pushed to give local authorities the power to mandate treatment for inebriates, this did not come to pass, and certainly would never have covered a man with the wealth and power of Ruck. O.C. Niessen, *Aristocracy, Temperance and Social Reform: The Life of Lady Henry Somerset* (London, 2007), pp. 4, 167–68.

79 The Slander of Women Act allowed women to sue for sexual slander without the need to prove damages; it applied to women only, as men had to prove a financial harm in similar suits. C. Shaw, 'Liberalizing Paternalism? Men and the 1891 Slander of Women Act', unpublished paper, permission to cite from author.

80 'Commission of Lunacy on Mr. Ruck', *Morning Post* (25 August 1858), p. 2.

81 After the legal drama was over, Mrs Ruck moved to London and the *Daily News* published an article on her untarnished reputation. The local people of her community, however, wanted her to know how loved and respected she was, presenting her with a lavish clock and a Bible engraved with a Welsh dedication. 'Presentation to Mrs. Laurence Ruck', *Daily News* (17 September 1859), p. 3.

82 'The Lunacy Commission on Mr. Ruck', *Daily News* (25 August 1858), p. 3.

83 'The Commission in Lunacy on Mr. Ruck', *The Times* (25 August 1858), p. 5.

84 'The Lunacy Commission on Mr. Ruck', *Belfast News-Letter* (28 August 1858), p. 4.

85 'Commission in Lunacy', *Daily Post* (25 August 1858), p. 3.

86 Wise, *Inconvenient People*, pp. 267–73.

87 'Commission of Lunacy', *Morning Post* (26 August 1858), p. 2.

88 'Lunacy Commission on Mr. Ruck', *Daily News* (27 August 1858), p. 3.

89 'Lunacy Commission on Mr. Ruck', *Daily News* (27 August 1858), p. 3.

90 'The Lunacy Commission on Mr. Ruck', *Daily News* (26 August 1858), p. 3.

91 NA, C 211/32B/57A, 1857–59; Wise, *Inconvenient People*, p. 274.

92 'Mr. and Mrs. Ruck', *Saturday Review* (4 September 1858), pp. 229–30.

93 'The Commission of Lunacy on Mr. Ruck', *The Standard* (25 August 1858), p. 7.
94 Seymour, *A Letter to the Right Honourable The Earl of Shaftesbury*, pp. 20–21.
95 'Action Against the Proprietor of a Private Asylum: Ruck versus Stilwell', *Medical News* (2 July 1859), pp. 534–35.
96 The article first appeared in *The Lancet* and was then reprinted in the *Daily News*: 'The Grievances of the Lunatic', *The Lancet* (21 August 1858), p. 209; 'The Grievances of the Lunatic', *Daily News* (23 August 1858), p. 2. It was not uncommon for experts to point out that doctors were not always qualified to sign certificates, and through ignorance rather than malice might sign certificates incorrectly. Granville, *The Care and Cure of the Insane*, p. 150.
97 P. McCandless, 'Dangerous to Themselves and Others: The Victorian Debate over the Prevention of Wrongful Confinement', *Journal of British Studies* 23:1 (1983), pp. 84–104. Each *cause célèbre* spurred a flurry of responses from the medical community and the Lunacy Commissioners defending themselves. For example, see J.J. Schwieso, '"Religious Fanaticism" and Wrongful Confinement in Victorian England: The Affair of Louisa Nottidge', *Social History of Medicine* 9:2 (1996), pp. 168–70.
98 J.M. Granville, letter to the editor, *The Times* (24 May 1880), p. 8.
99 J. Parkin, *Notice of the Establishment for the Treatment of Nervous and Mental Maladies* (London, 1843), p. 3.
100 E.L.H. Ash, *Mind and Health: The Mental Factor and Suggestion in Treatment, with Special Reference to Neurasthenia and Other Common Nervous Disorders* (London, 1910); W.S. Playfair, *The Systematic Treatment of Nerve Prostration and Hysteria* (London, 1883); Savill, *Clinical Lectures on Neurasthenia*.
101 J. Secord, *Visions of Science: Books and Readers at the Dawn of the Victorian Age* (Chicago, 2014), p. xcv.
102 H. Ellis, *Masculinity and Science in Britain, 1831–1918* (London, 2017).
103 Ticehurst House Hospital Papers, Case Records, MS 6381, 1875–1879, p. 15.
104 Ticehurst House Hospital Papers, Case Records, MS 6381, pp. 34, 15–17, 25–27.
105 Ticehurst House Hospital Papers, Case Records, MS 6382, p. 35.
106 Copy of letter to Dr Newington, 27 October 1875, Ticehurst House Hospital Papers, Case Records, MS 6382, p. 37.
107 Copy of letter to Dr. Newington, 27 October 1875, Ticehurst House Hospital Papers, Case Records, MS 6382, p. 38.

108 C. Merivale, *My Experiences in a Lunatic Asylum* (London, 1879), pp. 28–34.
109 Rev. John Richardson describes religious hypochondria as a self-centred view of religious life that can lead to melancholia but is not insanity in itself. J. Richardson, 'Personal Religion – Papers', in Rev. W. Wilks (ed.), *The Official Report of the Seventeenth Annual Meeting of the Church Congress Held at Croydon, 1877* (Croydon, 1877), p. 351. Another author describing patients at the Retreat classified their religious hypochondria as a mental disease. 'The Quakers', *Westminster Review* 92:182 (1869), p. 174.
110 Pedlar, 'The Most Dreadful Visitation', p. 82.
111 Merivale, *Experiences in a Lunatic Asylum*, p. 88.
112 Merivale, *Experiences in a Lunatic Asylum*, p. 33.
113 Copy of letter to Dr. Newington, 27 October 1875, Ticehurst House Hospital Papers, Case Records, MS 6382, p. 38.
114 J. Eigen, *Mad-Doctors in the Dock: Defending the Diagnosis, 1760–1913* (Baltimore, 2016).
115 Delusions (as opposed to hallucinations) were the key symptoms at Ticehurst Asylum for marking out madness. T. Turner, 'Rich and Mad in Victorian England', *Psychological Medicine* 19:1 (1989), p. 36.
116 Merivale, *Experiences in a Lunatic Asylum*, pp. 92–93.
117 Case notes of Merivale's patient history describe the cause of his illness as 'unknown' – the most common entry. MacKenzie, *Psychiatry for the Rich*, pp. 101–2. However, casebooks also noted he had a hereditary tendency to madness from both parents. Ticehurst House Hospital Papers, Case Records, MS 6381, p. 15.
118 A. Stiles, *Popular Fiction and Brain Science in the Late Nineteenth Century* (Cambridge, 2011), p. 121.
119 J. S*****R. *Ridiculous Fancies: An Allegory. Being the Lucubrations of a Madman* (London, 1872), pp. 2–3.
120 S.F. Richards, '"That Doctor and His Heartless, Bloodless Science!": Disembodied Rational Masculinity in Victorian American Culture', *Nineteenth-Century Contexts* 36:4 (2014), p. 368.
121 A. Tomkins, *Medical Misadventure in an Age of Professionalisation, 1780–1890* (Manchester, 2017), p. 200.
122 Much of the press coverage, and even Windham's counsel, sometimes forgot this fact, as they spoke as if his actual personal liberty, not only his decision-making abilities, were at stake.
123 The most detailed coverage of the case is a narrative overview and analysis of medical evidence. K. Jones, 'The Windham Case: The Enquiry Held in London in 1861 into the State of Mind of William Frederick Windham, Heir to the Felbrigg Estate', *British Journal of Psychiatry* 119:551 (1971), pp. 425–33; D. Degerman, '"Am I Mad?":

The Windham Case and Victorian Resistance to Psychiatry', *History of Psychiatry* 30:4 (2019), pp. 457–68.
124 'The Windham Affair', *Westmorland Gazette* (14 December 1861), p. 8.
125 Not all newspapers were equally fascinated. The solidly respectable *Illustrated London News* hardly gave the case more than a sentence of coverage. 'Metropolitan News', *Illustrated London News* (28 December 1861), p. 660.
126 Conspicuously missing from the list of petitioners was Windham's mother, who appeared neither for the petitioners nor the defence. NA, C211/34/61, Chancery: Commissions and Inquisitions of Lunacy, 1861–1863.
127 'The Windham Lunacy Case', *Lloyd's Weekly Newspaper* (15 December 1861), p. 7.
128 Windham's lawyers exploited popular misunderstandings of the lunacy law throughout the trial and conflated his Chancery trial with institutionalization.
129 'Gossip on the Windham Romance', *Freeman's Journal and Daily Commercial Advertiser* (6 January 1862), p. 3.
130 'Windham v. Giubeli – The Windham Affair – Motion to Commit', *Leeds Mercury* (6 December 1861), p. 3.
131 'The Windham Lunacy Case: Motion to Commit a Solicitor', *Sheffield & Rotherham Independent* (6 December 1861), p. 4.
132 *Commission de Lunatico Inquirendo, An Inquiry into the State of Mind of W.F. Windham, Esq., of Fellbrigg Hall, Norfolk* (London, 1861), p. 67. The fact that Winslow clarified his comment was not about the character of the laugh itself is significant in its context. Many doctors declared lunatics had a particular kind of laugh that marked them as such. Winslow was not declaring Windham was an actual lunatic, but rather suffering from moral insanity.
133 H.F. Augstein, 'J.C. Prichard's Concept of Moral Insanity: A Medical Theory on the Corruption of Human Nature', *Medical History* 40:3 (1996), pp. 311, 337, 342.
134 D. Skae, 'Remarks on That Form of Moral Insanity Called Dipsomania, and the Legality of Its Treatment by Isolation', *Edinburgh Medical and Surgical Journal* 3:9 (1858), p. 773.
135 J.C. Bucknill and D.H.Tuke, *A Manual of Psychological Medicine: Containing the History, Nosology, Description, Statistics, Diagnosis, Pathology, and Treatment of Insanity. With an Appendix of Cases* (London, 1862), p. 87.
136 H. Rimke, 'From Sinners to Degenerates: The Medicalization of Morality in the 19th Century', *History of the Human Sciences* 15:1 (2002), pp. 64–65, 71.

137 F. Winslow, *The Plea of Insanity in Criminal Cases* (London, 1843), p. 37.
138 'Legal Topics of the Week', *The Law Times* (11 January 1862), p. 137.
139 An article published less than two years later hoped that the idea of moral insanity could finally be erased from the medical and legal lexicon. 'Homicidal Mania and Moral Insanity', *Saturday Review* (21 March 1863), pp. 370–72.
140 Mayo went out of his way to state that the diagnosis should never be used as a way for a man with intellectual acuity but moral defect to avoid criminal prosecution. T. Mayo, *Medical Testimony and Evidence in Cases of Lunacy: Being the Croonian Lectures Delivered before the Royal College of Physicians in 1853: With an Essay on the Conditions of Mental Soundness* (London, 1854), p. 76.
141 'The Windham Case', *Dublin Evening Packet and Correspondent* (17 December 1861), p. 1.
142 'English Law Intelligence: The Windham Lunacy Commission', *Dublin Daily Express* (21 December 1861), p. 4.
143 'The Windham Lunacy Case – This Day', *London Evening Standard* (19 December 1861), p. 5.
144 'Mr. Windham's Case', *Edinburgh Evening Courant* (21 December 1861), p. 7.
145 'A Miserable Child of Fortune', *Belfast Morning News* (20 December 1861), p. 4.
146 'Commission of Lunacy on Mr. W.F. Windham', *Morning Chronicle* (17 December 1861), p. 3.
147 'Mr. Windham's Case', *Glasgow Herald* (18 December 1861), p. 6; 'Mr. Windham's Case – Commission of Lunacy', *Leeds Mercury* (18 December 1861), p. 1.
148 Correspondents wrote to the *Kendal Mercury* refuting Windham's attempts to equivocate his behaviour on the railway, testifying they witnessed him in a guard's uniform with a key to the carriages acting as a guard, and often in a radically disruptive way. 'Mr. Windham as a Railway Guard', *Kendal Mercury* (13 December 1862), p. 8.
149 One correspondent wrote in to testify he had personally witnessed Windham dressed as a railway guard, and that Windham had been allowed to drive the train. The author was horrified by the idea of Windham, whether mad or not, being able to drive the train. 'An Eastern Counties Traveller', letter to the editor, *The Times* (14 December 1861), p. 8.
150 'The Windham Case – Commission of Lunacy', *Daily News* (17 December 1861), p. 2.

151 'The Windham Romance', *Freeman's Journal and Daily Commercial Advertiser* (23 December 1861), p. 4.
152 'Mr. Windham's Case', *Caledonian Mercury* (3 January 1862), p. 4.
153 *Commission de Lunatico Inquirendo, Inquiry into the State of Mind of W.F. Windham, Esq.*, p. 4.
154 *Gloucester Journal* (21 December 1861), p. 6.
155 'Extraordinary Case of Alleged Lunacy', *Cheltenham Chronicle* (3 December 1861), p. 3.
156 The number of witnesses on both sides is remarkable. There were at least fifty for the petitioners and ninety for the defence. 'The Case of Mr. W. F. Windham', *The Times* (31 January 1862), p. 7. However, the main characters of the story did not appear on the stand. One author at the time thought it was ridiculous that they brought witnesses from St Petersburg, Spa, and Edinburgh, but did not call Windham's mother who sat in the courtroom. Nor did they call General Windham, seen as the key instigator of the action. 'The Case of Mr. W.F. Windham', *The Times* (3 January 1862), p. 5.
157 'Gossip on the Windham Romance', *Freeman's Journal and Daily Commercial Advertiser* (6 January 1862), p. 3.
158 Eigen, *Unconscious Crime*, pp. 105–18.
159 *Commission de Lunatico Inquirendo, Inquiry into the State of Mind of W.F. Windham, Esq.*, p. 108.
160 'The Case of Mr. W.F. Windham', *The Times* (8 January 1862), p. 5.
161 At these words in Windham's defence summary, the applause in the courtroom was ended with some difficulty. 'The Windham Lunacy Commission', *Leeds Intelligencer* (4 January 1862), p. 8.
162 The decision was split, however, with twenty-two jurors finding Windham sound to fifteen against. Public and media support was far more lopsided in support of Windham's freedom. C. Unsworth, 'Law and Lunacy in Psychiatry's "Golden Age"', *Oxford Journal of Legal Studies* 13:4 (1993), p. 491.
163 A Member of the Bar, 'Art. I. – The Windham Case', *Medical Critic and Psychological Journal* (July 1862), p. 422.
164 *The Times* (31 January 1862), p. 6.
165 Wise, *Inconvenient People*, p. 283.
166 Jones, 'The Windham Case', p. 428.
167 In a Chancery case almost thirty years later, counsel was at pains to highlight how their defendant was unlike Windham. In this case, a man had suffered a mental break but was on the road to recovery. The lawyer argued that were he released too early he could potentially destroy himself and his fortune like Windham. 'Remarkable Lunacy Inquiry', *Daily News* (13 February 1891), p. 7.

168 *Commission de Lunatico Inquirendo, Inquiry into the State of Mind of W.F. Windham, Esq.*, p. 174.
169 J. Tosh, 'Masculinities in an Industrializing Society: Britain, 1800–1914', *Journal of British Studies* 44:2 (2005), pp. 332–33.
170 'Law Intelligence', *Morning Post* (3 April 1884), p. 6. See chapter six for a fuller discussion of the connections between overwork and madness.
171 'Commission of Lunacy', *The Times* (2 April 1884), p. 4.
172 *Morning Post* (9 April 1884), p. 7.
173 *The Times* and to a lesser extent the *Morning Post* provided regular coverage. This is impressive given that Georgiana Weldon's incredibly high-profile case against Forbes Winslow for wrongful incarceration was winding through the courts on the same days.
174 'Mr George Gilbert Scott', *Edinburgh Evening News* (3 April 1884), p. 2.
175 *Morning Post* (9 April 1884), p. 7.
176 'Commission in Lunacy', *The Times* (9 April 1884), p. 4.
177 'Commission of Lunacy', *The Times* (2 April 1884), p. 4.
178 'Commission in Lunacy', *The Times* (8 April 1884), p. 3.
179 'Commission in Lunacy', *The Times* (10 April 1884), p. 3.
180 'Commission in Lunacy', *The Times* (10 April 1884), p. 3.
181 E. Walford, letter to the editor, *The Times* (12 May 1884), p. 14.
182 G. Stamp, 'Scott, George Gilbert (1839–1897)', *Oxford Dictionary of National Biography*, 23 September 2004.
183 See for example: 'The Alleged False Imprisonment in a Lunatic Asylum', *Daily News* (6 August 1879), p. 3; 'A Singular Lunacy Case', *Daily News* (8 December 1888), p. 7.

5

Media panics: stories of violence, danger, and men out of control

> They walk the town, they offend our decent instincts, they give occasion to the populace to say to one another 'See that mean dirty thing. It has escaped from a great house. All great houses have familiars such as this, but they are kept close at home.'[1]

The 'mean dirty thing' in this instance was a pair of *causes celèbres* about lunacy.[2] Thus *The Times* article both critiqued sensation journalism and reflected general feelings about Victorian lunatics. For those with little first-hand experience of mental disease, media stories would have been the most likely, and the most frequent, encounter with the issues of insanity. These stories helped shape cultural tropes of madness. While the most common types of article written on madness were narrative updates on local asylums, these would only attract the interest of those with a particular interest in the specific asylum.[3] Stories of violence and madmen, however, were a cornerstone of sensationalism, and a potent reinforcement of the trope of insanity.

Elaine Showalter argues that the Victorian archetype of the vulnerable and abused madwoman helped inspire public outrage and pushed forward legislation aimed at eliminating restraint and humanizing the care for the insane. This followed a larger argument where she outlines that the shift in humane treatment tracked an evolving icon of madness from the bestial eighteenth-century madman to the victimized Victorian madwoman.[4] The madwoman in the attic was a powerful archetype in the nineteenth century. Yet the bestial madman did not disappear from view; in fact, stories of violent and uncontrolled madmen kept this version of insanity firmly in the foreground.[5] Following Showalter's logic, if humane accounts of delicate madwomen helped spur the non-restraint movement, stories of violent madmen helped temper public pity with fear. Madmen should be treated humanely – but they should be contained lest the tragedies of this chapter should occur. The asylum continued even if it could not cure for fear of the madman on the loose.

There was increasing pressure for Victorian men to be non-violent, and to practise more self-discipline than ever before. 'And as the gospel of self-management spread, impulsive and violent behaviour became all the more threatening, by its actual growing rarity, at least in the circles frequented by self-improving persons, and by the increasing contrast it made with the self-improving way of life.'[6] But not all men could restrain their violence, and contemporaries worried about the inherent male trend towards irrational power and potential madness. Stories of men who lost control and unleashed unspeakable violence on strangers and loved ones could be used as a warning of the potential danger of unchecked male violence.[7] A madman was a source of potential and unrestrained violence, unleashing the darkest sides of masculinity. Dramatic stories in the media inscribed a typology of violent male madness that reinforced long-held stigmas about insanity.

The term 'moral panic' is sometimes used to describe sensational coverage that exaggerated potential dangers.[8] While the sociological concept of moral panic is typically used to understand contemporary events, recent scholarship suggests the term can usefully be pushed back to include nineteenth-century topics.[9] The classic moral panic draws on latent fears triggered by sensational events.[10] Such moments demonize those perceived as a threat to the social order and as an offence against basic human decency. David Garland reasons that a true moral panic must touch on an issue that typifies larger social anxieties and invokes moral reflection.[11] Fears of madmen demonstrated these qualities as a unified voice called out the potential threat of the issue, highlighting larger fears of failed masculinity and increasing rates of madness. Dramatic stories of violent madmen were a constant feature of the Victorian press and could cause a moral panic at specific moments of unease.

The British press was happy to supply a steady stream of murder and violence to a receptive audience.[12] They justified such stories early on as a civic responsibility; the public display of law and order was necessary so that the public had faith that justice would be served. In some papers this 'duty' occupied almost one-third of the total content.[13] These stories were often repeated verbatim across a number of papers, although actual incidents of crime were generally on the decline over the course of the nineteenth century. While some outlets did mock the hysterical fears of rising crime rates, few avoided reporting sensational stories in lavish detail.[14] When murder became the only capital offence of the nineteenth century, its trials tended to garner the most public attention, and could stir up a media or moral panic.[15] And when violent crime encompassed the threat of a madman, it was sure to garner widespread attention.

Victorian commentators understood theirs was an age of sensation, and that the media were always drawn to scandal. An increasingly competitive newspaper marketplace led to an aggressive news cycle with editors clamouring for ever more dramatic stories.[16] The more unusual the case, the more likely it was to receive widespread coverage. Certain sensational stories or court cases helped shape a mass reading audience in the last decades of the nineteenth century.[17] The constant string of narratives and use of emotional language helped stoke cultural anxieties.[18] Among tales of lady poisoners, East End ruffians, and artful dodgers, there was a steady flow of dangerous madmen. These stories covered madmen of all social situations and backgrounds, and took place in both domestic and public settings.[19]

The previous chapter detailed incidents of men finding their voice and protesting against wrongful confinement. These men attempted to take back the narrative of their experiences from doctors and asylum officials. And while wrongful confinement tales did make compelling copy, these individual stories were countered by a consistent flow of stories of madmen as dangerous, violent, and unstable figures. Such accounts reinforced a narrative that the madman was a figure to be feared, undermined the voices of lunatics themselves, and helped reinforce many of the worst stigmas of insanity. Scholars note how 'New Journalism' helped to delineate and direct government reaction to and public perception of major events.[20] While media coverage of changing laws and policies absolutely influenced public debate, it is important to look at the smaller scandals, and the everyday flow of sensational stories that shaped everyday stereotypes, if not public policy.

Sources for this chapter are grounded in research drawn from the British Newspaper Archive, starting with an initial database of over four thousand articles published on madness or insanity in over forty newspapers, and then expanded to include non-digitized medical journals, youth magazines, and leading periodicals. The most common stories were overwhelmingly about asylums, in particular about construction, expansion, finances, epidemics, and statistical data. However, the most sensational articles, those that were covered by multiple media outlets, centred on a few cases of wrongful confinement and violence such as those outlined in the last chapter.

While there were stories of madwomen committing acts of great violence, they were relatively rare. Women were less commonly charged with violent crimes than men. From 1843 to 1876 fifty-six women charged at the Old Bailey claimed some form of mental incapacity, and of those thirty-two were murder cases.[21] Broadmoor typically had a ratio of 4:1 male to female prisoners, and women had a much higher discharge rate.[22] Thus the source material for stories of madness and violence is heavily weighted towards men.

Violent madwomen were often seen as victims of tragedy rather than untapped sources of violence. The most common stories in the press of madwomen committing acts of violence were infanticide cases; these were covered in somewhat lurid detail. But these stories were represented very differently from other violent acts. Infanticide in general was understood by Victorians as a crime where both perpetrator and child were victims; and when the mother was found to have puerperal insanity, the empathy was even greater.[23] Not only were such stories less frequent, but the victims were also typically vulnerable and thus the perpetrators less imposing.[24] Such stories were generally framed as tragedies of poverty and circumstance, rather than the potential terror of madness. Madwomen were far more likely to be portrayed as victims of unlawful confinement or abuse than as sources of danger to the community.[25]

The publication of stories about madness continued consistently throughout the second half of the nineteenth century. There were gluts of interest around particular issues (shifting policies, the growth of madness, criminal responsibility) that occasionally became the subject of sensation. Violence and murder always made for dramatic reading, and a story with an extra twist or frisson of danger only helped sell newspapers.[26] The spectacle of male minds breaking down was a dominant trope of local and regional newspapers throughout the United Kingdom. This chapter will explore the various types of media stories of men and madness, and what such tales reveal about broader underlying fears. Domestic stories of violence in the home helped encourage families to send their loved ones to asylums lest such violence befall themselves. Stories of madmen in close quarters followed literary tropes of melodrama to reinforce the madman as a figure of terror. Stories of men on the boundaries of madness reinforced the stigma of madness as a type of disease inscribed on one's identity. And tales of criminal insanity fuelled confusion about criminal responsibility and questioned the meaning of incarceration and institutionalization. While previous chapters have overrepresented middle-class voices and experiences, here working-class men were often the focus of media sensations.

Domestic violence

One commonly reported type of story focused on male lunatics bringing violence and terror to their homes. Narratives of men no longer in control of their minds who enacted violence on those most dear were spellbinding. It is largely because of the valorization of the Victorian family home that when it was breached, the horror became all the greater. The home was characterized by its privacy and security.[27] And man's role as head of household was to be both provider and protector. As John Tosh notes, 'the man's duty to protect the home was more than an expression of power over his dependants; it implied collective measures alongside other householders, and thus underpinned the association of masculinity with physical self-reliance and personal bravery'.[28] When men failed to protect their families, and instead became the source of danger and fear, their actions were not only an abrogation of duty but also a betrayal. Stories of madmen turning on their families expressed deep underlying anxieties about working-class male violence in particular.

Stories that demonstrated a sudden act of male violence made for exciting media copy. Unlike in courtrooms, newspapers did not have to determine whether someone reached the level of insanity or not to use sensational terms. 'Madman' was used both in a technical sense and a colloquial one; when an act itself was seen as particularly barbaric, cruel, horrifying, or nonsensical, journalists were confident in naming the perpetrator as mad. Such was the case of an army sergeant who told two non-commissioned officers that his wife and children had been shot by unknown men who came down the chimney. When they followed the man home they found that, in fact, his wife and six children had been killed with a razor. The crime was horrific, and the sergeant eventually confessed to the murders and a plan to blow up the fort. The reporter had no need for a medical assessment:

> The unfortunate maniac, for it was evident that he could receive no other designation, as, although no thought was entertained of his being capable of committing such a deed, his manner had been for some time previously remarked as strange, appears, after destroying the lives of his wife and children to have made an attempt upon his own.[29]

A respectable man who would unleash such violence on his family was automatically dubbed a madman by a newspaper, before any legal or medical opinion intervened.

A murder in Preston was covered by a number of newspapers that emphasized how a family was transformed in an instant by a madman. A couple went to chapel leaving their daughter at home with her grandmother and a longstanding lodger. While their lodger had been out of sorts the last few days, they could not have imagined what would happen. The grandmother left the house and returned to find neither the child nor the lodger. The man was later found running down the street and surrendered to authorities. A more thorough search of the house found the girl in a corner nearly decapitated by a large knife.[30] The story was terrifying; papers emphasized the intense violence of the act and dubbed the perpetrator a madman.[31] The lodger explained at the coroner's jury that he killed the little girl to save her soul.[32] Press accounts did not have to determine whether the assailant met the legal threshold for insanity. Journalists presented such authoritative accounts of shocking and scandalous events as a way to explore and ultimately control the story.[33] The retelling of these and other incidents of sudden madness rather mimicked the patterns of a sensation novel.[34] The specific incidents were dangerous for the people involved; however, the level of media coverage and the degree of panic were disproportionate to the number of occurrences.

The more respectable the family situation, the more likely it was to make a sensational case when violence broke out. Nathanial Griffin had shown no indication of violence until his sudden attack against his family. He was the manager of the Sutton Works in Aston and had been told by his doctors to take a vacation to sooth his nerves. His family hired a nurse and did everything his doctor recommended. And yet without warning, he jumped out of bed, grabbed a poker, and began hitting the nurse with it. She screamed, bringing Mrs Griffin into the room; her husband struck her on the head several times causing serious injury and loss of blood.[35] The sensation here was the suddenness of the man's anger, and the violence unleashed within a well-respected family. The *Illustrated Police News* employed their visual format to emphasize how even the most respectable exteriors could contain chaos within. One could hardly imagine such an orderly house could contain such a scene as several men struggling to restrain a dangerous lunatic in his nightshirt (Figure 5.1).[36] The idea of horrors hiding beneath respectable exteriors was sure to capture readers' attention.

The extreme violence that a few madmen unleashed on their families and communities made for sensational, and horrific, reading. The *Cheshire Observer* reported a local tragedy with all the drama

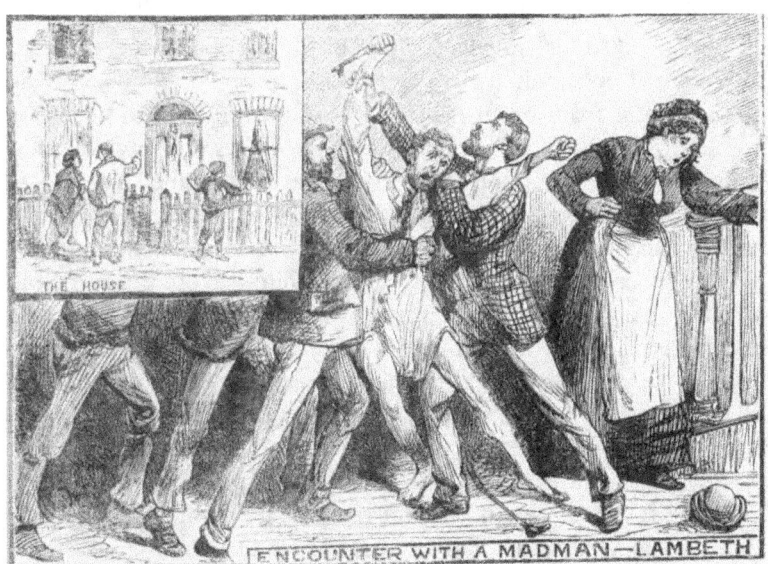

Figure 5.1 Interior and exterior scenes of a violent encounter

of a penny dreadful. John Shallcross, a brickmaker, attacked his family in a fit of acute mania. He first attacked his sister, punching and kicking her. When a neighbour tried to intervene, Shallcross picked up his sister's child and began using the baby to strike his sister again. He raised the child above his head, preparing to throw it to the ground before the neighbour stopped him. He then went after his father, hitting him with a rail and leaving him for dead. He ran and tried to hide when farm workers accidentally came across him. They rushed at him, struggled with him, injuring him severely, and when the man's brother tried to intervene, the madman grabbed his pikel and tried to stab him with it. When he was finally caught, the surgeon said the man was suffering violent madness of a kind so acute he had to be strapped to his bed. 'I never saw any one like him.'[37] The article emphasized the man's violence throughout, and the man's danger not only to his own family, but also to the entire community.

The potential physical power of a man out of his mind was a real threat, and these stories emphasized that a man without a mind was little more than a beast.[38] The sudden and intense violence unleashed by madmen on their own families made for terrifying reading.[39] In a village outside Derby, it was a father's worry over his son that seemingly led to his violence against his family. The father of seven children had been quite worried about his fifteen-year-old son, who was suffering from brain fever. He rose in the night to check on his delirious son before settling back to bed. His wife awoke a few hours later when her husband struck her and pushed her out of their bed. She screamed and woke the rest of the household. Her husband then turned on his son, trying to strangle him. A relative who was there helping to nurse the sick child tried to intervene but the man struck her, then managed to rip her jaw out of her mouth, throwing her to the floor and strangling her. This good-tempered, respectable farm labourer turned into a violent beast and murderer. All the reporter could surmise was that his son's illness preyed on the man's mind until he broke.[40] After he was arrested, he had another violent attack and it took seven men to restrain him.[41]

Some stories of violence could be used to encourage people to look for early warning signs and act without delay. James Smith had served ten years in the army in India and had returned home to work at a small arms factory in Birmingham. His employer noticed changes in his appearance, and recommended he take a few days off to recover. At home, however, his position deteriorated quickly as he began walking the streets with a stick, claiming he was a Fenian. When a doctor was called, he found him worse still, but did not yet seem dangerous enough to warrant an emergency lunacy order. He was put to bed but soon after got up raving, armed himself with a gun, and threatened anyone who came near him. He barricaded himself in his bedroom, and when police arrived, shot at them twice. They had to wait him out, and only secured him in the early hours of the morning after much resistance.[42]

Other stories captured the public imagination because of madmen's ability to sham sanity through 'cunning'.[43] The son of a publican attacked his seventeen-year-old sister in her bed, slitting her throat with a razor. The *Lancaster Gazette* implied this was the result of a secret, long-planned attack fuelled by his religious delusions.[44] The idea that the insane possessed a particular kind of guile to hide their plans or their delusions was particularly supported by lunacy doctors who believed they were the only experts who could see past such machinations.[45] This idea reinforced the need to be sceptical of those who seemed to be sane and could even fool legal authorities.[46] Such stories cast doubt on whether any man could truly recover from insanity.

Sensational stories of violence could help reinforce the idea that even the smallest delay in institutionalizing the insane could lead to devastating results. Stephen Dickenson, a shoemaker, was labouring under the delusion that a man was trying to shoot him. His widowed mother lived with him, and had tried to take care of him, but eventually she made the decision to send him to an asylum. Before that could happen, she was so concerned she asked a friend to sit up with her 'for she was very much frightened about her son, who did not seem right in his mind, and whose strange conduct had prevented her taking rest for the past three or four nights'.[47] When she went to bring her son some tea in the early hours of the morning, he met her on the stairs and hit her over the head with a post. After she died he was unrepentant, believing she had been conspiring with men to kill him. His jury found him insane at the time of the murder.[48] Such stories could act as a warning for families sceptical of seeking treatment and portrayed even mild-mannered lunatics as sources of potential danger.

In another story, a man suffering hydrophobia attempted to kill his wife and children. A watch was placed on him, but he still managed to set fire to his bed. He escaped with two knives to terrorize the neighbourhood. He shouted and threatened anyone who came near him before police constables caught up with him two hours later. Although the man was captured, the newspaper headline 'A Madman at Large' emphasized the few hours when he had escaped.[49] Domestic violence could quickly translate into community violence. In 'Exciting Chase after a Madman', a man threatened to kill his wife and sisters before leading police on a chase across both sides of the river Len and into a family home, where he terrified a couple in their bed. He was eventually caught by a constable and explained he was chasing Satan.[50]

Another popular narrative focused on families who tried to distance themselves from their mad relations and yet were still frightened by them. *The Times* told the story of 'A Lunatic at Large' who terrorized his family. A sergeant left the service in disgrace; his family rejected him, but he continued to harass them, causing them to call the police. It took five constables to get him to the station, and for his violent assault on one of the officers he was sentenced to a month's hard labour. While imprisoned he was declared mad and sent to the Kent Lunatic Asylum. The paper emphasized his threat to the community and, more specifically, his family, who were using special precautions as the man had a 'decided murderous tendency'.[51]

Much of the stigma associated with madness came from the fear that it was never fully cured.[52] Media stories seemed to reinforce that stereotype, and with tragic results. A miner who had recovered from a previous attack of suicidal insanity married and had four children. He seemed perfectly well until one evening when he started crying out in his bed that his life was over and there was no hope. His wife calmed him but did not notice he had hidden a rolling pin in the bed. He suddenly lashed out at her, hitting her in the mouth with his weapon before she managed to flee to the neighbours for help. By the time the police arrived he had injured many of his children and attempted to kill himself by placing his head in the fire.[53] One paper retold the basic facts of this case with the plea to create separate institutions for men such as this who were beyond help and should never be allowed to threaten their families or the public again.[54] Such stories undermined faith in the ability to cure mental disease.

Fictional tales reflected concerns about the dangers of lunatics outside the asylum that mimicked cases that were constantly being reported in the press. Such stories underscored contemporary worries about male violence and a broader civil project to control men's brutality.[55] In one short story, Captain Galton is introduced, held in a strait-jacket, under guard in his own house. His nephew arrives to find him pale and distraught, claiming to be held as part of a conspiracy. Released, however, the man transforms. Suddenly his face becomes distorted, and his mad fury is unleashed. Eric Ross's fictional madman displays both the ability to sham sanity, and the preternatural strength of the raving maniac. He then relates his history of love, betrayal, and revenge. Despite the man's breakdown and violence, there is a certain awestruck reverence for his character. In fact, in his madness his qualities as a man are put into greater relief. His nephew marvels that 'Even if he were mad, he appeared to be the wreck of a greater man than ever any of his family conceived him to be.'[56] Galton is delusional and violent and suffering from *delirium tremens*. He is only disarmed after his gun backfires in his hand, rendering him unconscious. The crisis of insanity passes after three months in hospital. In this case a domestic tragedy is averted only by chance; the story hardly recommends keeping a madman in the home, even for a short period.

Men's thwarted love could turn to the temporary madness of suicide, or madness and violence.[57] G.W. Walker exploited the idea of the dangerous lunatic kept at home for the stage. In his play 'The Madman', a young man is driven mad after financial setbacks and the betrayal of his marriage prospects. Upon seeing his beloved marry an evil man he loses his senses. His mother will not send him to an asylum, but instead keeps him secluded in her home with a keeper. But the maniac cannot be contained, and in his insane revenge he kills not only his evil rival but also his keeper.[58] One reviewer particularly praised the lead actor's ability to portray madness without melodrama and frenzy without hysteria.[59] The violent madman was a clearly recognized figure who could bring chaos to the home.

Scholars have pointed out that crime stories situated in specific locations made them particular, rather than universal. These stories contained the violence by naming a place and made it a specific problem of that area rather than a broad topography of inclusiveness.[60] That is how wealthy Londoners were predisposed to enjoy stories of violence and anxiety in the East End.[61] While some stories mentioned a town or village in their headlines, it was the home that was the central location, rather than any urban setting. Reports of sudden attacks within the private, intimate family home only reinforced anxiety and fear of the madman and underscored that a violent attack could happen anywhere.

Violence in close quarters

While most violence within the home was directed at family members, the story of a sudden mad stranger in any enclosed space could provide an even more intense feeling of danger. Newspaper stories of madmen terrorizing people in isolated spaces often took on literary qualities.[62] Melodramatic settings exemplified the dual purpose of Victorian crime reporting both to convey news and to provide entertainment. The stories outlined in this section underscored that madmen could come from anywhere. Dramatic reports of a madman in a railway carriage or on a ship, where the parties were sequestered by water or speed, were exhilarating because of their very strangeness. Stories of violence and murder were always popular, and the stranger the better.[63] Sensational language was always attractive to papers attempting to attract a wider audience.[64]

Until the twentieth century, the British railway carriage was typically a closed site without corridors or passages between cars or compartments. Once the train was in motion, there was also no easy way to signal for help or to exit the train.[65] Stories of madmen on the railways were so frequent in the mid-1860s that one can identify a media panic.[66] Brutal assaults were related in painstaking detail and consistent frequency for over a decade. Headlines like 'Another Madman in a Railway Train' could make it seem as though madmen were stalking every train in Britain.[67] In some cases, it seemed the train itself could cause the madness. On an express train from Carnforth to Liverpool travellers were terrorized by a man laughing maniacally outside their window. He would calm down when the train stopped at a station, only to be driven to a frenzy when the train moved and he clambered outside onto the carriage steps. He eventually brandished a pistol and threatened to shoot his fellow passengers.[68] Such tales reinforced doctors' warnings that the hustle and bustle of modern life, and railway travel in particular, could cause almost any man's mind to break.[69] The everyday process of travelling by train was rendered a dangerous and uncertain landscape.

Some of these stories detailed potential dangers only, but in others there was genuine blood to exploit. In Bedford, a lunatic suddenly attacked his keeper on a train in a brutal assault with a secreted razor. The lunatic attempted to slit his throat and when his keeper tried to intervene, the patient turned his violence outwards. The *Leicester Chronicle and the Leicestershire Mercury* detailed the scene at the next station when guards opened the doors to the third-class carriage and found two men covered in blood. The keeper lost his thumb in the struggle and was happy not to have lost his life.[70] The *Illustrated Police News* reinforced the nature of the violence in both image and description. The front-page illustration of the Bedford attack (Figure 5.2) portrayed an alarming scene of the event unfolding and varied from printed reports to increase the sense of danger. A knife is prominently displayed as if the guard had only managed to dislodge it from the lunatic's hand at the station.[71] The image shows bloody handprints while the copy reinforces that 'the floor and seats of the carriage had the look of a slaughterhouse'.[72] The story was told with a real sense of immediacy despite the fact no members of the public were in danger, and the attack was facilitated by not thoroughly searching the lunatic before he boarded the train.

Given that such sensationalized narratives were told with the pace and drama of a work of fiction, readers might not always have separated truth from imagination. Many news stories echoed the tropes of short stories published in the same newspapers, with only a first-person narrative to distinguish between fact and fiction. One such tale dramatized a sudden encounter with a madman in the kitchen. A former friend was now more beast than man and 'an expression of malignant terror stole over his features. If ever I saw murder, it was in his eye at that moment.'[73] Authors realized that to be trapped in a room with a madman made for a particularly tense dramatic situation. Some took their stories to even greater extremes, such as one tale that focused on being trapped at the top of a weather cock with a madman.[74]

196 *Out of his mind*

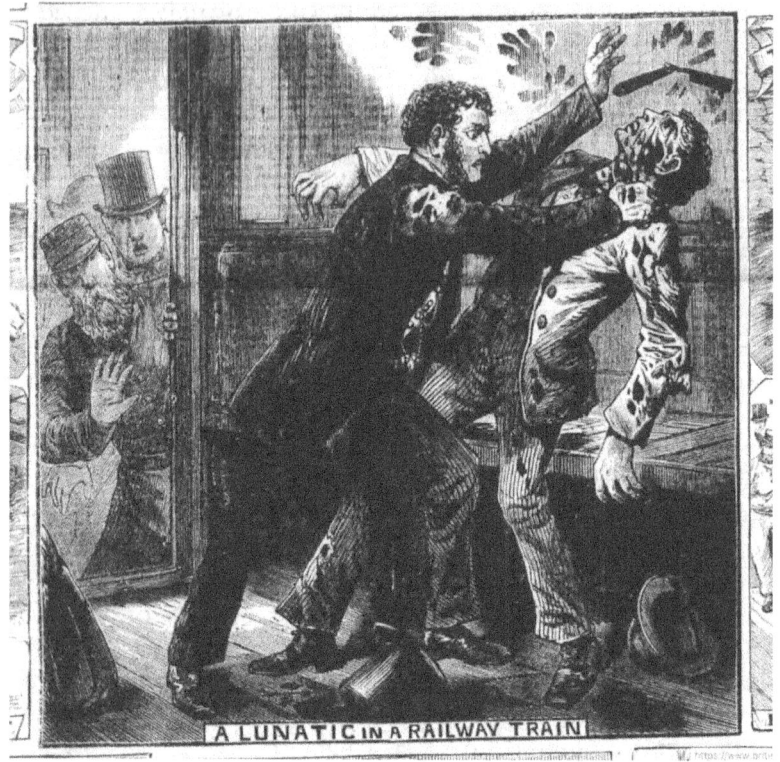

Figure 5.2 A lunatic in a railway train

And yet the drama of real-life situations could rival almost any fictional scenario. Violence on the open seas would always make for good media copy, and in the case of a madman's attack, incidents often occurred without warning.[75] A crew member who suddenly lost his senses on a voyage made for gripping reading.[76] Without having to provide much detail, these stories tapped into primal fears about the power of the ocean, the isolation aboard a ship, and the fragility of the human mind. While some articles gave only the barest elements, others outlined graphic, narrative features. One vessel from South America to Cork carried an Italian farmer on board who had travelled to seek his fortune. The reporter detailed how this man became despondent and paranoid on the journey, culminating in his grabbing a sword and attacking the crew. He wounded a couple of men and stabbed the captain through the heart, killing him. The man had no motive, no excuse, and no explanation, and the crime was explained as 'sudden mania'.[77]

Such stories rarely gave much characterization to the 'madman', and rarely offered any hope of prevention. The exception to this were stories of madness caused by *delirium tremens*; in such tales there was a clear cause of the mad outburst and a clear culpability with the perpetrator. In the case of one ship travelling from St John's to Liverpool, a sailor boarded the ship so inebriated he could not perform his duties for days. His alcoholic binge turned into an attack of *delirium tremens* by the fourth day, when he began frantically running around the ship and up the rigging. He then turned on the ship's crew; hoping to calm or frighten the man, the captain shot over his head. This only aggravated the man, who went after the captain. The carpenter grabbed the gun and shot the madman. The carpenter was charged with murder and was vindicated in his use of force. The title of the *York Herald*'s account, 'Justifiable Homicide', clearly exonerates the carpenter.[78]

Authors also set fictional stories in maritime settings.[79] Much like the real story of the Liverpool steamer, a tale appeared seven years later of a ship's engineer suffering a bout of *delirium tremens*. The flexibility of fiction allowed the author to detail the man's struggle with delusions and paranoid fantasies. Our narrator, the doctor, is the only one who seems to have a rapport with the madman and takes him into his cabin. The sense of confinement in the story only increases as it proceeds. The doctor drifts off to sleep and awakens to find the madman staring at him, clutching his knife. The author paints a vivid portrait of a man rendered beastly by his alcoholic indulgence. A man who before his illness was 'not only a manly, good-hearted fellow, but a wise and well-educated gentleman' is transformed into a dark and menacing animal circling his prey. Playing on the trope of the power of a doctor's eye, our narrator stares down the armed man and 'the devil in him was conquered'. A chase around the ship ensues, where the madman wreaks chaos on all before trying to kill himself.[80] The lunatic was unmanned in his delirium.

Stories of madmen on the seas were popular in juvenile publications as well. Desperate struggles aboard a ship made for an incredibly exciting narrative.[81] In one story a madman driven to despair by jealousy hides aboard a ship to surprise his rival at a vulnerable moment. Fuelled by revenge, he strangles the young man and threatens him with a revolver.[82] In another story, a madman loose aboard a ship terrorizes the crew. His strength is superhuman and his cunning intense; he is able to withstand an axe blow and twice escape.[83] Such stories made for thrilling reading and fit into broader trends in boys' literature emphasizing exotic locations.[84] Overcoming a madman was yet another way to demonstrate bravery and cleverness.[85] Such stories also reinforced the madman as a source of bestial violence.

These stories transformed the privacy and security of an enclosed space such as a railway carriage or ship into a scene of harrowing isolation. Tales of violence in such spaces, either real or fictional, were dramatic and compelling. These narratives also underscored the frailty of the human mind to modern life.[86] As one medical reviewer noted, 'No one can be indifferent to [madness] who considers his own liability to become insane in this crowding and jostling age, where men tread so closely upon each other's heels, where every nerve-fibre is at its highest tension, and the social wheels are made to revolve at the most terrific speed.'[87] Not only could such reports increase fear of strange madmen, but they also highlighted the incipient madness within all men.

The madness of strangers

Above all, stories of violent madmen reinforced a narrative that madmen were a potential threat and should be viewed with caution. Another genre of reports emphasized the mercurial nature of lunacy. Such stories of sudden, dangerous attacks reinforced the idea that early symptoms should be taken seriously, and that one should be cautious of rushing recovery. Anthony Carlton Cooke argues that in the twentieth century, fears of deinstitutionalization were associated with the idea of mental patients as embodiments of 'barely subdued violence'.[88] And it is clear to see this trope stretches back to the nineteenth century. If such stories resonated with the public in the twentieth century out of a fear of the mentally ill within the community, in the nineteenth century there was a strong narrative to keep patients in asylums even as their efficacy as a source of cure diminished.

Unchecked, unprovoked, and anonymous violence could make for some of the most terrifying stories of madness and crime. Of all the emotions that could prove troubling in excess, it is no surprise that anger might top the list. Anger's primordial and often violent expressions made it both a universal emotion, and one that most needed to be checked by civilized men.[89] In the case of Mr Dougan, a warrant was issued for his arrest which seemed to trigger a homicidal rage. When two constables tried to arrest him, he surprised them in a violent attack, struggling with them for over an hour. In the encounter 'Dougan displayed fiendish strength and tossed the officers off him like ninepins'.[90] Madmen were often represented as possessing supernatural strength. Dougan was finally subdued and tied with rope, but he subsequently could not be brought into court because he was so out of control.

In the early stages of the Whitechapel murders of 1888, as more women were horribly murdered and no credible leads were forthcoming, many wondered if a lunatic were to blame.[91] In fact, one of the most popular theories of the murderer at the time was that he must be an escaped or hidden madman:

> A homicidal lunatic possessed apparently of the superhuman cunning and force by which such unfortunate beings are sometimes characterised – a human tiger with no more moral responsibility than that huge and ferocious cat, his thirst for blood whetted with three successful crimes, is at large, according to this dreadful idea, in the midst of such a teeming hive of humanity as Whitechapel.[92]

Such explanations were a way to limit the horror of a series of gruesome murders; the actions of a madman had no deeper meanings, unlike theories that implicated misogyny, poverty, or police incompetence.[93] The association of violence and male madness was deeply entrenched in the public psyche.

Stories emphasized that madness could strike suddenly, and seemingly dissipate just as quickly. The more dramatic the contrast, the more impressive the story. James Fraser was a bank clerk enjoying his annual holiday when he attacked a neighbour. His neighbour, William Shadwell, opened the door when Fraser knocked. Fraser rushed in and immediately attacked Shadwell with a sword. The terrified man ran into the street and was pursued by Fraser, who continued to strike him. A young woman passed by carrying a pitcher of water and he turned his sword on her. Her screams attracted a crowd who attempted to stop him by throwing stones at him as he continued to attack the young woman until she was dead. Mrs Shadwell then returned home to see her husband lying severely injured on the ground; she fainted, and Fraser struck at her as well. Witnesses who had fled to a safe distance by this time noted he wiped off his sword on the grass and then returned to his home. When police arrived, he was calmly sitting with his sword in one hand and revolver in the other.[94] Fraser's fury dissipated as quickly as it appeared.

James Heslipp was a saddler who was institutionalized and released for madness after a short illness. For three years he seemed healthy, but then suffered a minor relapse. The following week he was again detained but no one would swear that he was truly insane. Magistrates released him to his friends. All seemed well until he walked to the next town with a billhook over his shoulder. Entering the town, he had a series of violent encounters with people, attacking strangers and becoming more enraged as he went. He killed an old woman and a young girl and left three people on the brink of death. He was only captured when he stopped for a swim in a pond and constables went into the water to fetch him. His crime had no motive, and he had no memory of his actions after the fact. However, while he later seemed calm, he would occasionally lash out in violence.[95] Heslipp's mind was known to be troubled, but because doctors were hesitant to swear that he was absolutely disturbed, he was not placed in confinement, and thus four people died.[96] One reason the wrongful confinement panic likely never led to a massive shift in legislative policy is that stories like these were such strong counter-arguments. Was it better to lock someone in a well-managed asylum for a short period of time to assess whether their mind was truly unsound or risk having them out and committing violence?

Stories of violence would always sell newspapers, and the sudden madman was a compelling genre. According to the papers, the moral of the story of Matthew Ackroyd was to be wary of trusting strangers. Ackroyd was a farmer, and when Samuel Edmunds moved to his area, the farmer gave him a job and a place to stay. After a good day's work and a meal with the family, all went to bed for the night. But half an hour later, when Ackroyd went to check on his beehives, he heard his new employee screaming. He quickly locked himself in the house and told his wife that the man 'appeared to be in the horrors'. Edmunds then appeared at the door naked, smashing the windows and threatening to kill the farmer. Ackroyd's servant, John Wilkinson, escaped out of the back door for help. He found aid and they followed Edmunds to an embankment where he wielded a large oak branch. They tried to corral him, but Edmunds struck out, hitting Wilkinson in the head, rendering him unconscious. The lunatic was subdued with difficulty and sent to the authorities.[97] When Wilkinson died of his injuries Edmunds was charged with murder. Authorities also discovered Edmunds had previously been discharged from the army and bore brands as a deserter.[98] First impressions of Edmunds hid a violence and bad character raging beneath the surface.

Stories of the sudden, violent lunacy of strangers underscored the associations of mental distress and danger. When stories of violence emerged, it was easy for journalists to label perpetrators as mad when there was no seeming cause for the outburst before they were ever evaluated by doctors or the courts. This easy association also helped to foster the connection that mad people were violent and criminal by nature. Modern research highlights that 'the constant revivifying of the intertextual commonsense about madness employed in news stories and other media productions contributes to the public's fear of those with a mental disorder'.[99] The constant flow of these stories reified stereotypes and stigmas about madmen.

Criminal insanity

Crime stories were a popular feature of the Victorian press, and newspapers had long justified their inclusion for the purpose of demonstrating justice in action. Even the most unsavoury or graphic crime could be printed if newsmen claimed it was in the public interest.[100] Stories of a crime, arrest, and sentencing could be quite satisfying to a sense of justice being served. And yet by the 1860s, there was a growing sense that the justice system was no longer working. Despite the fact that criminal statistics demonstrated falling crime rates, there were fears this was not the case. Much of that fear was driven by increasing coverage of violent crime in the media.[101] In most stories of violence, balance could be restored to the universe by the delivery of justice. Typically, this would be in the form of a trial and a decision of penal servitude or even death for the guilty. And yet in the case of the mad criminal, there was little sense of clear justice. To punish a man who was not responsible for his actions was cruel; yet many worried that sending a brutal murderer to an asylum provided no justice.

The laws on criminal insanity evolved significantly over the course of the nineteenth century. What did not change, however, were public fears that those who were detained at her majesty's pleasure did not face justice. As Anthony Trollope explained, people's sense of justice and the law did not always connect:

> There is perhaps no great social question so imperfectly understood among us at the present day as that which refers to the line which divides sanity from insanity ... We know that the sane man is responsible for what he does, and that the insane man is irresponsible; but we do not know, – we only guess wildly, at the state of mind of those, who now and again act like madmen, though no court or council of experts has declared them to be mad. The bias of the public mind is to press heavily on such men till the law attempts to touch them, as though they were thoroughly responsible; and then, when the law interferes, to screen them as though they were altogether irresponsible.[102]

Feelings around criminal insanity as a defence stimulated a number of complex and contradictory emotions, and the press was not immune from stirring both sides. In between the most sensational trials that helped define criminal law were everyday sensations that spoke to society's great fear: that lunatics were 'getting away' with their crimes.[103] In particular, in cases of violent madmen there was little empathy for perpetrators, who were seen as hardened sources of violence rather than suffering patients.

The M'Naghten rules (1844) helped define criminal insanity for generations and have been ably detailed by legal historians.[104] However, this decision did little to settle lunacy law definitively either in the courts or in the court of public opinion. As issues like provocation or drunkenness were less accepted by judges, the insanity defence was increasingly used in the courtroom.[105] Such a shift left some to worry about the course of justice. There was concern that an insanity defence might undermine broader cultural attempts to make men responsible for their own actions.[106] Concerns over the lack of accountability in insanity verdicts led to legislation like the proposed 1874 bill to outline what kind of insanity would render a homicide not criminal.[107] The emergence of the sentence 'guilty but insane' points to the deeply held belief that criminal madmen ought to be held responsible in some way for the damage they caused.

If legal authorities were not able to come to any clear consensus, medical experts exhibited an even greater variety of opinions on criminal insanity and responsibility. Doctors believed their role in determining mental soundness was key to the administration of justice. Forbes Winslow urged that courts bring in the most qualified doctors, and that the judge and jury needed to be informed on the details of insanity.[108] Yet throughout the century, medical experts continued to debate the meaning and best practices of criminal lunacy findings.[109] Henry Maudsley believed it was impossible to determine moral responsibility until society could get past 'the theological notion that vices and crimes are due to the instigation of the devil'.[110] And this uncertainty whether even the greatest experts could get it right, coloured reporting of criminal insanity trials. Many papers were happy to report that they doubted doctors' diagnoses and they feared that medical men were being manipulated by cunning murderers in a perversion of justice.

Matt Cook believes that criminal trials 'define the boundaries of normality and ... rearticulate ideologies of gender, class and nation'.[111] The cases discussed below were problematic precisely because they did not help define boundaries, but rather highlighted the uncertainty and ambiguity of insanity. Popular writings on the problem of criminal insanity were divided on whether justice was or could be done for those who claimed an insanity defence. Writing for the *Leisure Hour*, one author confidently stated that many cases of supposed insanity were shammed. In relating several cases of 'pretended mental disease' of men within prisons, the author blurs the line between criminality and lunacy and admits some might suffer some mental problems while still insisting such men deserved punishment.[112] Almost two decades later, an author for *Macmillan's* attempted to defend the efficacy of criminal asylums while having to admit there were likely exceptional cases where a man feigned insanity to escape the noose. However, this author reasoned 'it is surely much better that a man should occasionally escape the punishment he deserves, than that any should be punished who labour under mental disease'.[113] Not all observers were content with this logic, however.

In 1864 a case of suspected criminal insanity divided legal and medical experts, and they fought it out in the popular and medical press. George Victor Townley was tried for the murder of his former fiancée. His case was a local sensation with crowds of people clamouring around the courthouse. Reports on the day of his sentencing discussed onlookers 'eagerly discussing the chances of the prisoner's escape'.[114] Thus, to at least some observers, the possibility of a decision of insanity would have been a miscarriage of justice. He was found guilty and sentenced to death; however, the judge had doubts, and further inquiries into his mental soundness continued.[115] Three medical experts, four Derbyshire magistrates, and three Commissioners in Lunacy all agreed that Townley was not of sound mind; his execution was cancelled and he was sent to Bethlehem hospital.[116] Once hospitalized he was examined by four further experts in insanity, including the medical superintendent of the newly founded Broadmoor and the resident physician at Bethlehem. They found him sound. He was then sent back to prison.

Thomas Laycock, Professor of Medicine at Edinburgh University, understood that this case could be a significant blow to his chosen specialty. 'If men so eminently qualified differ, how can less experienced practitioners be expected to sign certificates of lunacy which shall not be open to doubt? And how will they fare in courts of law?'[117] Debates over Townley's level of responsibility became 'the engrossing subject of conversation in this country'.[118] His transfer to Pentonville prison hardly settled the question of whether justice was served in this case. He jumped over a bannister to his death less than a year after his transfer.[119] Such stories undermined confidence in the ability of medical and legal experts to get at the truth of a defendant's sanity.[120] There was little sense that justice was served in this case.

The M'Naghten case was supposed to provide some clarity in Victorian insanity trials. In the decades that followed, medical experts fleshed out the details of criminal responsibility; however, this did little to simplify or clarify a boundary between madness and sanity.[121] Two cases in 1875 highlighted how the public sense of justice was unsatisfied where issues of criminal responsibility were at stake. In one a man committed a senseless murder but then seemed to try to cover his crime. In another, a lunatic in an asylum carried out a long-planned murder.

John Tierney was working in a coal pit and murderously attacked a fellow worker, Peter Campbell, with his pick.[122] He then smashed the man's head with a heavy object several times, fracturing the bones in his face. Early reports of the event emphasized the violence and senselessness of the killing. Headlines proclaimed it a 'Brutal Murder', 'Shocking Murder', and a 'Mysterious Murder'.[123] The men had worked alone together for two years. They were steady, temperate, and none of their co-workers had noticed anything peculiar about Tierney. Several witnesses had seen the two men together before the violence and there seemed to be no trouble. When someone heard moaning shortly thereafter, they went to investigate and found Peter Campbell lying on the ground with two stones on him and Tierney holding his pick with his face covered in blood. When asked who had hurt Campbell, Tierney admitted it was he and then left. He met several other witnesses as he left and explained to them all calmly that he was leaving; no one noticed anything unusual in his behaviour. It was only when he went looking for his wife at a neighbour's house that he began acting strangely. He asked his neighbour where he might hide as he had 'put the pick in Campbell'. He got a change of clothes and some money and left. He was arrested that evening on his way to Glasgow. When he was charged before the sheriff he was seen as peculiar but not unsound.[124]

Early reports suggested this was not a simple act of murder and an attempt to flee. There were stories among the neighbours that Tierney's mind had been unwell for some time, and there were rumours he had been treated for lunacy and never truly recovered. Media reports did not quite label him a madman but acknowledged this was a strange and seemingly motiveless crime.[125] At trial, numerous coalminers who worked with the two men testified the two had no serious quarrels, and that Tierney seemed quite normal and in control of himself up to and including the day of the murder. Doctors brought in to examine the prisoner found him sane at the moment they examined him and yet 'of peculiar temperament, being suspicious and indifferent'.[126]

Tierney's defence put forward evidence to claim lingering insanity as the cause of his unmotivated attack. In the year 1860 Tierney had lost a child, and multiple witnesses testified that it deeply affected his mind. He had visual delusions, became deeply suspicious, and once cut up a cat claiming it was a witch. His wife was afraid of him and neighbours came in to watch him and protect her. He was removed to Ireland as a lunatic, though he eventually escaped and lived with his mother-in-law. When he returned home he continued to be eccentric, and his family did not trust him, evidenced by the fact that his wife had only agreed to live with him again ten days before the murder.[127] His clergyman refused to give him 'the privileges of religion' because he believed Tierney's intellect was so weak he could not use his judgement, and was a danger to his wife.[128] Whether he was actually insane or not at the time of the crime was the question left in the hands of the jury. In his instructions to the jury, Lord Ardmillan was clear that insanity was defined by 'the deprivation of reason, that shattering of the powers of the mind' and should not extend to a man who was simply irascible, strange, or sullen.[129]

In this case, the jury did not find Tierney met the threshold of insanity and found him guilty, and yet recommended mercy on the grounds that he had formerly been insane.[130] The case divided media outlets just as it had apparently divided the jury. There was enough controversy that the Secretary of State intervened with a special medical inquiry. Tierney's death sentence was commuted to penal servitude for life. While this might have been what the jury ultimately wished, it did not satisfy a sense of justice. A reporter for the *Dundee Courier* believed that Tierney had simply killed a man on a small provocation.[131] In his opinion, Tierney's past lunacy had no bearing on his callous act. Rather, this was a brutal man, quick to anger, who had never mastered self-control.

The *Waterford Standard* thought the jury's decision was 'unfortunate, and indeed, indefensible. Tierney was either mad, or not mad.' The man should have been sent to the gallows or an asylum. The author understood the jury's confusion, however as:

> The law of this country recognises no intermediate states of partial mental impairment between insanity and soundness of mind; and grave difficulties cannot fail to arise, and to complicate still further the already entangled and knotty question of criminal responsibility, if the principle be once admitted that there are graduations in the power of will, and, therefore, in culpability for offences.[132]

Such a decision satisfied no one and left the impression that either a madman was being punished for something he did not understand, or that a dangerous murderer was avoiding the noose because of overly sympathetic doctors and jurors.

There was equal frustration in the medical press about the case, and about what role doctors and the media should play. Forbes Winslow wrote to *The Times* angry at what he perceived as a miscarriage of justice. He believed the miner never recovered from his former attack of lunacy and committed an impulsive act of violence. At this point an execution date had been set and Winslow was pleading for authorities to intervene.[133] This in and of itself caused a furore in the medical community. One doctor wrote to *The Lancet* frustrated that doctors were 'rushing into the daily press' to undermine the case.[134] These were not simply esoteric medical debates, but happened against the backdrop of very real stakes in murder trials. When a trial became a media sensation, it drew on larger contemporary issues and concerns. As Roger Smith explains, 'Trials have the form of theatre; profound issues of human concern become concrete in the individuality of participants and in the shape of the plot as the trial unfolds.'[135]

Other cases directly highlighted the inconsistencies in defining lunacy via medical versus legal means. A patient at the Leicester Borough Asylum stabbed and killed an attendant. The case was sensational as it appeared the murder had been planned. The patient, George Fordham, was a sixty-two-year-old lunatic pauper who had been transferred from a workhouse to an asylum after he became violent and dangerous. At the asylum, authorities noted he made a number of complaints that were found to be exaggerations or fabrications. He was known to start quarrels, and at Christmas had a fight with attendant John Smith over a trivial matter. Witnesses remembered Fordham saying 'he would hunt him to the death, even if it were fifty years to come'.[136] Eight months later Fordham stabbed Smith, gloried that he had his revenge, and declared he was happy to hang for it. At the trial he was charged with murder and found sane enough to plead not guilty. As a patient in an asylum at the time, it is no surprise his counsel urged the man to be acquitted on the grounds of insanity. However, the trial judge instructed the jury that just because a man suffered delusions that were strong enough to require his detention, that did not preclude him from being held criminally responsible for his actions. Fordham was found guilty and sentenced to death.[137] It is no surprise this unusual case reached the papers.

The debates this trial spurred, however, went far beyond the particulars of the case and became a stand-in for larger arguments about criminal responsibility. In a letter to *The Times* before the case came to trial, John Manley argued that there had been an increase in patient attacks on their attendants in asylums, and that this had inspired Fordham. Manley pointed to a contemporaneous case where a patient named M'Kave had murdered an attendant and at trial the judge had stopped proceedings after the asylum owner testified the man was *non compos mentis*. Manley believed that Fordham should face the full criminal justice system and not simply be transferred to Broadmoor as a criminal lunatic. He worried that 'the inmates of asylums possessing strong criminal intentions may learn that their confinement in an asylum does not necessarily exempt them from punishment for offences they know to be wrong'.[138] As the medical superintendent of the Hampshire County Lunatic Asylum, he felt confident in his knowledge of the nature of lunatics.

Manley's letter sparked definite outrage. The idea that lunatics in asylums had been inspired to commit acts of murder against their keepers after reading of M'Kave's case in the newspapers seemed rather far-fetched to the *Daily Telegraph and Courier*. The author mocked Manley's simplistic interpretation and marvelled at the supposed close reading of the newspapers on the part of his inmates. 'If Doctor Manley's murderous madmen are such curiously appreciative reasoners, it might be a moot point whether the physician would not be justified – at least during assize time – in keeping the newspapers out of their way altogether.'[139] The doctor for Fisherton House Asylum was even more outraged by Dr Manley's assertions. To treat the insane as if they were mentally and morally competent was to undermine both the mental health and criminal justice systems. 'The idea of making insane persons responsible for their actions, either in asylums or outside, seems to me preposterous, and can never be carried out.'[140] Yet the outrage surely touched on underlying concerns about madmen not 'paying' for their crimes.

The *British Medical Journal* weighed in with a balanced opinion. The benchmark of mental capacity was a thorny issue, and they knew it. They acknowledged that the nature of the mental disturbance that could justify putting a man in an asylum might not be enough to spare him criminal responsibility. There were lunatics who were judged competent enough to draft a will or sign a contract. Yet the number of certified lunatics who could be called legally responsible was a tiny minority. Criminal acts performed by lunatics were typically the result of 'blind exuberant violence, from hallucinations of the senses, from definite delusions, or from morbid impulse, the veritable character of which is shown by its mode of development and by collateral indications of mental derangement'. The problem with determining guilt of an asylum inmate was that it assumed they had a rational motive and were capable of self-control.[141] Fordham might have had a motive to kill his attendant – but that motive was irrational and he did not possess the normal amount of self-control to stop himself.

Dr Forbes Winslow reached out to the media to express his concern about the precedent set by this case. While all individuals were assumed of sound mind unless legally proved not to be, an inmate of an asylum was by definition not of sound mind. 'A patient in an asylum must be regarded as irresponsible for his actions; he is placed there by his friends for protection and care, and he need not be dangerous to himself or others to be so confined.' Winslow railed against the standard of criminal responsibility that simplified the measure to knowing the difference between right and wrong; he stated that the vast majority of patients would, in fact, know this difference. However, he stressed that 'homicidal insanity is generally impulsive, and the murderer who has no control over his actions for the time being may imagine that a sudden command is given him to destroy a certain person, and after the act he will express contrition and remorse for the crime'.[142] Yet Winslow must have known that it was not so simple to outline a universally accepted definition of criminal insanity.

Despite the negative press, Manley was insistent in his position. He wrote to *The Times* again that he had personally witnessed patients under his care specifically reference cases where lunatics had not been charged for violent crimes.[143] He feared this emboldened their actions and felt there were no consequences to their potential violence. The chaplain of the borough asylum where Smith was killed must have agreed to some extent; he warned patients there not to indulge their 'passionate and revengeful feelings'.[144] Such statements implied that even asylum patients could control their violent urges, and thus were to some degree responsible when such efforts failed.

William Orange, superintendent of Broadmoor, was perhaps uniquely suited to write on the issue of criminal insanity. He felt often the wrong questions were being asked by the court in trying to untangle the difference between moral depravity and insanity. In particular, he doubted the ability of anyone to know whether at the time of committing the act, an insane person would know it was wrong. He also believed courts needed more closely to examine how delusions could interfere with decision-making abilities; an insane person might know something was against the law and yet still commit the act because of their delusions.[145] But doctors continued to disagree about the specific working out of criminal law into the twentieth century.[146]

Given the wealth of opinions among legal and medical experts on criminal responsibility, it should come as no surprise that when sensational cases made their way through the courts the press exploited these ongoing tensions to sell papers. There is evidence of defendants' increasing willingness to plead insanity after mid-century.[147] There was not, however, any evidence that the insanity defence was more effective. The reasons why juries chose to accept or reject an insanity plea were more opaque in the nineteenth century than they are today.[148] There was often a gap between the technical evolution of the insanity acquittal and how this played out in practice.[149] And yet media coverage of the 1870s could certainly lead readers to think there was a problem with the law and its application. All of these stories underscored the inherent violence of men, whether they reached the legal threshold of insanity or not. Such public stories made clear that men who were out of control could strike out at any time as the result of seething resentment or momentary impulse.

The introduction of the verdict 'guilty but insane' in 1883 appears almost oxymoronic. This attempt to hold defendants responsible for their actions even when they were insane demonstrates a lingering feeling that the law should have some punitive force even to those not in control of their actions.[150] Media coverage of such cases seemed to balance the desire for culpability and justice.[151] This verdict satisfied the public in ways that the plea of not guilty by reason of insanity did not.[152] As the *Pall Mall Gazette* explained in 1896, the new verdict made it much riskier to advise a plea of not guilty. When found guilty but insane, 'such a prisoner is sent to Broadmoor, and it is quite uncertain when his discharge will be granted'.[153] The indefinite nature of the asylum stay felt like a penalty and thus satisfied the need for rehabilitation and punishment.

Conclusion

As this chapter demonstrates, the figure of the violent madman was a common trope of Victorian newspapers. Fear of the potential violence of madmen continued into the twentieth century. One article, reprinted in at least two publications, worried about the creation of institutions like the After Care Association which helped lunatics transition from asylums to normal life. The authors worried if they could deal with the 'large class' of patients likely to be driven mad again once back in the world:

> The question of the premature discharge of lunatics is a serious one. To this premature discharge are due many of the daily tragedies which startle the newspaper reader. A certain number of homicidal maniacs are let loose upon society every week, are allowed to return to their families, and remain with them until a fresh outburst of insanity once more compels their removal.[154]

The bombardment of stories, both lengthy and brief, about violent madmen terrorizing their families and complete strangers certainly helped reinforce some of the more negative stereotypes about insanity in the nineteenth century. While doctors might have pleaded for insanity to be seen as a form of illness like any other, it is clear that the public did not see things the same way. Men who fought against their diagnosis were also fighting against these narratives. And calm, peaceful lunatics who were more likely to be victims than perpetrators of violence saw the stigma of their illness only rise. Stories of violent madmen also played on deeper fears of the unstable nature of masculinity more generally, to be outlined in the final chapter.

Notes

1 *The Times* (21 June 1858), p. 8.
2 One case centred on a potentially insane aristocratic woman harassing her nephew; the other detailed a family fighting for the inheritance of a mentally incapacitated man and his infant son.
3 Topics included descriptions of individual asylums, administrative functions, finances, construction projects, and so on. The style of such stories did not lean into sensation and tended to be local stories reported in a matter-of-fact style.

4 Showalter, *The Female Malady*, p. 10.
5 Vicky Long also identifies the trope of the dangerous male lunatic in the early twentieth century. Long is trying to counter the notion that this stereotype largely emerged only in the 1980s through tabloid reporting on violent offenders suffering mental breaks in the 1980s. Unfortunately, her chapter on gender does not extend into the nineteenth century. V. Long, *Destigmatising Mental Illness? Professional Politics and Public Education in Britain, 1870–1970* (Manchester, 2014), pp. 137–39.
6 Wiener, *Men of Blood*, p. 13.
7 S. Sullivan, 'Spectacular Failures: Thomas Hopley, Wilkie Collins, and the Reconstruction of Victorian Masculinity', in M. Hewitt (ed.), *An Age of Equipoise:; Reassessing Mid-Victorian Britain* (Aldershot, 2001), p. 85.
8 P. King, 'Moral Panics and Violent Street Crime 1750–2000: A Comparative Perspective', in B.S. Godfrey, C. Emsley, and G. Dunstall (eds), *Comparative Histories of Crime* (London, 2011), pp. 53–70. The term 'moral panic' is a rich one and largely originates in Stanley Cohen's work. S. Cohen, *Folk Devils and Moral Panics* (New York, 2011), pp. vi –xliv.
9 J. Springhall, *Youth, Popular Culture and Moral Panics: Penny Gaffs to Gangsta-rap, 1830–1996* (New York, 1998).
10 C. Emsley, 'Violent Crime in England in 1919: Post-war Anxieties and Press Narratives', *Continuity and Change* 23:1 (2008), p. 174.
11 D. Garland, 'On the Concept of Moral Panic', *Media Culture* 4:1 (2008), pp. 10–11.
12 L.P. Curtis, *Jack the Ripper and the London Press* (New Haven, 2001), p. 79.
13 A. Rodrick, 'Melodrama and Natural Science: Reading the "Greenwich Murder" in the Mid-Century Periodical Press', *Victorian Periodicals Review* 50:1 (2017), pp. 68–69.
14 C. Pittard, '"Cheap, Healthful Literature": The *Strand* Magazine, Fictions of Crime, and Purified Reading Communities', *Victorian Periodicals Review* 40:1 (2007), pp. 1–23.
15 M.J. Wiener, 'Judges v. Jurors: Courtroom Tensions in Murder Trials and the Law of Criminal Responsibility in Nineteenth-Century England', *Law and History Review* 17:3 (1999), pp. 467–506.
16 This situation was created, in large part, through technological advances and the repeal of the stamp duty. J. Rowbotham, K. Stevenson, and S. Pegg, *Crime News in Modern Britain: Press Reporting and Responsibility, 1820–2010* (Houndmills, 2013), p. 39.

17 M. Hewitt, 'The Press and the Law', in J. Shattock (ed.), *Journalism and the Periodical Press in Nineteenth-Century Britain* (Cambridge, 2017), p. 154.
18 R.J. Barrow, 'Rape on the Railway: Women, Safety, and Moral Panic in Victorian Newspapers', *Journal of Victorian Culture* 20:3 (2015), p. 347.
19 Typical stories of interpersonal domestic violence among the working class were often overlooked unless they featured a gruesome crime, children, or cases of madness. B. Walsh, *Domestic Murder in Nineteenth-Century England: Literary and Cultural Representations* (London, 2016).
20 N. O'Ceallaigh Ritschel, *Bernard Shaw, W. T. Stead, and the New Journalism: Whitechapel, Parnell, Titanic, and the Great War* (New York, 2017), p. 9.
21 Eigen, *Unconscious Crime*, p. 69.
22 Men were discharged at a rate of 1 in 5, and women 1 in 3; many were sent to other institutions, not home. M. Stevens, *Broadmoor Revealed: Victorian Crime and the Lunatic Asylum* (Barnsley, 2013).
23 The popular trope of infanticidal mothers as a tragic by-product of illegitimacy was not borne out by actual court cases. A.R. Higginbotham, '"Sin of the Age": Infanticide and Illegitimacy in Victorian London', *Victorian Studies* 32:3 (1989), pp. 322, 324.
24 For example: 'Horrible Murder in America', *Dublin Evening Packet and Correspondent* (8 September 1859), p. 3; 'Terrible Scene with a Madwoman', *Londonderry Sentinel* (14 June 1888), p. 3; 'Murderous Freak of a Madwoman', *Gloucester Citizen* (18 January 1889), p. 4.
25 One case of a violent madwoman kept in a basement got particular media attention. 'Shocking Case of Lunacy: A Female Imprisoned for Twelve Years', *Belfast News-Letter* (24 December 1866), p. 4; 'Extraordinary Imprisonment for Lunacy', *Birmingham Daily Post* (27 December 1866), p. 5; 'Shocking Lunacy Case', *Liverpool Mercury* (22 December 1866), p. 8; 'Extraordinary Imprisonment for Lunacy', *Manchester Times* (29 December 1866), p. 2.
26 K. Williams, *Get Me a Murder a Day! A History of Mass Communications in Britain* (London, 1997), pp. 47–65.
27 Walsh, *Domestic Murder in Nineteenth-Century England*, p. 3.
28 Tosh, *A Man's Place*, p. 3.
29 'A Wife and Six Children Murdered by a Madman at Sandown', *Hampshire Telegraph and Sussex Chronicle* (19 May 1860), p. 4.
30 'Murder by a Madman at Preston', *Liverpool Mercury* (19 March 1877), p. 6.

31 In this case the exact story was reproduced. 'Murder by a Madman at Preston', *York Herald* (20 March 1877), p. 6; 'Murder by a Madman at Preston', *York Herald* (24 March 1877), p. 2.
32 'Murder by a Madman', *Dundee Courier* (20 March 1877), p. 5.
33 D. Liddle, 'Anatomy of a "Nine Days' Wonder"', in A. Maunder and G. Moore (eds), *Victorian Crime, Madness and Sensation* (London, 2004), p. 99.
34 A. Gabriele, *Reading Popular Culture in Victorian Print: Belgravia and Sensationalism* (New York, 2009), pp. 2–3.
35 'Murderous Attack by a Madman at Erdington', *Birmingham Daily Post* (13 December 1884), p. 6; 'Murderous Attack by a Madman at Erdington', *Western Mail* (15 December 1884), p. 2.
36 In this case, a widow had been looking after a fellow lodger while his wife inquired about sending him to St Thomas's Hospital. He attacked her violently with a knife, and her screams attracted people to her aid. 'Encounter with a Madman', *Illustrated Police News* (2 August 1884), p. 2; 'Encounter with a Madman – Lambeth', *Illustrated Police News* (2 August 1884), p. 4.
37 'Fatal Encounter with a Madman at Kingsley', *Cheshire Observer* (3 August 1872), p. 7.
38 Pedlar, *'The Most Dreadful Visitation'*, p. 15.
39 In one story a man threw his young daughters out of a window. 'A Madman's Crime', *Aberdeen Journal* (10 June 1896), p. 5.
40 'Murder by a Madman Near Derby', *Leeds Mercury* (12 March 1886), p. 8.
41 'The Murder by a Madman Near Derby', *Leeds Mercury* (15 March 1886), p. 3.
42 'Besieging a Madman at Small Heath', *Birmingham Daily Post* (14 March 1868), p. 4.
43 This was a longstanding popular idea. 'A Lunatic's Cunning', *Morning Post* (24 July 1823), p. 4; 'Singular Case of Alleged Insanity: Commission of Lunacy', *Daily News* (21 May 1858), p. 6; S.E. De Vere, letter to the editor, *Daily News* (30 August 1878), p. 6.
44 'Shocking Murder by a Madman', *Lancaster Gazette* (9 April 1879), p. 4.
45 The idea that lunatics could possess a particular kind of cunning was generally accepted by medical experts. H. Landor, 'Cases of Moral Insanity', *British Medical Journal* 4:1 (1857), p. 542; Noble, *Elements of Psychological Medicine*, p. 215.
46 Eigen, *Unconscious Crime*, p. 96.
47 'Murder by a Madman', *Morning Chronicle* (15 August 1860), p. 8.
48 'Murder by a Madman', *Morning Post* (15 August 1860), p. 5.

49 'A Madman at Large', *Lancaster Gazette* (27 September 1873), p. 7.
50 'Exciting Chase after a Madman', *Lancaster Gazette* (7 August 1875), p. 3.
51 'A Lunatic at Large', *The Times* (13 September 1886), p. 6.
52 In some ways this parallels the stigma of the tubercular man who was an essentially feminized figure. K. Byrne, *Tuberculosis and the Victorian Literary Imagination* (Cambridge, 2011), p. 174.
53 'Attempted Murder by a Madman', *Illustrated Police News* (13 March 1880), p. 2; 'Attempted Murder by a Madman at Haswell', *Daily Gazette* (2 March 1880), p. 4.
54 'Attempted Murder of a Family by a Madman', *Lancaster Gazette* (21 April 1880), p. 4. This was long after the creation of Broadmoor that at least allowed the possibility of cure and release.
55 Wiener, *Men of Blood*, p. 9.
56 E. Ross, 'Sketches from Life: The Strange Story of a Madman, Or, a Night of Horror', *North-Eastern* (11 December 1885), p. 3.
57 'A Madman's Story of a Lost Love', *Trewman's Exeter Flying Post* (2 May 1866), p. 6.
58 'The Madman', *The Era* (14 May 1881), p. 7.
59 'Mr. George Leitch as the Madman', *The Era* (22 October 1881), p. 9.
60 Walsh, *Domestic Murder in Nineteenth-Century England*, p. 24.
61 J.R. Walkowitz, 'Jack the Ripper and the Myth of Male Violence', *Feminist Studies* 8:3 (1982), p. 544.
62 M. Cook, *Narratives of Enclosure in Detective Fiction: The Locked Room Mystery* (London, 2011), p. 172.
63 Williams, *Get Me a Murder a Day!*.
64 Barrow, 'Rape on the Railway', p. 346.
65 P. Bailey, 'Adventures in Space: Victorian Railway Erotics, or Taking Alienation for a Ride', *Journal of Victorian Culture* 9:1 (2004), pp. 5–6.
66 A. Milne-Smith, 'Shattered Minds: Madmen on the Railways, 1860–1880', *Journal of Victorian Culture* 21:1 (2016), pp. 21–39.
67 'Another Madman in a Railway Train', *Scotsman* (25 February 1865), p. 7; 'Another Madman in a Railway Train', *The Era* (5 March 1865), p. 5.
68 'A Madman on a Railway: Perilous Position of Two Travellers', *Belfast News-Letter* (11 January 1865), p. 3.
69 K.M. Odden, '"Able and Intelligent Medical Men Meeting Together:" The Victorian Railway Crash, Medical Jurisprudence, and the Rise of Medical Authority', *Journal of Victorian* Culture 8:1 (2003), p. 37.

70 'Struggle for Life in a Midland Railway Carriage', *Leicester Chronicle and the Leicestershire Mercury* (29 July 1877), p. 11.
71 In fact, the keeper managed to throw the razor out of the window before they reached the station. 'A Madman in a Railway Carriage', *Illustrated Police News* (4 August 1877), p. 2.
72 'A Lunatic in a Railway Train', *Illustrated Police News* (4 August 1877), p. 1.
73 'Murder by a Madman', *Glasgow Herald* (16 August 1860), pp. 1–2.
74 'A Ride on a Weather-Cock: An Adventure with a Madman', *Daily Gazette for Middlesbrough* (3 May 1887), p. 4.
75 'A Night with a Madman', *Bradford Observer* (16 June 1870), p. 6.
76 A lieutenant in the Indian Army suddenly turned violent and attempted to kill the steward of a ship. *Daily News* (18 November 1862), p. 3. In the case of the ship the *Jessie Osborne*, a madman began cutting at the rigging of the ship and the crew struggled to contain him. The captain finally shot at him, wounding and subduing him. 'The Alleged Shooting of a Madman', *Lancaster Gazette* (7 August 1875), p. 3.
77 'Murder by a Madman on Board Ship', *Nottinghamshire Guardian* (20 May 1881), p. 2.
78 'Justifiable Homicide', *York Herald* (22 August 1863), p. 1. Another paper lists the same conclusion and provides a plot summary of the events. 'A Ship's Crew Chase by a Madman: Justifiable Homicide', *Sheffield & Rotherham Independent* (17 August 1863), p. 3.
79 'A Night with a Madman', *Bradford Observer* (16 June 1870), p. 6.
80 The story was reprinted in other sources: 'A Night with a Madman', *Trewman's Exeter Flying Post* (3 August 1870), p. 6.
81 R.M. Ballantyne's novella *The Madman and the Pirate* was serialized in the *Union Jack* and published as a novel in 1883.
82 'Charlie, Mike and Don; or, the Comic Adventures of Three Boys', *Boys of England: A Journal of Sport, Travel, Fun and Instruction for the Youths of All Nations* (11 May 1877), p. 371.
83 The title of this instalment was 'A Madman's Freak'. 'The Boys of Kingswood', *Boys of England and Jack Harkaway's Journal of Travel, Fun and Instruction* (15 December 1893), p. 39.
84 L. Honaker, '"One Man to Rely On": Long John Silver and the Shifting Character of Victorian Boys' Fiction', *Journal of Narrative Theory* 34:1 (2004), p. 27.
85 K. Boyd, *Manliness and the Boys' Story Paper in Britain: A Cultural History, 1855–1940* (Basingstoke, 2003), p. 125.
86 Fabrega Jr, 'Culture and History of Psychiatric Stigma', p. 110.
87 'Mad Folk', *Belgravia: A London Magazine* (10 December 1869), p. 206.

88 A.C. Cooke, *Moral Panics, Mental Illness Stigma, and the Deinstitutionalization Movement in American Popular Culture* (Basingstoke, 2017), p. 2.
89 A. Bain, *The Emotions and the Will* (London, 1875), p. 172.
90 'Struggle with a Madman', *Daily Telegraph* (31 January 1908), p. 4.
91 'Horrible Murder in Whitechapel', *Sheffield & Rotherham Independent* (1 September 1888), p. 3.
92 '"Murder Will Out," Says a Time-Honoured Proverb', *Northern Echo* (1 September 1888), p. 3.
93 'The Whitechapel Murder', *Bristol Mercury and Daily Post* (3 September 1888), p. 5; S.A. Barnett, 'What is to be Done?' *The Times* (16 November 1888), p. 4.
94 'Murders By a Madman in Scotland', *The Times* (28 July 1892), p. 7.
95 A billhook in this context is likely the agricultural cutting tool with a sickle-shaped blade used to prune branches. 'A Madman Runs amuck with a Billhook', *Freeman's Journal and Daily Commercial Advertiser* (11 July 1887), p. 5; 'Murders by a Madman in Ireland', *The Star* (14 July 1887), p. 4.
96 'Four Persons Murdered by a Madman', *Royal Cornwall Gazette Falmouth Packet, Cornish Weekly News & General Advertiser* (15 July 1997), p. 7.
97 'Shocking Murder at Kildale-in-Cleveland', *Evening Gazette* (21 August 1871), p. 3.
98 'Shocking Event at Kildale', *York Herald* (26 August 1871), p. 10.
99 J.H. Coverdale, S.M. Coverdale, and R. Nairn, 'Behind the Mug Shot Grin: Uses of Madness-Talk in Reports of Loughner's Mass Killing', *Journal of Communication Inquiry* 37:3 (2013), pp. 202–3.
100 C. Upchurch, *Before Wilde: Sex Between Men in Britain's Age of Reform* (Berkeley, 2013), p. 133.
101 C. Casey, 'Common Misperceptions: The Press and Victorian Views of Crime', *Journal of Interdisciplinary History* 41:3 (2011), pp. 368–69.
102 Trollope, *He Knew He Was Right*, vol. 1, p. 213.
103 At mid-century, fears centralized around debates over puerperal insanity in infanticide cases. The idea that such women were 'getting away with murder' was a longstanding fear. Marland, *Dangerous Motherhood*, p. 197; A.M. Kilday, *A History of Infanticide in Britain c. 1600 to the Present* (Houndmills, 2013), pp. 183–217.
104 R. Moran, *Knowing Right from Wrong: The Insanity Defense of Daniel McNaughtan* (New York, 1981); J. Eigen, *Witnessing Insanity: Madness and Mad-Doctors in the English Court* (New Haven, 1995).

105 Judges were far more sceptical of the plea for far longer than lawyers. Wiener, 'Judges v. Jurors', pp. 499–500.
106 Wiener, 'Judges v. Jurors', pp. 477–78.
107 After a select committee it was eventually abandoned. W. Orange, 'An Address on the Present Relation of Insanity to the Criminal Law of England', *British Medical Journal* (13 October 1877), p. 509.
108 Winslow, *The Plea of Insanity*, p. vi.
109 H. Maudsley, 'Criminal Responsibility in Relation to Insanity', *Journal of Mental Science* 41:175 (1895), pp. 657–65; 'Discussion', *Journal of Mental Science* 41:175 (1895), pp. 665–74.
110 Maudsley, *Responsibility in Mental Disease*, p. 34.
111 M. Cook, 'Law', in H.G. Cocks and M. Houlbrook (eds), *Palgrave Advances in the Modern History of Sexuality* (Houndmills, 2006), pp. 64–86.
112 'Phenomena of Criminal Life: Insanity amongst Criminals, and Simulated Disease', *Leisure Hour* (10 September 1857), pp. 581–84.
113 'Broadmoor, and our Criminal Lunatics', *Macmillan's Magazine* 38 (1878), p. 139.
114 'Trial of George Victor Townley for the Wilful Murder of Miss Goodwin', *Leicestershire Mercury* (19 December 1863), p. 2.
115 'George Victor Townley', *Tipperary Vindicator* (18 December 1863), p. 3.
116 Under proofs of insanity his admission book notes: 'As to there being a conspiracy and justification of his act – and a disposition of mind which would lead him to repeat the act had he the power, also many religious absurdities.' Incurable & Criminal Patient Casebooks, Bethlem, CBC-05, p. 40.
117 'Professor Laycock on the Medico-Legal Relations of Insanity, with reference to the Townley Case', *Journal of Mental Science* 10:50 (1864), p. 293.
118 'The Respite of the Convict Townley', *Derbyshire Times and Chesterfield Herald* (23 January 1864), p. 3.
119 'Suicide of George Victor Townley', *Glasgow Herald* (18 February 1865), p. 3. His admission to Bethlem did note a family history of insanity. Incurable & Criminal Patient Casebooks, Bethlem, CBC-05, pp. 40–41.
120 'Justice to Criminal Lunatics', *Journal of Mental Science* 11:55 (1865), pp. 431–33.
121 J. Eigen, 'Lesion of the Will: Medical Resolve and Criminal Responsibility in Victorian Insanity Trials', *Law & Society Review* 33:2 (1999), pp. 453–57.
122 It is not clear why, but papers were unsure whether his name was Tierney or Middleby. See 'The Cambuslang Murder', *Waterford Standard*

(13 October 1875), p. 4; 'The Cambuslang Murder', *Renfrewshire Independent* (18 September 1875), p. 1.
123 'Brutal Murder in a Coal Mine', *Bradford Observer* (23 April 1875), p. 4; 'Shocking Murder at Cambuslang', *Glasgow Herald* (22 April 1875), p. 4; 'Mysterious Murder', *Dewsbury Reporter* (24 April 1875), p. 3.
124 C.T. Couper, *Reports of Cases Before the High Court and Circuit Courts of Justiciary in Scotland*, vol. 3 (Edinburgh, 1879), pp. 154–57.
125 'Shocking Murder at Cambuslang', *Edinburgh Evening News* (22 April 1875), p. 2.
126 'The Cambuslang Murder Case', *Hamilton Advertiser* (18 September 1875), p. 2.
127 Couper, *Reports of Cases Before the High Court*, pp. 158–59.
128 'The Cambuslang Murder Case', *Hamilton Advertiser* (18 September 1875), p. 2.
129 Couper, *Reports of Cases Before the High Court*, p. 165.
130 'Murder in a Coal Mine', *Bradford Bail's Telegraph* (17 September 1875), p. 4.
131 'The Cambuslang Murder', *Dundee Courier* (27 April 1875), p. 3.
132 'The Cambuslang Murder', *Waterford Standard* (13 October 1875), p. 4.
133 L.S. Forbes Winslow, 'Homicidal Lunacy', *The Times* (24 September 1875), p. 12.
134 J. Crichton Browne, letter to the editor, *The Lancet* (2 October 1875), p. 509.
135 R. Smith, 'The Victorian Controversy about the Insanity Defence', *Journal of the Royal Society of Medicine* 81 (1988), p. 73.
136 *Thirteenth Annual Report of the Commissioners in Lunacy* (London, 1876).
137 There was a strong appeal for mercy and the death sentence was commuted to a life of penal servitude. *Thirteenth Annual Report of the Commissioners in Lunacy*, pp. 40–41.
138 J. Manley, 'Murderous Lunatics', *The Times* (31 August 1875), p. 4.
139 *Daily Telegraph* (4 September 1875), p. 5.
140 W. Corbin Finch, letter to the editor, *The Times* (3 September 1875), p. 9.
141 'Murderous Lunatics', *British Medical Journal* (4 September 1875), pp. 303–4.
142 'The Humberstone Murder', *Leicester Chronicle and the Leicestershire Mercury* (11 September 1875), p. 2.
143 J. Manley, 'The Insane', *The Times* (9 September 1875), p. 8.
144 'The Late Murder at the Borough Asylum', *Leicester Chronicle and the Leicestershire Mercury* (11 September 1875), p. 2.

145 W. Orange, 'An Address on the Present Relation of Insanity to the Criminal Law of England', *British Medical Journal* (20 October 1877), p. 553.
146 C. Mercier, 'Insanity and Murder', *British Medical Journal* (11 February 1905), p. 331.
147 There is some disagreement about when the insanity plea became more successful. White places it 'late' in the century. S. White, 'The Insanity Defense in England and Wales Since 1843', *Annals of the American Academy of Political and Social Science* 477:1 (1985), pp. 45–46. Eigen contends that the success of the insanity plea in the courtroom was more directly linked to the building of Broadmoor. Eigen, *Unconscious Crime*, p. 161.
148 Eigen, *Mad-Doctors in the Dock*, p. 22.
149 J.N. Ainsley, '"Some Mysterious Agency": Women, Violent Crime, and the Insanity Acquittal in the Victorian Courtroom', *Canadian Journal of History* 35:1 (2000), p. 39.
150 S. Walton, *Guilty but Insane: Mind and Law in Golden Age Detective Fiction* (Oxford, 2015), p. 97.
151 'The Clifton Sensation', *South Wales Daily News* (2 December 1896), p. 5; 'Incendiarism in South London: Pascall's Great Fire', *South London Chronicle* (22 January 1898), p. 9; 'Guilty but Insane', *Sheffield Evening Telegraph* (22 November 1898), p. 4; 'Guilty, But Insane', *South Devon Advertiser* (18 February 1899), p. 6.
152 The Queen was one of its biggest supporters, writing to Gladstone that she was happy the new law had been passed and that it would be 'a great security'. Queen Victoria to Mr Gladstone, 23 August 1883, in G.E. Buckle (ed.), *The Letters of Queen Victoria: A Selection from Her Majesty's Correspondence and Journal between the Years 1862 and 1885 v. iii* (London, 1928), p. 439.
153 'Silk and Stuff', *Pall Mall Gazette* (12 November 1896), p. 1.
154 'From the "Referee"', *Worcestershire Chronicle* (22 February 1902), p. 3.

6

Degeneration and madness: inheritance, neurasthenia, criminals, and GPI

> The modes of living which have raised us, so to speak, to the heights of civilization, have carried with them those aids to early degenerative changes which we meet with in everyday life, and which, it is only fair to assume, have resulted from an hereditary transmission, which has taken its origin from some cause, and at some period in the history of man, of which we are bound to confess our ignorance, but which makes itself manifest in many ways in those multifarious conditions of disease and decline which assail us on all hands.[1]

In his text on neurasthenia, Rumler identified a common feeling at the turn of the twentieth century: British men were not what they used to be. More troubling still, all of the civilizing practices of modern life were opening the door to some long-dormant vulnerability to madness. Insanity was a resonant issue in Victorian culture because it touched on larger inherent concerns. Mainly, what was the state of British manhood, was it tenable, and what did this say about the health of the nation? The articulation of such questions in both medical and popular literature points to a deepening pessimism about British manhood, one that coexisted with celebrations of the soldier-hero, the skilled worker, and the idea of the British gentleman as the apex of civilization.

The mental collapse of men troubled a society obsessed with fears of degeneration and national decline. Particularly worrying were those who were struck down in their prime, falling prey to an inherited defect, succumbing to the strains of the modern world, or dissolving under the excesses of their lives. The numbers of patients in asylums increased at seemingly exponential rates. When asylum figures rose at mid-nineteenth century they were dismissed as reflecting those now in care who once would have been ignored.[2] Over time, however, such arguments became less effective as the number of certified lunatics under asylum care greatly outstripped the rising general population, and the problem seemed to increase every year. It appeared that more men were becoming insane, and fewer were being cured. As the century progressed, many worried whether madness was curable at all.[3] And when preventative measures seemed to fail, theorists looked to endemic, inherited, and obdurate causes.

When no other explanation could be found, the weakening fibre of British manhood was blamed for the apparent increasing rates of insanity and the intransigence of mental disease. As Andrew Smith notes in his study of gothic fiction, 'the dominant masculine scripts came to be associated with disease, degeneration, and perversity... from within that masculine culture'.[4] Fears of degeneration embodied larger anxieties about men, about class, and about sexuality. This final chapter focuses on the deep strain of pessimism that ran through medical psychiatric thinking, the real-world implications of this shift, and the echoes of these changes in the culture at large. This dangerous negativity opened the door to the 'hopes' of eugenicists and the age of 'heroic' medicine in the twentieth century.

Daniel Pick defines 'degeneration' as the ultimate Victorian pathology. It was at once a medical and political philosophy that could be used in a number of contexts, from poverty to alcohol abuse, to military power, to crime and insanity. It also connected with broader ideas of evolution and race theory that were central to theories of empire.[5] Not all of these issues are within the purview of this study; yet it is impossible to study nineteenth-century psychiatry and not see the shadow of degeneration. 'Degeneration' was a medical term in the nineteenth century, but it referred to a disease that had moral effects.[6] Medical texts justified popular ideas of disease, and conferred legitimacy on the idea of diseases of modern life.[7]

While degeneration theories exploded in the 1880s, there is a longer history of hereditary thinking that is an important point of origin for histories of insanity. Such narratives crossed medical and popular genres; madness was a key through-line in debates about the functions and meanings of inheritability. These debates took multiple forms, but the figures of the neurasthenic and the degenerate criminal became prominent tropes to underscore the dangers of degeneration. These icons were particularly salient as they highlighted how doctors believed class and gender influenced patients' susceptibility to madness, the factors that caused their breakdown, and the forms it would take.[8] The chapter ends with a discussion of General Paralysis of the Insane, a mental and physical ailment that embodied fears of degeneration, over-civilization, and uncontrolled sexual excess.

Medical and popular theories of inheritance

Concepts of degeneration blurred and conflated medical conditions, behaviour, and action in one theory.[9] Its origins, however, began in models of inheritance developed much earlier. As Theodore Porter points out, 'Heredity had the feel of a deep cause and yet seemed to be supported by ordinary experience. It was similarly scientific and popular, and it worked well with statistics.'[10] Mid-century medical practice recognized the importance of heredity in understanding insanity. The acceptance of the role of inheritance in a diagnosis of insanity was inscribed into the foundational practice of asylums. Lunacy Commissioners were interested in statistics on the potential inheritance of insanity from the outset, and asylums tracked family history along with other demographic data. Such ideas were not limited to medical experts but were also baked into the popular culture of the time. While non-medical dialogues did not always contain the most up-to-date or comprehensive reflections of medical thinking, there was a clear general familiarity with issues of inheritance and disease on the part of the general population. Such ideas were the bedrock of fears that took on a renewed urgency in the 1880s when they were linked to a series of perceived social crises in London.[11]

Theories of inheritance were always gendered, and the implications could be devastating to men and women. Most doctors assumed women were more likely to pass on insanity, as they did all hereditary weaknesses.[12] Such theories tie into larger fears about women's bodies as sites of transmission and disease.[13] Neurological theories often pointed out that the 'insanity of the mother, as regards transmission, is more serious than that of the father'.[14] However, such primary statements often contained more complicated sub-clauses. In the case of the oft-cited Jules Baillarger quotation about women as the key transmitters of insanity, he also stated that a father's illness was most dangerous to male children.[15] Biologists always emphasized that both sexes were necessary for humanity's ascent from savagery to civilization.[16] And as the one sex whose brain was not fully tied to their animal nature, men had a duty to preserve and pass down a healthy mind to the next generation of boys.[17] Men, especially of the middling classes, were held to a higher expectation of self-control in terms of indulging in behaviour that could increase the possibility of passing on an inherited illness. Therefore, to indulge in any behaviour that could threaten mental stability could be framed as selfish and unmanly.[18] Theories of acquired facets of degeneration remained a potent force to argue for controlling behaviour of men and women through the end of the nineteenth century.[19]

Theories of biometry and Mendelian genetics proclaimed their novelty at the turn of the twentieth century, and yet they were in many ways the continuation of approaches standardized in the previous decades.[20] As early as 1846, Forbes Winslow had pointed out that insanity caused by a hereditary disposition or of congenital origin was the most difficult to treat.[21] Winslow's emphasis on heredity, and its negative prospects, would be a consistent theme of psychiatric thought in the second half of the nineteenth century. Daniel Noble's influential 1853 textbook outlined a number of hereditary factors and value-laden causes that could lead to insanity. The range of inheritable traits that could lead to madness was quite broad, and included 'the moral conduct of the parents'.[22] A full-scale theory of heredity and degeneration, *Treatise on the Degeneration of the Human Species*, was published by Bénédict Morel in 1857. He saw madness as a key mechanism in the destruction of families, passed down the generations in increasingly destructive forms.[23] Some of these early treatises argued that characteristics acquired during a person's life could be transmitted to future generations; by changing such habits, there was still hope for change.

Such ideas were not limited to medical textbooks, and by the 1850s many believed that physical and moral qualities ran in families. And both men and women were portrayed as the vehicles and victims of inherited madness.[24] In Jane Margaret Hooper's story, insanity of a most insidious and cruel kind is detected in a young boy. His parents were healthy, but varying types of mental disease lurked in other branches of the family. As one character explains, 'Those who have studied the mysterious laws by which hereditary disease works, have observed that the scourge often passes over one generation, or touches it.'[25] One of Wilkie Collins's early short stories demonstrates how the shadow of inherited madness could cause havoc. The hero explains that his 'family had suffered for generations past from the horrible affliction of hereditary insanity, and the members of it, in my time, shrank from exposing their calamity to others'.[26] The trope of inherited madness was firmly established in popular culture.

One could also find ideas of constitutional inheritance woven into popular advice literature and stories for men and women. The author of one dialogue between father and daughter in the 1850s on her choice of husband centres on monetary, religious, and hereditary arguments. Her father advises her to look out for a mentally healthy partner above all.[27] A fictionalized story of what happens when a man overlooks his wife's constitutional weakness was a thinly disguised piece of didactic literature.[28] It is only after he has four sickly children that the protagonist realizes the danger of his poor choice. He worries that if they survive adulthood, 'these children will have others again, and so their hereditary defects will pass down from them to the latest generation ... I may, for anything I know, become the very means of deteriorating the human race to the very end of time.'[29] The fatalism of these works is poignant.

At mid-century, such bleak pronouncements were at least significantly balanced by hopes for potential cures for insanity, particularly for those whose symptoms were noticed early. As one medical attendant of a large poorhouse in Scotland noted, 'we cannot prevent insanity from making its inroads; but we can, by judicious treatment, allay its evils, and even produce a cure'.[30] Others reasoned that if there were cultural or social pressures increasing the likelihood of insanity, such features could be changed.[31] However, even at the most optimistic of times, there was always a dark shadow over any inherited illness. John Waller argues that the very notion of hereditary disease was the product of a desire to rationalize doctors' inability to treat chronic illness. Building off ancient ideas of individuals' inborn constitution, when doctors could not cure a patient a heritable flaw became a logical explanation.[32] In an era with rising asylum rates and lowering hopes of cure, inheritance provided an explanation as to why cure rates continued to stagnate at the reformed asylum. Men's hope of recovery appeared even more elusive than women's through the public asylum (Figure 6.1). Insanity fit perfectly into larger debates about hereditary determinism.[33]

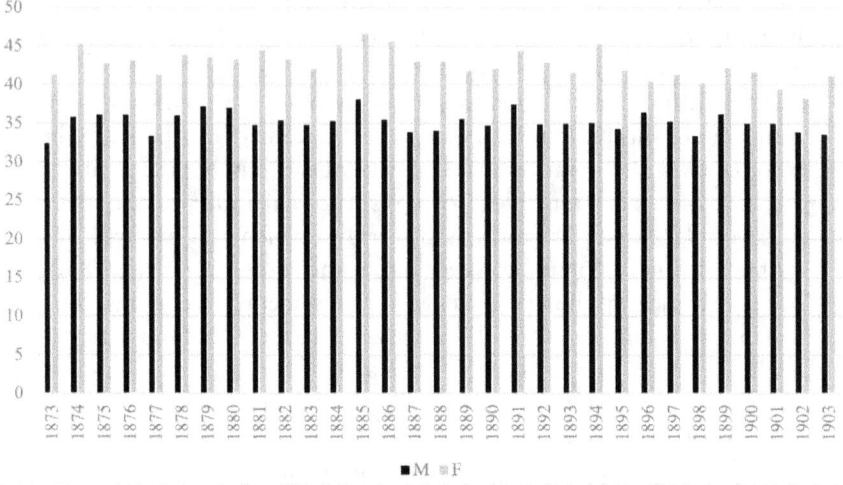

Figure 6.1 Percentage of recoveries vs admissions to asylums

Henry Maudsley was one of the most persistent, and increasingly pessimistic, voices pointing to the dangers of inheritance. Over the course of his career, one can trace a man gradually losing his faith in alienists' curative powers.[34] In an article for the *Journal of Mental Science* in 1867, he traced the history of fifty lunatics, and found half of them had evidence of an inheritable predisposition. He believed that bad habits could also deteriorate the mind, but believed hereditary predisposition was the main cause of insanity. He also began to use the language of degeneration as he outlined the 'predisposing causes of the degeneracy of the race'.[35] One reviewer who was critical of some of Maudsley's more essentialist somatic theories agreed that bloodlines often predicted destiny:

> We cannot escape from the great overhanging cloud of hereditary influences, the fact that moral intellectual traits follow down a race from father to son, or reappear in more remote descendants, exactly as do peculiarities of feature or diseased states of bodily constitution, such as scrofula and gout.[36]

In placing insanity in concert with other physical diseases known to be hereditary, the reviewer reinforced Maudsley's claims.

Samuel Strahan was a barrister with a deep interest in medical theories in the 1890s.[37] He believed that the general public's ignorance about the laws of inheritance and the ability of disease to pass through families was leading to the weakening of the British populace. In particular, he argued that insanity was increasing because people did not understand how the predisposition to madness could be passed down. Strahan saw almost all cases of breakdown as evidence of an inborn nervous temperament or predisposition to mental decay. He worried particularly about men who might recover from madness temporarily, and in their periods of lucidity, marry and beget even more children doomed to insanity.[38] Men who inherited a parent's weak disposition might be less blameworthy than their intemperate brothers, but their outlook was far bleaker. He did, however, believe that for some men with mild ailments a marriage with a woman of solid pedigree could prevent insanity. Women were not so lucky according to Strahan, as the experience of motherhood itself could instigate madness.[39] In a later work he was even more extreme in his recommendations, stating that anyone whose hereditary constitution was so flawed it would end in madness or death should not 'be allowed to contaminate the race and increase suffering and misery by propagating his or her unfitness'.[40]

As Robert Nye notes, by the end of the nineteenth century ideas of degeneration had spilled out far beyond strictly medical thinking. 'By 1900, like a giant whirlpool, degeneracy theory had pulled into its vortex a huge area of individual and social behaviour.'[41] One story in the *Gentleman's Magazine* told of siblings whose mother died insane and whose father was driven insane after he developed monomania. The brothers swore themselves to bachelorhood as 'the likelihood of our ending our days in a lunatic asylum is too strong'.[42] Max Nordau most famously associated fin de siècle literature and culture with mental debility and moral and physical degeneration.[43] One writer for the *Review of Reviews* in 1894 drew attention to Nordau's comparison between the Decadents and insane patients to ask, as many other periodicals would, 'Is Europe going mad?'[44] The spectre of madness was haunting European culture.

Doctors continued to see the connections between urban lifestyles and mental instability, while emphasizing there were typically inherited weaknesses at play. According to J. Michell Clarke, those least likely to recover were those with a 'hereditary taint or sexual troubles'.[45] Some still held out hope that early intervention could provide solutions; but given that that had been the advice for over a century, it seemed unlikely.[46] Degeneracy was a permanent stain, and those labelled as such had no hope. As Albert Wilson explained, while some normal people might suffer temporary insanity and return to normal, a degenerate person could never be normal.[47] Over time, theories of degeneration built off earlier ideas of inheritance in increasingly negative and deterministic ways.

Not made of strong stuff: drunkards, criminals, and neurasthenics

There was no English equivalent to Bénédict Morel or Cesare Lombroso, and without pressing continental fears of revolution, it would be easy to downplay anxieties about British degeneration. Concerns about the state of the British stock did not lead to specific policy changes.[48] However, this does not mean such fears were not prevalent and significant. From the 1880s degenerationalist fears crystallized around two theories of insanity linked to class. While some experts believed civilization was fraying people's nerves, others pointed towards the grinding conditions of poverty.[49] Concerns over particular types of male lunatics became acute: the drunk pauper, the degenerate criminal, and the neurasthenic professional. Doctors debated which group was more prevalent, or more dangerous to the nation; none provided much comfort about the state of British manhood. It is clear, however, that the poor were far more likely to be held accountable for their own demise. While some did note the environmental reasons for working-class illness, many pinpointed a choice of alcohol as the root cause of serious insanity and crime. For the middle classes, hard work was the inevitable, if more excusable, cause of disease. Yet this problem would also prove destabilizing as its cause was woven into the very fabric of middle-class masculinity.

A full understanding (and sometimes misunderstanding) of Darwin's statements on evolution led many to fear that the human species was degenerating into its earlier, more brutal incarnations among the poor.[50] The decades that followed the evolutionary debates were shadowed by fears that society was regressing, and men and women backsliding to inferior forms.[51] This was particularly pointed when discussing the urban working classes.[52] Dr James Cantlie believed that city life itself was destroying its inhabitants' bodies and minds; he pleaded for fresh air and exercise as a balance to hard work as the only hope to fight off the spectre of degeneration.[53] Another doctor from Salford believed his practice proved that the conditions of the industrial poor were significantly undermining their health. He alleged that both environmental and moral causes were driving this degeneration, and that they were interrelated.[54] Statistical surveys seemed to demonstrate that British subjects showed marked physical weakening. Many indicators seemingly signalled a perilous decline, such as that one-third of those who attempted to sign up for the Boer War were refused on health grounds. While recent historians note that many of these sensational statistics rested on problematic data sources, this was not generally known at the time.[55] Anecdotal and qualitative evidence was taken by many as fact.

Echoes of these fears spread far beyond medical advisors. When addressing the issue of endemic poverty in London, William Booth felt compelled to document that there were some people who were beyond help or reform. According to him, this was 'a residuum of men and women who have, whether from heredity or custom, or hopeless demoralisation, become reprobates'.[56] Such beliefs by medical and social reformers helped fuel both degenerationist and eugenicist ways of thinking. The two communities influenced each other, although they were distinct discourses.[57] To the general public, the degenerate was a reprobate who suffered his fate due to his own moral failures. The archetype of degeneration was a 'man of bad moral tendencies and habits, a profligate, spendthrift, gambler, drunkard, opium fiend, libertine, and the like'.[58] Even fellow inmates of asylums could pass judgement on men whose illness could be traced to moral failings. John Weston, an inmate of the Bristol Asylum, had no sympathy for his fellow patient, a grocer who could not break his drinking habits even as they destroyed his mind. Because the man could not stop his drinking, Weston dismissed him, writing that 'he was no man at all, but a donkey and a fool!'[59]

Fears of the self-made degenerate manifested in various ways and were primarily dealt with by social reformers, criminal justice activists, and religious authorities. The most salient strands of this discourse of mental disease among the poor focused on connections to alcohol abuse and criminality. Alcohol was deeply implicated in the stigma of mental illness, as demonstrated in chapter three. However, by the end of the century alcoholic insanity was being reframed from a personal failure to a family curse. And while such failings could cross class boundaries, much of the degenerationist literature focused on the working classes and alcohol.[60]

John Edward Morgan, an early proponent of hereditary pessimism, found alcohol abuse to be one of the top three reasons leading to the unfitness of the working man in cities. Alcohol abuse was particularly worrying as the consequences spread beyond 'the guilty sufferers, [and] are passed on to the offspring, and thus become, year by year, more generally diffused among the great mass of the people'.[61] In his chapter on 'The Curse Entailed on Descendants by Alcohol', Axel Gustafson quotes both Greco-Roman dictums and up-to-date medical experts to underscore the dangers of alcohol on the next generation. He concludes that alcohol abuse is the most likely disease to transmit to the next generation, and its chronic nature makes it incredibly difficult to treat.[62]

Doctors agreed that the alcoholism of either parent could lead to intemperance or even madness in their children. One can find this reinforced in asylum care. In one case a wild and violent boy of fourteen was sent to Colney Hatch Asylum. His father had abused alcohol and abandoned the family, and his mother was designated an intemperate. These facts were enough of an explanation for the young boy's disease. His doctor hoped that 'under care and discipline he will stamp out his terrible inheritance and merge into a healthy and unfettered manhood'.[63] The moral of such cases was clear, however; without intervention, drinking could send the next generation to the madhouse. Later doctors pointed out a susceptibility to alcohol abuse as a sign of degeneracy itself.[64] To Caleb Saleeby, alcoholism could be both a symptom of degeneracy and a cause. In either instance he believed that any man or woman who had trouble with alcohol should not be allowed to marry and procreate.[65] Eugenicists often saw the issues of imbecility, feeble-mindedness, and insanity as inexorably linked through alcoholic excess.[66]

A man who broke down as a result of alcohol was unfortunate, but the results were understandable according to medical logic of the time. And these men could be an enormous source of shame to their families. One can see this reflected in popular culture through novels with a temperance theme. While many stories reaffirmed Victorians' obsession with women's problematic drinking, men remained central to these concerns. Novelists detailed how the slow descent into alcoholic excess and death crossed gender boundaries.[67]

In one temperance novel, the central character, Lucy, plunges into alcoholic despair after a doctor's poor prescription and sadness at her husband's life at sea. Her loneliness leads to drinking that ruins her own life, that of her sister, and of her husband. However, the novelist is very clear in explaining that Lucy's predilection to alcohol was inherited. It was 'her father's failing'.[68] Thus even women's drinking could sometimes be explained by a degenerate father.

Alcoholic insanity could also lead to criminal actions, and courts and asylums alike were unsure of the best treatment in such cases. *Delirium tremens* was used to defend cases of temporary insanity in seemingly random crimes.[69] However, when alcohol was introduced as part of an insanity defence, it was rarely effective unless combined with other exciting causes such as head trauma.[70] Edward Smith was a shoemaker first institutionalized at Macclesfield Asylum in 1876. Authorities believed his troubles stemmed from drink. He was released and managed on his own for over five years. But then his madness returned and he stabbed his wife in the neck. He was admitted to Northamptonshire Asylum in 1883. Once in the asylum he seemed to recover himself quickly, and while authorities knew he was dangerous to others, within a week he was working in the shoemaker's shop making good progress. The medical superintendent explained his decision to so quickly transition him into the workshop as a way to promote his recovery. Believing the man's insanity to stem mostly from drink, once it was free of his system they hoped for a quick recovery. In fact, he was on a list for potential early discharge. This did not happen: on 6 September 1883 he stabbed and killed another inmate with his work knife.[71] Even when patients were weaned off alcohol, the madness could remain.[72]

There was a longstanding idea that crime and insanity were attendant problems growing at similar levels.[73] The idea of the hereditary criminal was a common trope in mid-century medical and popular thought. Such an ideation fed into dominant theories of degeneration by the end of the century.[74] And while Cesare Lombroso's theories were not wholeheartedly embraced in Britain, there was an appreciation for his theory of the born criminal as atavistic throwback.[75] Such ideas were not limited to medical journals but seeped into popular culture, like the *Gentleman's Magazine* author who believed criminality and civilization progressed hand in hand and asserted that the most violent crimes were the result of insane perpetrators.[76] There was a reluctance to codify any action against the 'criminal classes', or embrace the more radical elements of continental criminology; such policies were a direct threat to liberal thinking. Perhaps unsurprisingly, the one area that did have early and aggressive legislation against criminals was Ireland, where the Dangerous Lunatic Act of 1838 specifically linked insanity and criminality.[77] Racialized fears of potential Irish criminality led to more extreme legislation. While the seasoned criminal was never seen as a real source of revolution in England, he was understood as a threat to civilization.[78]

Fears of degeneration were very real in families who believed they were touched by a hereditary curse of madness. Such fears became concrete in criminal cases. Robert Thomas Rippingale was a bookkeeper at a small plaster company who was accused of embezzling from his employer. His defence admitted to the crime but argued mental incapacity. He had a family history of insanity, had suffered a previous fall, and had had a brain fever. The conditions were ripe for mental collapse, and his defence suggested that overwork had triggered his incipient madness. A surgeon called to examine Rippingale stated: 'I found him in a state of intense mental distraction; he was lying on the bed with his hands convulsively clutched round his brow; he described himself as though he felt something in his head ready to burst, and seemed as if he was grasping to prevent it.'[79] In this case, the jury accepted that the man was not in control of his actions, and had not wilfully embezzled funds. In fact, the money was found largely unspent still in his possession.[80] Such everyday stories and experiences made fears of degeneration resonate with a large group of people who wanted to understand how and why happy, reliable family men could become criminal madmen.

Henry Maudsley supported the idea that some habitual criminals were in fact true 'moral imbeciles'. He believed such men were beyond hope of cure, and that they were examples of a degenerate version of humanity. Such men had no sense of morality and their families were populated with the insane, though he made no claims about the level of criminal responsibility such types should face.[81] It is not difficult to find cases that support such ideas, and a system that was not sure whether to treat such offenders as criminals or lunatics. Wilson John was a twenty-one-year-old labourer sent to Millbank prison for larceny. While there he was found to be insane and transferred to Broadmoor. With a history of chronic epilepsy, doctors were not surprised to see his mind deteriorate; his delusions eventually spurred violent actions.[82] William Davis Aen was arrested for housebreaking and sent to prison. He was eventually transferred to Broadmoor after he was diagnosed with insanity caused by a congenital defect. He was calm, well behaved, and worked well at the prison. But his mental state was weak, and he never recovered.[83] Such men blurred lines between criminality and insanity and were classic examples of degenerates.

Men who committed crimes and were found to be insane at trial were held at the discretion of medical and legal authorities. For patients detained as criminal lunatics, their families suffered the double-edged stigma of insanity and criminality in their families. And increasingly, blood relatives were well aware they could now be seen as degenerate stock, as criminal insanity left 'a sort of physical stigma on the family, damaging the chances of its members in marriage, which it is only natural that they would wish to conceal'.[84] This explains why some families were eager to find another explanation for mental disease, such as an accident or sunstroke. The family of Frederick Duggar, a plasterer committed to Broadmoor after an act of criminal arson, was insistent that no member of their family suffered from insanity.[85] While he first showed symptoms after the death of their father, they speculated the actual cause of the disease was a fall in America.[86] While the doctors believed an emotional crisis had triggered an inherited weakness in Duggar, the family was keen to blame a physical accident that had occurred years previously. An accident or illness were the only causes of mental disease that did not carry a slew of dangerous implications for the rest of the family.

Some families preferred the idea that their criminal relative was a drunkard and not insane, believing this distinction carried less stigma (although, as we have seen, experts often disagreed[87]). Philip Dawe, aged fifty-three, beat his wife to death out of the blue. When police reached the scene, Dawe was kissing her before he laid down on the floor. At trial, the man's history of committal to a lunatic asylum was the most relevant piece of evidence as to his mental state. The prisoner's brother, Julius Dawe, reluctantly confirmed that there was a slight family history of madness. He testified that Dawe had recently been released from a lunatic asylum, and that over his lifetime he had tried to commit suicide at least five times. However, his stepson did not believe he was insane but rather morally weak. He testified 'I believe him to be a man of sound mind when the drink is out of him – the reason he was taken to a convalescent home, or lunatic asylum, was through drink – he has been ever since more or less of unsound mind.' He admitted there were eccentrics in the family, yet he believed Dawe's madness should be traced to two causes: 'laziness and drink'.[88] Philip Dawe's family was clearly ashamed of him, but they construed his problems as personal weakness for indulging in alcohol. They rejected the idea of a familial taint and instead found Dawe to blame.

David Elderage was admitted as a pauper to Glasgow Royal Lunatic Asylum in a violent and dangerous state after he tried attacking his mother. Once there he became suicidal, trying to strangle himself. He was released as cured but quickly relapsed and was admitted again after a failed suicide attempt. The cause of his disease was listed as hereditary, with both his sister and mother listed as insane.[89] Authorities would have been glad to see such a man had no children. Family history could pop up and affect even the most seemingly stable citizens. Arthur John Haseler was a respectable watchmaker who suddenly shot a detective for no apparent reason. The official police report noted his grandfather had died of paralysis and his father of 'cerebral softening'. Two of his brothers were dead of consumption and hydrocephalus. To observers it was no surprise his doomed family heritage had led to insanity.[90] These men's insanity and criminality were intimately related.

In deciding on a convict patient's cause of disease and potential release, medical authorities considered the patient's health, the safety of the community, and the class background of the patient. Rowles Pattison was a solicitor, married with children, with no family history of insanity, but he suffered from the effects of drink. He was in and out of criminal asylums as he struggled with his sobriety.[91] What to do next was a negotiation between family members, government officials, and the medical staff. His wife wrote to the medical superintendent after his second detention, hoping that he could be released as she believed his stay had cured him of his drinking. In his response, Dr Orange could not express such confidence. The doctor feared that he was prone to relapse, having relapsed so many times before.[92] Asked to intervene on Pattison's behalf, Charles

Murdoch from the Home Department wrote to Dr Orange about the possibility of an early release. 'I should be very sorry to stand in the way of his earning his bread, but I doubt whether such a skittish animal who has shied so very often should be ridden without a martingale.'[93] In this case, authorities seemed more inclined to give Pattison the opportunity to prove himself as his crimes were non-violent and he was a member of the middle class. Murdoch was right in his assumptions eventually; after almost two decades of independence, Pattison ended up in court again charged with theft.[94] Pattison was given multiple chances to prove he was not a hopeless degenerate because of his class background and pristine family history.

The archetype of the degenerate drinker or criminal was largely classed as a phenomenon of the urban poor. And yet degenerationalist fears were not limited to the working class. Perhaps most troubling to some theorists in the latter decades of the century was the prospect that insanity was disproportionately affecting those of the middle and upper classes. Such thinkers worried that the requirements of modern life led to damaged stock; 'a weak-nerved race of men, in process of degeneration, forms the sign-manual of our times'.[95] A focus on the nerves was a common trait of such theorists, who believed sedentary lifestyles and too much brain work put a stress on the middle classes. Such thinking intermingled hereditary and situational factors, wrapping both in the cloak of degeneration.[96] For the aristocracy, there was an added concern that the combination of close relations marrying and a lifestyle of overindulgence led to mentally weak children.[97] While working-class men were often blamed for alcoholic indulgence or degenerate stock, middle-class men's demise was blamed on the circumstances of modern life.

As John Tosh notes, bourgeois Victorian masculinity was essentially rooted in 'a punishing work ethic' balanced only by the reputed comforts of domestic bliss.[98] Influential educators argued that manliness could only be achieved through hard work starting in boyhood.[99] Hard work as a cause of illness represented a specific gendered and classed problem in the nineteenth century. Unlike many other causes of madness that could be avoided or mitigated, hard work was something only the very wealthy could evade. Moreover, few doctors or public moralists recommended a life of indolence. Early signs of nervous disease included a lack of energy. A sufferer would be marked by '[t]he absence of manly confidence, courage, fortitude, self-possession, [and] a command of the will and the affections, are sufferers from this class of organic disease'.[100] For those who might be found lacking in manly vigour the solution was strenuous, dangerous, and difficult work. This bracing message was particularly resonant for the middle classes, who were receptive to such assertions, often backed by religious authorities, that urged them to channel their masculine energy into the world of work and productivity.[101] Yet few middle-class professions offered the opportunity for any physical activity. Nervous disease was dangerous to the sufferer and threatened the next generation just as much as the animalistic criminal.

The high stress of men's working lives was often identified as a reason for their susceptibility to insanity, whereas for women it was more often linked to their physical, bodily responses.[102] Women were typically advised to slow down, avoid brain work, and regather their energies in the safety of the home that social commentators and medical authorities assumed was their 'natural space'.[103] For middle-class men, by contrast, hard work and intellectual stimulation were part of their expected activities and thus advising their avoidance was more problematic. William Julius Mickle, a physician writing in the 1880s, believed men were exposed to more dangers owing to careers in the military and industrial jobs (where they might suffer physical injury), and the 'intellectual overwork' of professional and literary life; thus they were more vulnerable to diseases of the mind.[104] A man who overworked his muscles would exhaust his body; a man who overworked his brain could destroy his mind. Gilbert M'Murdo, a surgeon at Newgate prison, testified as early as 1850 that *any* healthy man who pushed himself too hard, and who suffered setbacks in his professional life, could be driven insane.[105] Physician John Charles Bucknill argued in 1885 that the wealthy were more likely to end up in an asylum than their working-class counterparts due to their radically different experiences of modern life.[106] Men of the 'respectable' classes put a high priority on self-control and restraint with few opportunities for release.[107] Much of a family's social status was tied up with men's economic labour, and any failure to live up to expectations tended to be interpreted as a failure of character.[108]

The stresses of modern life seemed endemic for the middle classes, and doctors created new categories of diagnosis to address the effects on the body and mind. Neurasthenia, as described by American physician George Beard in the 1860s, and popularized in Britain in the 1880s, was specifically a disease of 'modern' life linked to, among other things, enhanced pressures in the education system.[109] Some railed against the imprecision of the term, with one doctor calling it a 'diagnostic wastebasket'.[110] Its flexibility could also be expedient, however, and it continued to be used in Britain through the First World War and beyond. By the 1880s, psychiatrists across Europe and the United Kingdom had become increasingly interested in the variety of disorders of the 'nerves' that needed their care.[111] Undue pressure of work or study, it was generally understood, could damage men and women's mental and physical health; however, medical authorities were far more concerned about men's overburdened minds.[112]

Victorian diagnoses of mental breakdown were typically differentiated by gender and by proximate cause: women were more likely to be diagnosed with hysteria, while men were more likely to be labelled neurasthenic.[113] Neurasthenia was a divisive diagnosis among brain specialists, as it was both broad and somewhat vague.[114] Symptoms could include headaches, overactive senses, insomnia, distraction, irritability, and general pain.[115] It was a frustrating and often chronic condition, but in itself did not count as insanity. However, physicians specializing in neurasthenia wanted the disease taken more seriously precisely because they considered it made patients vulnerable to absolute mental collapse. In his medical text covering hysteria and neurasthenia, J. Michell Clarke could write as late as 1905 that the dread of madness was so profound that it constituted one of the exciting causes that could turn a neurasthenic into a lunatic. He cautioned that patients' greatest anxiety was 'the fear of breaking down in some part of [their] professional work, which especially affects such avocations as those of the priest, the barrister, schoolmaster, or lecturer'.[116] Hard work could push a man to neurasthenia, and if he continued in that overwork, or simply gave in to fears about overwork, he might be driven to madness. Specialists cautioned their patients, and other doctors, to take symptoms seriously and to treat the disorder in its early stages.[117] At their core, these concerns reflect a perceived vulnerability in men's nervous systems.[118]

William Evans Pope was an early proponent of the fact that nervous disorders were rapidly increasing, particularly among 'the educated and refined'. He believed the 'artificial' way of life and constant uncertainty led to nervousness and insanity.[119] By the latter decades of the nineteenth century, doctors who recognized such problems believed all modern urban men were vulnerable to nervous debility, and any precipitating cause could push them over the brink into madness.[120] Such concerns were echoed over the next decades, with some doctors stressing that advancing civilization was to blame for rising rates of insanity. Anxiety acted 'like a grain of sand in a delicate watchwork'.[121] As one fatalistic reviewer noted, 'we are all too busy, and try too much. Unhappily, there is but little choice in the matter.'[122] According to such logic, successful men could scarcely avoid some degree of mental or physical breakdown as a by-product of their accomplishments. The harder they worked to establish their lives and careers, the greater the risk of destroying all they worked for.[123]

Patient experiences were used to directly echo such points. In the case of one patient, minor symptoms caused by overwork soon became a serious problem. His first symptoms included anxiety, weakened powers, and body pain; the local surgeon recommended rest for a few weeks. He improved and went home but his condition worsened. His family eventually intervened and sent him to Clifton Hall Asylum, where doctors witnessed his further descent. He thought he was going to be sent to the gallows, and later grew terrified of the dark, and believed that wild beasts would attack him in the yard of the asylum. Describing these symptoms to his former doctor in a letter, he explained that laying 'on my sleepless bed at night, I saw, and sometimes felt, as it were, bears hugging me, and demons appearing to me'.[124] An anxious disorder led to serious mental debility in this case.

Popular culture was littered with representations of men living lives on the brink of collapse. The two male antagonists of Wilkie Collins's *Basil* both suffer mental breakdowns after great mental anguish. Basil discovers that his wife is unfaithful and has an almost immediate physical and mental breakdown. Basil overhears to his horror two men debating whether he is drunk or mad:

> 'MAD!' – that one word, as I heard it, rang after me like a voice of judgment. 'MAD!' – a fear had come over me, which, in all its frightful complication, was expressed by that one word – a fear which, to the man who suffers it, is worse even than the fear of death; which no

human language ever has conveyed, or ever will convey, in all its horrible reality, to others.[125]

His rival, after a vicious physical confrontation with Basil, develops what his doctors fear might be a dangerous monomania. The doctor speculates 'there has been madness in his family'.[126] Theories of acquired weakness or congenital flaws were woven seamlessly into theories of the degenerate middle-class man.

Fears of corrupted stock and toxic workplaces helped explain to many observers why the modern man seemed a pale comparison of his ancestors. A former patient of the Glasgow Royal Lunatic Asylum offered his own life experience at mid-century as an example of how insanity could develop. He believed all madness rested on some physical weakness or inherited deficiency; the pressures of the middle-class lifestyle allowed this weakness to manifest. He predicted that 'the more artificial and luxurious our habits of living become', the more madness would take root.[127] He spoke from personal experience as his breakdown occurred after he suffered some family tragedies and became 'obsessed by science'. He was filled with uncontrollable impulses to kill his loved ones, and he was haunted by voices of his starving children. Recognizing the problem, he handed himself into the authorities.[128] His narrative echoed many people's suspicions that a mental collapse revealed a pre-existing inherited weakness that overwork could trigger.

The very habits and lifestyle proscribed to the middle-class man could lead to his destruction. The requirements of middle- and upper-class masculinity included supporting a wife and children in a respectable home through labour in the public sphere. As scholars have noted, Victorian manhood entailed meeting challenges, and pushing oneself to physical and emotional limits.[129] Many commentators argued that the dangers of overwork were greater for the present generation than for their ancestors. Herbert Spencer worried that, despite the fact that his contemporaries lived more sober and sensible lives than their fathers and grandfathers, the pace of modern life and the pressures it exerted were making them weaker. 'We are continually breaking down under our work', he wrote, and he worried that the overworked man might pass on a weaker constitution to his children even if he showed no actual signs of madness himself.[130] Many high-profile men suffered such breakdowns to some degree, including John Stuart Mill, John Ruskin, Francis Galton, Arnold Toynbee, and John Bright, and yet none was so serious that it required an asylum.[131] They would have been considered the lucky ones.

Doctors at Bethlem certainly noticed overwork as a cause of illness in many patients across a variety of professions. The stresses of a bank clerk and police inspector might have been very different, but doctors judged both men to be suffering from insanity caused by overwork.[132] Even in cases where the 'supposed cause of insanity' was left blank or stated as unknown, overwork was often suspected as a potential problem. Thomas George Callaghan was seventeen when he was admitted to Bethlem in 1888. Before his confinement he was working from 9 to 7 every day, and he had been responsible for large sums of money.[133] Other men were classified as suffering from business anxiety specifically, rather than overwork.[134] Families also saw men crumble in the face of financial losses, both real and imagined.[135] The problem of overwork was a familiar refrain of doctors, teachers, and social commentators in the second half of the nineteenth century. It was an idea that preoccupied many Victorians, who worried that the speed and requirements of modern professional expectations could lead to broken nerves, low spirits, or nervous collapse. The masculine work ethic so prized in nineteenth-century culture threatened to slip into a pathology that could lead to madness and death. Such tensions mirror Herbert Sussman's description of Victorian masculinity as 'barely controlled energy that may collapse back into the inchoate flood or fire that limns the innate energy of maleness'.[136] The very habits and lifestyle prescribed to the middle-class man could lead to his destruction.

Nerve specialist Thomas Stretch Dowse compared the modern Briton with 'primitive' societies and found that the latter suffered far fewer physical and mental diseases. He also dubiously stated that Russian labourers and Indian brahmins lived to over a hundred years healthily.[137] Much like the drunken or criminal urban underclass, theorists speculated that the middle-class neurotic was also produced by city life, although he was much less culpable in his demise. There was a broad consensus among the medical community that modernity, and civilization itself, lay at the root of many psychological ailments in the late Victorian era.[138] In his later writings, Henry Maudsley warned that when a society reached a certain level of complexity in its evolution it was bound to sow the seeds of its own destruction. Despite the potential of upward ascent, when any organism 'has reached a certain state of complex evolution it inevitably breeds changes in itself which disintegrate and in the end destroy it'.[139] Maudsley's fears of the dark side of progress echoed psychiatric, biological, and medical theories of degeneration.[140] In most cases, it was impossible to distinguish between inherited and acquired illness.

GPI, syphilis, and degeneration

In his *Introduction to the Study of Insanity* of 1899, John Macpherson defined General Paralysis of the Insane as 'essentially a disease of modern civilization'.[141] GPI was a specific diagnosis created by Victorian medical personnel based on their clinical experience, their scientific knowledge, and, above all, their contemporary prejudices. The ailment is a prime example of Charles Rosenberg's theory about the cultural construction of disease.[142] The diagnosis of GPI was a mixture of symptoms and character evaluation. The evolution of the purported cause of the disease proves Rosenberg's thesis. Early theories of the cause of GPI identified too much work, strain, and doing too much. Such patients were rarely stigmatized, and in fact there was a belief that such a form of insanity only appeared in moral but overworked or over-extended men.[143] And manliness was key. As Henry Maudsley explained, 'General paralysis is emphatically the disease of manhood ... the sole cause of the disease may sometimes lie in the agitation and anxieties incident to the most active period of life.'[144] And yet by the final decades of the century, GPI had become the disease of degeneration *par excellence*, linked to excesses of debauchery rather than productive work. The evolution in thinking about GPI traces evolving fears about men's behaviour and the greatest threats to the nation.

Most physicians believed they understood the symptoms and general prognosis of GPI. Individual doctors disagreed on some of the variances of the disease; however, GPI was understood as a deadly illness that destroyed the mind and body. GPI was officially recognized as a distinct disease in 1869 by the Medico-Psychological Association.[145] It progressed in three phases. First symptoms would include facial and ocular problems, as well as speech problems coupled with exalted and excited ideas. The second stage introduced more widespread mental enfeeblement, and paralysis. The third stage was a complete mental and physical breakdown leading to certain death.[146] British doctors generally agreed that GPI patients demonstrated an expansive form of insanity marked by delusions of grandeur. This florid final phase of madness could also be identified by the general public.[147]

At mid-century, the GPI patient was often understood as exemplifying a mind overworked and overtaxed. Such patients were believed to have too much energy and ambition. Thomas Stretch Dowse believed general paralysis was related to other forms of bodily exhaustion, and that an overworked nervous system led to an incurable organic disease. To Dowse and others like him, GPI was a value-neutral disease, caused by overstraining the mind through work or pleasure:

> We meet with professional and business men, as well as men of pleasure, such as the gambler, and the débauché, who reach the zenith of manhood with a splendid physique, but who, probably from circumstances, are impelled to lead a life of overstrain, and in consequence of this their reserve forces are constantly being overtaxed, brain function becomes disturbed, and rapid exhaustion of the nervous system is frequently the inevitable sequence.[148]

The full spectrum of potential causes of GPI made it an even more dangerous disease to the health of the British nation. Much like neurasthenia, GPI could also be described as a diagnostic wastebasket.[149] The outcome of the disease, however, was almost universally grim.

GPI patients proved tragic figures in the asylum, suffering marked delusions and increasing physical debility and death. Supposed recoveries often relapsed. Robert Connor was a general labourer admitted to Glasgow Royal Lunatic Asylum in August 1868 with a diagnosis of GPI. He was excited and incoherent, and believed he had vast wealth and could make more selling herring. He made a seeming recovery, but within a year he was dead.[150] A lithographer admitted in February 1875 had only been suffering for a few days but his symptoms were pronounced. Alongside tell-tale stuttering, he believed he had untold riches and that he was able to talk to God. He was likely a difficult patient to manage as he ripped up his clothes believing they would be remade into suits of gold.[151]

While asylum doctors had little success treating such patients, the more doctors learned of the causes and types of men who most suffered from the disease, the more they worried.

In the more detailed casebooks of Manor House, patients' delusions were often outlined with meticulous care. The delusions of grandeur were so marked that when patients began proclaiming themselves kings and emperors, doctors immediately looked for signs of paralysis to confirm GPI. Eleazar Henry Moses was admitted in 1882 with what doctors classified as 'typical' delusions of a general paralysis patient. Moses believed his wealth surpassed that of the Rothschilds and that he owned half of St James Square. He claimed to have bought the famous elephant Jumbo and was going to exhibit him for a great profit. He also swore he had eleven wives, and eventually that he had bought the universe itself. He was generally quite happy at the asylum and he detailed his great plans and massive wealth almost to the end.[152] But not all GPI patients were so even-tempered. William Harry Sandy was admitted in 1886 with GPI after an attack on his wife. He too had delusions of grandeur but became angry when they were challenged. Apart from grand plans for hunting and foot racing, he eventually related that he had the power to raise the dead and would do so.[153]

William Julius Mickle, medical superintendent of Grove Hall Asylum, wrote a full-length treatise on GPI. He found disturbing results when looking at the demographics of the disease from the Lunacy Commissioners' data. He identified men suffering at a rate of 4 or 5 to 1 woman, and he believed the progression of the disease to be much faster in hard-working men like soldiers and miners.[154] Most troubling for the future of the nation, Mickle found that the highest percentage of registered lunatics who suffered from GPI were those involved in governing the nation (Table 6.1).

Mickle also believed the disease was hitting an even younger demographic than it had in previous generations, and that it was striking the exact men who were vital to national security. All of this combined to prove to him disastrous conclusions:

> The above impression, if correct, would speak ill for the vitality of the peoples of the West of Europe, as far at least as the disease may be deemed analogous to a prodigal wasting of vital power, and premature senility; the early attainment of old age in the individual members of a race being the forerunner and prophet of its imminent decay.[155]

Table 6.1

Orders of persons	Percentage of general paralytics among the insane
Government of country	24.1
Commercial conveyance	21
Commerce	18.6
Mineral workers	18
Mechanists	17.5
Workers in food, drink, etc.	16.8
Entertaining, performing personal offices	14.5
Textile fabric-workers	14.2
Defence of country	13.6
Learned professions, literature, art, science	12.8
Agriculture	10.1
Aristocrats & plutocrats	7.9
Various	3

Source: W.J. Mickle, *General Paralysis of the Insane*, London: H.K. Lewis, 1880, p. 97.

GPI incapsulated perhaps more than any other diagnosis the fear of degeneration. Many doctors directly linked GPI to over-civilization and degeneration.[156] A disease that could be inherited or acquired through excess was potentially dangerous and destabilizing. With a wide range of recognized physical and mental symptoms, it was easy to confuse with other diseases, particularly in the early stages, and experts eventually admitted it was difficult to distinguish from other forms of dementia even through autopsy.[157] GPI represented up to 20 per cent of British male admissions to asylums, and its results were typically fatal.[158]

Over time, descriptions of the disease increasingly shifted characterization of the sufferer from one who was overly energetic or ambitious to one who was deeply flawed. By the end of the century, more and more doctors saw the GPI patient as a problematic case.[159] And while some researchers have retroactively linked GPI to a fatal complication of neurosyphilis, this was not generally accepted in the nineteenth century.[160] Sexual excess crept into the list of causation, but its connection to syphilis was tenuous and complicated. Doctors only began making direct links between syphilis and GPI in the 1880s; few, however, were prepared to see it as an exclusive link.[161] GPI was commonly listed, along with alcoholism and epilepsy, as an example of a disease of degeneration.[162] There was also an increasing belief that GPI could only appear in a man who already had an underlying condition of weakness, and did not take root in 'healthy stock'.[163]

Because of the value-laden nature of Victorian mental health treatment, doctors could pick and choose diagnoses and their causes based on the general impressions they had of patients. Alfred Downing Everington was a married man of forty-nine with six children admitted to Manor House Asylum in 1882. Doctors noted a case history of sexual excess and syphilis. However, this was all noted in the past tense. The medical staff showed no moral judgement of a patient they described as being 'powerfully' built with a 'well shaped head'. They noted he had all the symptoms of general paralysis, and his delusions included talk of harems and concubines. Yet there was little disdain for the patient they described as being in good spirits.[164] When he was transferred to Bethlem asylum, despite his classic signs of GPI and a history of syphilis, the cause and type of illness were left blank. And he was noted as being of sober habits. Syphilis and chronic rheumatism were listed as equally weighted pre-existing conditions in Everington's case notes. His death several months later was listed as a result of 'natural causes'.[165] In 'respectable' male patients, syphilis was dismissed as the result of youthful indiscretion, and was unlikely to be named the sole cause of mental disease.[166]

Identification and treatment methods varied according to how and where a patient sought out treatment. Bethlem generally tended to classify mental disorder according to traditional definitions of mania and melancholia. In the 1860s and 1870s one begins to see patients diagnosed with 'general paralysis' and 'mania with paralysis' at admission; official causes ranged from money worries to business to a 'hard life in India'.[167] GPI is mentioned in the case of one farmer suffering symptoms of unknown origin for three months in 1877; but it is couched with a general mania diagnosis as well.[168] By the 1890s officials were increasingly listing GPI as a form of disorder, yet the cause of the disease was still not clear; business and financial anxieties continued to be stated as the leading causes. In the case of John Charles Hudson, there were so many causes doctors could not decide. Clearly Hudson led a lifestyle with multiple triggers, including overuse of 'narcotics, alcohol, worry and overwork'.[169] GPI was often simply understood as a disease of excess.

Bethlem was not alone in categorizing multiple causes of GPI. Patients at Hanwell Asylum had business worries listed as the most common cause of GPI through the 1880s; by 1880 almost 60 per cent of Hanwell paralytic patients had ambition, business anxieties, and overwork listed as the cause. There was a real reticence to characterize such patients in the prime of manhood as dissipated, nor did many doctors recognize syphilis as a major cause of GPI before the 1890s.[170] The middle-class general paralytic was understood as a tragic character, whose energy for life and desire to work eventually pushed a man to insanity. However, within asylums that catered to a broader class of patients, one can trace earlier efforts to place the blame on patients even before connections to syphilis were cemented. In her study of Scottish asylums, Gayle Davis found alcohol to be the number one stated cause of GPI between 1880 and 1910.[171]

One reason doctors were hesitant to make an exclusive link between syphilis and GPI is because both diseases were misunderstood. Syphilis had its own long history, identified and named since the early modern era.[172] Yet, despite this fact, syphilis was always a difficult disease to treat and 'cure', as it could often lie dormant for ten to thirty years. Until the 1906 Wassermann blood test, it was not always clear who had syphilis once the tell-tale lesions disappeared.[173] Because of this, many doctors had faith that they could cure syphilis given the right conditions. Therefore, a doctor treating GPI might not think their patient's 'cured' syphilis from a decade earlier was the cause. As Henry Maudsley explained, the disease was understood to have several causes in the 1860s. 'General paralysis is usually the result of continued excesses of one sort or another, but it may unquestionably occur without any marked excesses, and when it does so there will mostly be discoverable an hereditary taint in the patient.'[174] By the 1880s, Alfred Cooper was still insisting that syphilis rarely produced nervous disorders on its own; he believed it required another cause to trigger the secondary illness.[175]

Even at the end of the century, doctors were hesitant to link GPI to syphilis because of their faith in their ability to cure syphilis. Mercury was the most common treatment of syphilis throughout the nineteenth century, and its toxic effects were believed not only to help clear up sores, but also to actually treat the underlying illness.[176] One specialist believed that the majority of cases could be treated successfully if done well; his treatment methods included ointments and bedrest.[177] A Harley Street practitioner with a special interest in GPI left his personal reflections and handwritten commentary on the most recent German medical discoveries. He believed that patients who were thoroughly treated with mercury during the early phases of syphilis were unlikely to suffer GPI. Whether they did or did not develop GPI was also dependent on whether they had underlying chronic diseases, heart conditions, or were alcoholics. Those who were young and healthy he believed would be spared this fate, and therefore could resume sexual intercourse with their wives.[178] He also praised an article from *Monde Medical* in 1913 on the importance of hygiene in the treatment of syphilis.[179] The transition to understanding syphilis as the cause of GPI was a gradual shift rather than a radical break.

Several British physicians are credited with finally cementing the link between syphilis and GPI, including Frederick Mott and Thomas Clouston. George Savage identified syphilis as a potential cause of GPI in the 1880s, but it was one of many potential causes, and he was sceptical of its being the primary cause. He continued to see the main cause as worry, and its classic case that of the 'anxious-minded, conscientious man'.[180] Hideyo Noguchi discovered the *spirachaete pallidum* of syphilis in the autopsied brain of GPI patients that might have ended debates in 1913. And yet theories of multiple causes continued throughout the 1920s. As Gayle Davis notes, 'alienists developed and then clung to a complex and multi-causal concept of GPI which drew heavily on issues of blame and respectability, and on the wider Victorian medico-social concepts of civilisation and degeneration'.[181] General Paralysis of the Insane was a diagnosis that shifted dramatically over the course of the century. Yet throughout it maintained the idea of an inheritable disease that could be brought on by the curses of civilization.

As links between syphilis and GPI became more pronounced, if not exclusive, links to degeneration only increased. The syphilitic GPI patient was seen as a potential threat to the health of the nation because of the fear that he might have passed on his syphilis before his GPI emerged, affecting one, if not two generations of children.

John Edward Morgan in his classic work on degeneration wrote of syphilis that 'wherever the blood of the community is extensively contaminated by this poison, there likewise fears may be entertained respecting the future vigour of the race'.[182] Yet there was real reticence to install any policies to restrict men bringing venereal disease into the family beyond the Contagious Diseases Acts' clumsy attempts to police prostitutes' bodies.[183] There were limits on how public, and how explicit, one could be when discussing sexual disease.[184] At the Campbell divorce trial, when the lawyer exposed that Colin Campbell suffered from syphilis, his father left the court and newspapers refused to print details of the specifics.[185] Even doctors were reticent to counsel men to disclose their venereal disease.

Venereal disease was often particularly gendered as female; Mary Spongberg argues that 'the question of male responsibility in the spread of the disease was generally ignored in the medical literature'.[186] While men's role in spreading disease was certainly ignored in policy, and in practice by many doctors, this was not due to a misunderstanding of methods of transmission. Dr Arthur Allbutt was an early pioneer in advocating for women to be educated about the dangers of syphilis and believed families should inquire about the health of prospective bridegrooms.[187] More commonly, doctors would discreetly deal with their male patients without informing potential or current spouses. The Royal Commission on Venereal Disease (1913–1916) found that middle- and upper-class men went to their doctors for assurance they could safely marry and were free from disease.[188] The medical profession's belief they could successfully treat syphilis led to its continued spread.

Feminists pushed back against this medical culture, and identified venereal illness as a significant problem. They were able to find sympathetic ears among some eugenicists. Combined, this movement shifted the blame of inherited syphilis from women onto men.[189] Such rhetoric reached its peak in the work of Frances Swiney, who framed men as the perpetrator of inherited violence onto women and their children through sexual indiscretion. She writes that woman is:

> The martyr of organised and systematic sexual wrong-doing on the part of the man who should have been her mate ... In his own enfeebled frame, in his diseased tissues, in his weak will, his gibbering idiocy, his raving insanity, and hideous criminality, he reaps the fruits

of a dishonoured motherhood, an outraged womanhood, an unnatural abnormal stimulated childbirth, and a starved, poison-fed infancy.[190]

Such conversations broadened into larger attacks on men's sexuality and the problems of male lust.[191] Elaine Showalter contends that the syphilitic man stood as the archetypal villain in feminist fiction, a figure of contamination and degeneration, and a potent symbol of women's struggle.[192]

While early authors tended to caution that knowledge of hereditary illness could become a curse, by the end of the century there were strong voices countering any support of ignorance. Authors such as Sarah Grand were livid at the very idea that women needed to be protected from the idea of inherited syphilis, and clearly understood its connection to some form of mental illness (if not GPI specifically). While some male critics found her book *The Heavenly Twins* vulgar or offensive, it became a sensation.[193] Two of its heroines end up marrying rakes who threaten to pass on the mistakes of their dissolute lives to their wives. In the case of Edith Beale, she ignorantly marries a syphilitic man, although the novelist leaves some physical clues. Within a year she becomes infected and gives birth to a child with congenital syphilis. Suffering dementia, on her deathbed she is aware enough of her situation to rave against the cruelty of a society that would keep her wilfully ignorant of her husband's illness. Evadne Colquhoun, learning of her husband's illness before her marriage is consummated, refuses to follow Edith's fate and lives chastely with her husband to protect herself and any future children. It is only after her husband's death that she reads on the heredity of vice and truly mourns her doomed husband and rails against women being raised in ignorance of such matters.[194] In such feminist literature, women are painted as society's sacrificial lambs to men's vice and secrecy.

Early twentieth-century feminists pointed to the dangers of marital transmission of syphilis as yet another example of the cruelties of marriage and its dangers to national health. The dangers of marital syphilis were not only a hazard to an unsuspecting wife but also a scourge on a new generation of children. The source of degeneration was clearly placed with husbands' vice as women were rendered sterile or gave birth to deformed or idiot children. In the case of Emma Brooke's *A Superfluous Woman*, the doomed heroine marries into one of the most aristocratic families in England. The reader is only later introduced to the full extent of the 'secrets of the House of Heriot', when Lord and Lady Heriot's two undisclosed children are revealed. They are both seriously deformed, and the little girl is so amoral she one day kills her little brother. The woman's death after yet another childbirth can only be presented as a release. The author not only points towards syphilis, but also to a broader idea that the moral bankruptcy of generations could be passed along. This was beyond simply the sins of the father being visited on his sons. When looking at the children, the knowing doctor in Brooke's novel sees that 'On those frail, tiny forms lay heavily the heritage of the fathers. The beaten brows, the suffering eyes, expiated in themselves the crimes and debauchery of generations.'[195]

Doctors believed that men who were sexually promiscuous could be a great danger not only to their own mental stability, but also to their entire family. Doctors held that a man could transmit any serious lack of control to his children. This played out in a dramatic form in one secret family drama revealed in a partial family archive. Roberta von Rigal (née Nuttall), the daughter of an Irish doctor, married Baron von Rigal Grunland, a groom to the German Emperor.[196] It was a high-society marriage, and the Baroness von Rigal continued to keep her social obligations in England though the family spent much time in Germany. However, the marriage was challenged when their young daughter began masturbating excessively. While this might have been a story of over-policing a young girl's sexuality, it was also a story of her father's problematic sexual acts.

Roberta von Rigal (and her doctors) believed that her daughter's masturbatory problems were the result of her husband Franz's sexual indiscretions. He admitted to his wife that he had contracted syphilis, visited brothels, partaken in 'all kinds of perverse practices', and threatened to do those same practices with his wife.[197] Their daughter's illness brought to light issues that were typically kept secret.[198] Roberta wrote to her mother-in-law in 1912 to try to explain what had happened; she couched her news by saying she knew her husband had been raised well and that she knew his mother would be shocked to hear of her son's actions. Exactly what these were is unclear, but Roberta von Rigal wrote to her mother-in-law that if only he had taken up with a 'demi-mondiane' in a normal way she might have forgiven him. She writes 'But it is the places to which he has gone, the degrading things which he has done, and the lowest of the low levels to which he has sunk, which has dealt such a cruel blow.' [199] She believed that her husband could or would not stop his perversions, that reconciliation was impossible, and that he had doomed their daughter.

Franz later swore a sacred oath at his mother-in-law's grave to stop his activities; yet he did not stop. Roberta von Rigal wrote to defend her choice to leave her husband and take her children away as the only way they 'will at least have the chance to fight against their hereditary curse'.[200] Franz von Rigal took some form of responsibility for his daughter's condition and wrote to the doctor asking when she could return home. Her doctor wrote acknowledging that while von Rigal might feel guilty, his daughter was not to be trusted as she had clearly already 'contaminated your other children'.[201] Roberta, her husband, and the doctor all clearly agreed that his daughter's institutionalization was the direct result of her father's sexual indiscretions. While Franz von Rigal was never institutionalized, and his sexual indiscretions never hampered his freedom of activity, his shame clouded his entire family. This story is a family tragedy, but it also highlights how sexual perversions could be inscribed in the body and become tangled into ideas of inheritance.

At one point or another, the syphilitic and GPI patient stood in for all of the great fears of degeneration: he could be working class or middle class, his disease caused by inherited weakness, overwork, or excess sexuality. Whether acquired or inherited, medical thinkers entranced by the idea of degeneration looked to the future with worry. Many authors emphasized women's bodies as susceptible to disease and vectors of degeneration.[202] Such a focus on women absolutely existed, and yet doctors and members of the public understood men could pass down inherited illness, and madness could travel along the male and female line.

Conclusion

As a government report noted as early as the 1850s, British men's inherited weakness and stressful lifestyles put them at particular risk of breakdown:

The mental activity which belongs to eager competition in a crowded and ambitious country is a frequent cause of cerebral disorder to persons who from parentage or other circumstances are pre disposed to it; and this special influence is, of course, likely to develop itself in proportion as the particular period is fraught with occasions of excitement and fatigue.[203]

Fears of madness, and its potential danger to the nation, did not dissipate over time. The popularity of degeneration theories in the 1880s brought with them intense scrutiny of the health of the British nation, and of British manhood.[204] Theories of inheritance made family tragedies part of the national discourse.

In the midst of seemingly exponential growth in new technologies and the shifting social landscapes of the mid-Victorian era, there were always voices worried about what the rapid pace of modern life was doing to the everyday citizen. What this chapter reveals is a general anxiety that surrounded conversations on progress and civilization, and how later fears of degeneration were tied to much earlier fears of inheritance. Doctors and authorities pointed to two key problematic figures that defined the degenerate male based on disparate class fears: the neurasthenic and the criminal. The general paralytic was assumed by many as an example of the middle-class man who pushed himself too far – the neurasthenic could become the paralytic. Yet, as increasing fears of the link between syphilis and GPI were played out, the icon of the disease became the syphilitic/alcoholic who brought his disease on himself.

Notes

1 Rumler, *Causes, Nature, and Cure of Neurasthenia*, p. 80.
2 Justitia, letter to the editor, *Daily News* (4 March 1851), p. 2.
3 A. Scull, *Social Order/Mental Disorder: Anglo-American Psychiatry in Historical Perspective* (Berkeley, 1989), p. 229.
4 A. Smith, *Victorian Demons: Medicine, Masculinity and the Gothic at the Fin-de-Siècle* (Manchester, 2004), pp. 1–2.
5 D. Pick, *Faces of Degeneration: A European Disorder, c. 1848–1918* (Cambridge, 1989), pp. 2–3, 8, 11, 15, 21.
6 K. Hurley, 'Hereditary Taint and Cultural Contagion: The Social Etiology of Fin-de-Siècle Degeneration Theory', *Nineteenth-Century Contexts* 14:2 (1990), p. 198.

7 A. Bonea, M. Dickson, S. Shuttleworth, and J. Wallis, *Anxious Times: Medicine and Modernity in Nineteenth-Century Britain* (Pittsburgh, 2019), pp. 4, 7.
8 L. Walsh, 'A Class Apart? Admissions to the Dundee Royal Lunatic Asylum 1890–1910', in Andrews and Digby (eds), *Sex and Seclusion, Class and Custody*, pp. 249–70.
9 M. Hawkins, 'Durkheim's Sociology and Theories of Degeneration', *Economy and Society*, 28:1 (1999), p. 120.
10 T.M. Porter, *Genetics in the Madhouse: The Unknown History of Human Heredity* (Princeton, 2018), pp. 58, 60–61.
11 Pick, *Faces of Degeneration*, p. 201.
12 See especially bibliography of: J.W. Ballantyne, 'Teratogenesis: An Inquiry into the Causes of Monstrosities', *Transactions of the Edinburgh Obstetrical Society* (31 December 1895), pp. 281–96.
13 R. Boddice, *The Science of Sympathy: Morality, Evolution, and Victorian Civilization* (Baltimore, 2016), p. 44; P.K. Wilson, 'Eighteenth-Century "Monsters" and Nineteenth-Century "Freaks": Reading the Maternally Marked Child', *Literature and Medicine* 21:1 (2002), pp. 1–25.
14 Quoted in: Bucknill and D.H. Tuke, *A Manual of Psychological Medicine*, 1862, p. 269.
15 D. Clark, *Notes on Mental Diseases* (Toronto, 1892), p. 20; S. Worcester, *Insanity and Its Treatment: Lectures on the Treatment of Insanity and Kindred Nervous Diseases* (New York, 1882), p. 86.
16 R. Jann, 'Darwin and the Anthropologists: Sexual Selection and its Discontents', *Victorian Studies* 37:2 (1994), pp. 287–306.
17 R. Boddice, 'The Manly Mind? Revisiting the Victorian "Sex in Brain" Debate', *Gender & History* 23:3 (2011), pp. 334–35.
18 A.C.J. Gustafson, *The Foundation of Death: A Study of the Drink-Question* (London, 1884), pp. 168, 179–80.
19 C. Lawrence, 'Degeneration under the Microscope at the Fin de Siècle', *Annals of Science* 66:4 (2009), pp. 467–68.
20 T.M. Porter, 'Asylums of Hereditary Research in the Efficient Modern State', in S. Müller-Wille and C. Brandt (eds), *Heredity Explored: Between Public Domain and Experimental Science, 1850–1930* (Cambridge, 2016), p. 82.
21 Winslow, *On the Incubation of Insanity*, p. 4.
22 Noble, *Elements of Psychological Medicine*, p. 234.
23 An early excerpt from the work was translated for the *Medical Circular* in Britain in 1857. Hurley, 'Hereditary Taint and Cultural Contagion', pp. 193, 207.
24 T. Boyle, *Black Swine in the Sewers of Hampstead: Beneath the Surface of Victorian Sensationalism* (New York, 1989), pp. 154, 149.

25 J.M. Hooper, *The House of Raby or, Our Lady of Darkness*, vol. 1 (London, 1854), p. 219.
26 W. Collins, 'The Monktons of Wincott Abbey', *Fraser's Magazine* (November 1855), p. 485.
27 Anon., *Prudent Marriages and Their Effects on Posterity; or A Father's Advice to his Daughter Against Forming an Alliance with a Plain and Sickly Family* (London, 1858).
28 Perhaps too thinly disguised for one reviewer. 'Review of *The Lancashire Wedding*', *Athenaeum* (15 June 1867), p. 788.
29 Anon., *The Lancashire Wedding, or Darwin Moralized* (London, 1867), p. 74.
30 Mather, *Thoughts and Suggestions*, p. 164.
31 Williamson, *Thoughts on Insanity and Its Causes*, p. 26.
32 J. Waller, '"The Illusion of an Explanation": The Concept of Hereditary Disease, 1770–1870', *Journal of the History of Medicine and Allied Sciences* 57:4 (2002), pp. 414–15.
33 H.G. Stewart, 'On Hereditary Insanity', *Journal of Mental Science* (April 1864), pp. 50–66; and Tuke, *A Manual of Psychological Medicine*, 1862, p. 264.
34 M. Pantelidou and A.K. Demetriades, 'The Enigmatic Figure of Dr Henry Maudsley (1835–1918)', *Journal of Medical Biography* 22:3 (2014), pp. 180–88; Lawrence, 'Degeneration under the Microscope', pp. 455–71.
35 H. Maudsley, 'On Some of the Causes of Insanity', *Journal of Mental Science* (January 1867), pp. 495–97.
36 'Physiological Psychology', *Westminster Review* (January 1868), p. 29.
37 Strahan was a member of the council of the Medico-Psychological Association of Great Britain and Ireland and New York, and author of two books on psychological disease.
38 S.A.K. Strahan, *Marriage and Disease: A Study of Heredity and the More Important Family Degenerations* (London, 1892), pp. 4, 85–86.
39 Strahan, *Marriage and Disease*, pp. 112–14.
40 S.A.K. Strahan, *Suicide and Insanity: A Physiological and Sociological Study* (London, 1893), p. 79.
41 R.A. Nye, *Crime, Madness, & Politics in Modern France: The Medical Concept of National Decline* (Princeton, 1984), p. 250.
42 'L'Homme Propose: Dieu Dispose', *Gentleman's Magazine* (July 1892), pp. 1, 3.
43 M. Nordau, *Degeneration* (London, 1898).
44 'Is Europe Going Mad?' *Review of Reviews* (February 1894), pp. 148–49.

45 Clarke, *Hysteria and Neurasthenia*, p. 262.
46 Ash, *Mind and Health*, p. 88.
47 A. Wilson, *Unfinished Man: A Scientific Analysis of the Psychopath or Human Degenerate* (London, 1910), p. 14.
48 Pick, *Faces of Degeneration*, pp. 176–78.
49 Porter, *Genetics in the Madhouse*, pp. 87–88.
50 Coxe, *Lunacy in Its Relation to the State*, p. 32; J. Gayon, 'Natural Selection, Regression, and Heredity in Darwinian and Post-Darwinian Evolutionary Theory', in Müller-Wille and Brandt (eds), *Heredity Explored*, pp. 174–78.
51 A. Maunder, '"Stepchildren of Nature": *East Lynne* and the Spectre of Female Degeneracy, 1860–1861', in Maunder and Moore (eds), *Victorian Crime*, p. 59.
52 The feeble-minded were a particular focus of authorities as the source of crime, illegitimacy, disease, poverty, and the general degeneration of the race. The specific study of feeble-mindedness is largely beyond the purview of this book; however, there was often significant overlap. M. Jackson, *The Borderland of Imbecility: Medicine, Society and the Fabrication of the Feeble Mind in Late Victorian and Edwardian England* (Manchester, 2000), p. 2.
53 J. Cantlie, *Degeneration Amongst Londoners* (London, 1885), p. 42.
54 J.E. Morgan, *The Deterioration of Race from the Too Rapid Increase of Great Cities* (London, 1866), pp. 5, 25–26.
55 E.J. Smith, 'Class, Health and the Proposed British Anthropometric Survey of 1904', *Social History of Medicine* 28:2 (2015), pp. 308–9.
56 W. Booth, *In Darkest England and the Way Out* (New York, 1890), p. 204.
57 B. Luckin, 'Revisiting the Idea of Degeneration in Urban Britain, 1830–1900', *Urban History* 33:2 (2006), p. 237.
58 A. MacDonald, 'Moral Stigmata of Degeneration', *The Monist* (1 January 1908), p. 112.
59 Weston, *Life in a Lunatic Asylum*, pp. 24–25.
60 C.W. Saleeby, 'The Discussion of Alcoholism at the Eugenics Congress', *British Journal of Inebriety* (October 1912), pp. 58–65; *Report of the Royal Commission on the Care and Control of the Feeble Minded*, vol. 8 (Cd 4202, London, 1908).
61 Morgan, *The Deterioration of Race*, pp. 25–26.
62 Gustafson, *The Foundation of Death*, pp. 171–79.
63 Sheppard, *Lectures on Madness*, p. 104.
64 W. Pickett, 'A Study of the Insanities of Adolescence', *Journal of Mental Science* (January 1901), p. 440.

65 C.W. Saleeby, *Parenthood and Race Culture: An outline of Eugenics* (London, 1909), pp. 206, 217.
66 *Report of the Royal Commission on the Care and Control of the Feeble Minded*, vol. 8 (London, 1908).
67 R.R. Warhol, 'The Rhetoric of Addiction from Victorian Novels to AA', in J.F. Brodie and M. Redfield (eds), *High Anxieties: Cultural Studies in Addiction* (Berkeley, 2002), p. 101.
68 F. Spenser, *Lucy's Temptation: A Temperance Story for Young Men and Women* (London, 1896), pp. 30, 40.
69 See, for example: Charles Martin, 22 November 1869, t18691122–76, OBP; James Daniel Rogers, 19 August 1872, t18720819–630, OBP; James Hayes, 11 January 1875, t18750111–145, OBP. As Joel Eigen notes, *delirium tremens* was rare as a defence, however, featuring in only twelve trials from 1844 to 1913. Eigen, *Mad-Doctors in the Dock*, p. 82.
70 Thomas Lidbetter, 13 July 1863, t18630713–957, OBP.
71 *Thirty-eighth Annual Report of the Commissioners in Lunacy* (London, 1884), pp. 79–80.
72 Another patient at Hoxton House whose cause of delusional insanity was listed as alcohol turned violent after a seemingly rapid recovery. He was home on trial pending discharge and suddenly attacked his wife, fracturing her skull and jaw. He had no previous history of violence. *Fifty-Second Annual Report of the Commissioners in Lunacy* (London, 1898), p. 40.
73 Barlow, *On Man's Power over Himself*, p. 67.
74 H. Ifill, *Creating Character: Theories of Nature and Nurture in Victorian Sensation Fiction* (Manchester, 2018), pp. 98, 109.
75 J. Dunnage, 'The Work of Cesare Lombroso and its Reception: Further Contexts and Perspectives', *Crime, History & Societies* 22:2 (2018), p. 6.
76 W.C. Sullivan, 'The Psychology of Murder in Modern Fiction', *Gentleman's Magazine* (November 1904), p. 487.
77 Such extensive legislation was never extended to England or Scotland. M.K. Bachman, '"Furious Passions of the Celtic Race": Ireland, Madness and Wilkie Collins's *Blind Love*', in Maunder and Moore (eds), *Victorian Crime*, pp. 183–84.
78 It would be a Liberal government in England that first introduced the Habitual Criminals Act in 1869, though its implementation was somewhat weakened. The 1871 Prevention of Crimes Act placed more powers in the court for dealing with habitual offenders. Pick, *Faces of Degeneration*, pp. 182–84.
79 'Newark Borough Sessions', *Nottinghamshire Guardian* (15 April 1864), p. 12.

80 While murder is the most high-profile example of defendants being found insane, out of eighty-two Old Bailey trials where men were found *non compos mentis* between 1850 and 1913, only sixteen were for murder. Assault was the most common charge (37), with others ranging from arson (6), theft (20), sexual offences (4), and fraud (2). *Old Bailey Proceedings Online*.
81 H. Maudsley, *Body and Mind* (London, 1873), pp. 128–31.
82 Berkshire Record Office, Broadmoor Asylum, D/H14/D2/2/1/504/1, Schedule A.
83 Berkshire Record Office, Broadmoor Asylum, D/H14/D2/2/1/1320/4, D/H14/D2/2/1/15, p. 17.
84 'American Lunatic Asylums from Within', *Saturday Review* (20 January 1872), p. 88.
85 Berkshire Record Office, Broadmoor Asylum, D/H14/D2/2/1/376/3, 31 March 1872, letter from B.T. Lepaght.
86 Berkshire Record Office, Broadmoor Asylum, D/H14/D2/2/1/376/6, 28 November 28 1877, letter from Henry Duggar.
87 Most medical authorities would have seen little distinction in terms of the hereditary damage.
88 Philip James Dawe, 2 August 1881, t18810802-713, OBP.
89 29 April 1867, David Elderage. Records of Glasgow Royal Lunatic Asylum, HB 13/5/58. .
90 Berkshire Record Office, Broadmoor Asylum, D/H14/D2/2/1/808/1526/4, 24 July 1891, D/H14/D2/2/1/808/1526/11–16.
91 Berkshire Record Office, Broadmoor Asylum, D/H14/D2/2/1/1189.
92 Berkshire Record Office, Broadmoor Asylum, D/H14/D2/2/1/1189, 28 January 1886, letter from Dr Orange to Mrs Pattison.
93 Berkshire Record Office, Broadmoor Asylum, D/H14/D2/2//1189, 21 February 1891, Charles Murdoch to Dr Orange.
94 Berkshire Record Office, Broadmoor Asylum, D/H14/D2/2/1/1189, 22 August 1903, W.H. Nicholls to medical superintendent.,
95 Rumler, *Causes, Nature, and Cure of Neurasthenia*, p. 5.
96 Milne-Smith, 'Shattered Minds', pp. 21–39.
97 Ifill, *Creating Character*, pp. 103–5.
98 J. Tosh, 'Hegemonic Masculinity and the History of Gender', in Dudink, Hagemann, and Tosh (eds), *Masculinities in Politics and War*, p. 48.
99 H. Ellis, 'Thomas Arnold, Christian Manliness and the Problem of Boyhood', *Journal of Victorian Culture* 19:4 (2014), pp. 425–41.
100 Moseley, *Twelve Chapters*, p. 23.
101 Sussman, *Victorian Masculinities*.
102 D.D. Hovell, *On Some Conditions of Neurasthenia* (London, 1886), pp. 3–17.

103 L. Appignanesi, *Mad, Bad and Sad: The History of Women and the Mind Doctors from 1800 to the Present* (London, 2008).
104 Mickle was specifically interested in the diagnosis of GPI. W.J. Mickle, *General Paralysis of the Insane* (London, 1880), pp. 89–96.
105 George Bishop, 6 May 1850, t18500506-1011, OBP.
106 For example, he believed that a poor man could be partially insane and continue at his profession with little effect. J.C. Bucknill, 'Recovery From Lunacy', *The Times* (21 August 1885), pp. 13–14.
107 Tosh, 'Masculinities in an Industrializing Society', pp. 331, 334.
108 Oppenheim, *'Shattered Nerves'*, pp. 150–51.
109 A. Crozier, 'What was Tropical about Tropical Neurasthenia? The Utility of the Diagnosis in the Management of British East Africa', *Journal of the History of Medicine and Allied Sciences* 64:4 (2009), p. 525. David Schuster ably tracks the medical and cultural context of American neurasthenia. D.G. Schuster, *Neurasthenic Nation: America's Search for Health, Happiness, and Comfort, 1869–1920* (New Brunswick, 2011).
110 Shorter cites Conrad Rieger classifying neurasthenia as a wastebasket diagnosis as early as 1896. E. Shorter, *From Paralysis to Fatigue: A History of Psychosomatic Illness in the Modern Era* (New York, 1992), pp. 220–32.
111 J. Slijkhuis and H. Oosterhuis, '"Paralysed with Fears and Worries": Neurasthenia as a Gender-Specific Disease of Civilization', *History of Psychiatry* 24:1 (2013), pp. 79–80. For the most comprehensive overview of neurasthenia see M. Gijswijt-Hofstra and R. Porter (eds), *Cultures of Neurasthenia from Beard to the First World War* (Amsterdam, 2001).
112 Appignanesi, *Mad, Bad and Sad*; J. Kennaway, 'The Piano Plague: The Nineteenth-Century Medical Critique of Female Musical Education', *Gesnerus* 68:1 (2011), pp. 26–40.
113 Clarke, *Hysteria and Neurasthenia*, p. 171.
114 Dowse, *On Brain & Nerve Exhaustion*, p. 2.
115 Savill, *Clinical Lectures on Neurasthenia*, p. 22.
116 Clarke, *Hysteria and Neurasthenia*, p. 206.
117 Ash, *Mind and Health*, p. 88.
118 R. Browne, *Neurasthenia and Its Treatment by Hypodermic Transfusions* (London, 1894), p. 27.
119 W.E. Pope, *Nervousness: Its Causes, Symptoms, and Cure*, 2nd edn (London, 1855), pp. 3, 5, 6.
120 A. McLaren, *Impotence: A Cultural History* (Chicago, 2007), p. 116.
121 Dowse, *The Brain and the Nerves*, p. 3.
122 Review of 'High-Pressure Business Life; its Evils, Physical and Moral, by Henry Smith', *The Spectator* (21 October 1876), p. 1320.

123 S. Colella, *Charlotte Riddell's City Novels and Victorian Business: Narrating Capitalism* (New York, 2016), p. 36.
124 Quoted in Noble, *Elements of Psychological Medicine*, pp. 116–18.
125 W. Collins, *Basil* (London, 1862), p. 166.
126 Collins, *Basil*, p. 281.
127 *The Philosophy of Insanity*, p. 12.
128 *The Philosophy of Insanity*, pp. 21, 27.
129 B. Griffin, *The Politics of Gender in Victorian Britain: Masculinity, Political Culture and the Struggle for Women's Rights* (Cambridge, 2012), pp. 171–72.
130 H. Spencer, *Education: Intellectual, Moral, and Physical* (New York, 1896), p. 259.
131 Scull, *Hysteria*, p. 97.
132 Charles William Brown (1865), Admission register, Bethlem, ARA 26; William Faulkner (1896), Admission register, Bethlem, ARA 37.
133 Male Patient Casebook, Bethlem, 1888, CB 134, p. 14.
134 For example: William Draper (1876), Admission register, Bethlem, ARA 29; Frederick Samuel Roberts (1897), Admission register, Bethlem, ARA 37; Thomas Hough (1877), Admission register, Bethlem, ARA 29.
135 Henry Hall (1876), Admission register, Bethlem, ARA 20; John Jolly (1866), Admission register, Bethlem, ARA 26; Thomas Crosland (1897), Admission register, Bethlem, ARA 37.
136 Sussman, *Victorian Masculinities*, p. 13.
137 Dowse, *On Brain & Nerve Exhaustion*, pp. 16, 18.
138 T. Loughran, *Shell-Shock and Medical Culture in First World War Britain* (Cambridge, 2017), p. 55; M. Micale, 'Jean-Martin Charcot and les *névroses traumatiques*', in M.S. Micale and P. Lerner (eds), *Traumatic Pasts: History, Psychiatry, and Trauma in the Modern Age, 1870–1930* (Cambridge, 2001), p. 139.
139 H. Maudsley, *Body and Will* (London, 1883), pp. 238–39.
140 Bonea et al., *Anxious Times*, p. 200.
141 J. Macpherson, *Mental Affections: An Introduction to the Study of Insanity* (London, 1899), p. 256.
142 C.E. Rosenberg, 'Framing Disease: Illness, Society, and History', in Rosenberg and Golden (eds), *Framing Disease*.
143 J. Hurn, 'The History of General Paralysis of the Insane in Britain, 1830 to 1950' (PhD dissertation, University College London, 1998), p. 75.
144 Maudsley, *Physiology and Pathology of the Mind*, p. 411.
145 Hurn, 'History of General Paralysis of the Insane in Britain', p. 46.
146 G. Davis, 'The Most Deadly Disease of Asylumdom: General Paralysis of the Insane and Scottish Psychiatry, c.1840–1940', *Journal of the Royal College of Physicians of Edinburgh* 42:3 (2012), p. 267.

147 Hurn, 'History of General Paralysis of the Insane in Britain', p. 39.
148 Dowse, *On Brain & Nerve Exhaustion*, pp. 2, 9–10.
149 Shorter, *From Paralysis to Fatigue*, pp. 32, 222.
150 Robert Connor, House surgeon's notes for physician: Male, Records of Glasgow Royal Lunatic Asylum, HB 13/5/58, 1868.
151 James Campbell, House surgeon's notes for physician: Male, Records of Glasgow Royal Lunatic Asylum, HB 13/5/61, 1875.
152 Manor House Asylum Case Notes, Male Patients, MS 5725, 6222. He died in September 1888.
153 Manor House Asylum Case Notes, Male Patients, MS 6222. He died two months after admission.
154 Mickle, *General Paralysis of the Insane*, pp. 89, 66.
155 Mickle, *General Paralysis of the Insane*, pp. 93–94.
156 J. Wallis, 'Looking Back: This Fascinating and Fatal Disease', *The Psychologist* 25:10 (2012), pp. 790–91.
157 Wallis, *Investigating the Body in the Victorian Asylum*, p. 191.
158 Davis, 'The Most Deadly Disease of Asylumdom', p. 266.
159 Hurn, 'History of General Paralysis of the Insane in Britain', p. 71.
160 C.E. Lens et al., 'The Clinical Spectrum of General Paralysis of the Insane: A Historical Cohort Study', *European Psychiatry* 30:1 (2015), p. 1.
161 A.R. Hanley, *Medicine, Knowledge and Venereal Diseases in England, 1886–1916* (Basingstoke, 2017), p. 86.
162 W.F. Bynum, 'Alcoholism and Degeneration in 19th Century European Medicine and Psychiatry', *British Journal of Addiction* 79:4 (1984), p. 63.
163 Strahan, *Marriage and Disease*, p. 107.
164 Manor House Asylum Case Notes, Male Patients, MS 5725, pp. 430–31.
165 Alfred Downing Everington (1884), Male Patient Casebook, Bethlem, CB 124, p. 73.
166 J. Townsend, '"Unreliable Observations": Medical Practitioners and Venereal Disease Patient Narratives in Victorian Britain', *Nineteenth-Century Gender Studies* 9:2 (2013), pp. 3–9.
167 Thomas Lewis Applegate (1877), Admission register, Bethlem, ARA 29; Richard Watson (1866), Admission register, Bethlem, ARA 26; Count Angelo Francois Joseph de Brignola (1866), Admission register, Bethlem, ARA 26.
168 Colin Carmichael (1876), Admission register, Bethlem, ARA 29.
169 John Charles Hudson (1897), Admission register, Bethlem, ARA 37.

170 Maudsley did see some connection to sexual excess, but rather as an early symptom of GPI than a cause. Hurn, 'History of General Paralysis of the Insane in Britain', pp. 85–89.
171 'Unknown' was still listed as cause in the overwhelming majority of cases. G. Davis, *'The Cruel Madness of Love': Sex, Syphilis and Psychiatry in Scotland, 1880–1930* (Amsterdam, 2008), pp. 216, 219.
172 K. Siena (ed.), *Sins of the Flesh: Responding to Sexual Disease in Early Modern Europe* (Toronto, 2005).
173 Even the Wassermann test had problems with false positives. A. Scull (ed.), *Cultural Sociology of Mental Illness* (Los Angeles, 2014), p. 475.
174 H. Maudsley, 'On Some of the Causes of Insanity', *Journal of Mental Science* (January 1867), p. 497.
175 Given that such causes could include alcohol, sex, overtaxing the body or mind, extreme temperatures, heredity, or 'any damaging influences', it is easy to see why it was difficult to pinpoint causation. A. Cooper, *Syphilis and Pseudo-Syphilis* (London, 1884), p. 224.
176 Davis, *'The Cruel Madness of Love'*, pp. 160–61.
177 H. Head, *Syphilis of the Nervous System within Six Years of Infection* (London, 1910), pp. 2–12.
178 F. Parkes Weber, PP/FPW/B.314, Book of Dr F. Parkes Weber, 13 Harley Street. Wellcome Library, London.
179 F. Parkes Weber, PP/FPW/B.314, Book of Dr F. Parkes Weber, 13 Harley Street. Wellcome Library, London.
180 He seemed more inclined to believe it could be caused by sexual excess by men whose wives were particularly voluptuous or amatory. G. Savage, *Insanity and Allied Neuroses: Practical and Clinical*, 2nd edn (London, 1886), pp. 282–84.
181 Davis, *'The Cruel Madness of Love'*, pp. 203, 204, 199.
182 Morgan, *The Deterioration of Race*, pp. 33–34.
183 K. Gleeson, 'Sex, Wives, and Prostitutes: Debating Clarence', in J. Rowbotham and K. Stevenson (eds), *Criminal Conversations: Victorian Crimes, Social Panic, and Moral Outrage* (Columbus, 2005), pp. 221–24.
184 E. Showalter, 'Syphilis, Sexuality, and the Fiction of the Fin de Siècle', in R.B. Yeazell (ed.), *Sex, Politics, and Science in the Nineteenth-Century Novel* (Baltimore, 1986), p. 105.
185 A. Jordan, *Love Well the Hour: The Life of Lady Colin Campbell* (Leicester, 2010), p. 92.
186 She does note a brief moment when feminists and eugenicists highlighted men's role in the transmission of disease; however, she claims it was short-lived. M. Spongberg, *Feminizing Venereal Disease: The Body of*

the Prostitute in Nineteenth-Century Medical Discourse (New York, 1997), p. 143.
187 E. Liggins, 'Writing Against the "Husband-Fiend": Syphilis and Male Sexual Vice in the New Woman Novel', *Women's Writing* 7:2 (2000), p. 179.
188 L. Bland, *Banishing the Beast: Feminism, Sex and Morality* (London, 2002), p. 236.
189 Spongberg, *Feminizing Venereal Disease*, pp. 143–44.
190 F. Swiney, *The Bar of Isis, or The Law of the Mother* (London, 1907), pp. 38–39.
191 L.A. Hall, 'The Next Generation: Stella Browne, the New Woman as Freewoman', in A. Richardson and C. Willis (eds), *The New Woman in Fiction and Fact: Fin-de-Siècle Feminisms* (Houndmills, 2001), pp. 233–34.
192 Showalter, 'Syphilis, Sexuality, and the Fiction of the Fin de Siècle', p. 88.
193 M. Bonnell, 'The Legacy of Sarah Grand's *The Heavenly Twins*: A Review Essay', *English Literature in Transition* 36:4 (1993), pp. 470–74.
194 S. Grand, *The Heavenly Twins* (Leipzig, 1894), pp. 398–99.
195 E.F. Brooke, *A Superfluous Woman* (New York, 1894), pp. 270–78.
196 'Town and County News', *Cambridge Independent Press* (13 December 1901), p. 5.
197 Declaration from Hilda F. Chater, 3 March 1914, GC/76/9. Wellcome Library, London.
198 Letter from Franz von Rigal, 10 December 1913, GC/76/8. Wellcome Library, London.
199 Copy of letter from Roberta von Rigal to her 'Omi', 16 February 1912, GC/76/7. Wellcome Library, London.
200 Copy of letter from Roberta von Rigal to her 'Omi', 16 February 1912, GC/76/7. Wellcome Library, London.
201 Copy of Dr Harry Corner's letter to Franz Rigal, 26 January 1913, GC/76/6/8. Wellcome Library, London.
202 Spongberg, *Feminizing Venereal Disease*, p. 1.
203 General Board of Health, *Papers Relative to Sanitary State of People in England* (Cm 2415, 1857–8), pp. xl–xli.
204 M. Härmänmaa and C. Nissen (eds), *Decadence, Degeneration, and the End: Studies in the European Fin de Siècle* (Houndmills, 2014); D.L. Silverman, *Art Nouveau in Fin-de-Siecle France: Politics, Psychology, and Style* (Berkeley, 1989); E. Sutton, *Aubrey Beardsley and British Wagnerism in the 1890s* (Oxford, 2001).

Epilogue

'There's, of course, shell shocks', he said. 'General collapse. Nerves simply give way – can't stand it. The wear and the strain, and the noise, the horror and the rest of it–'

'They come home like this–' We had stepped by one of the cots where a man was lying with his face turned straight toward the light. His eyes were closed, his thin, nerveless hands lay, palms upward, on the gray blanket. The slender veins in his wrists showed very clear.

'He's been like that perhaps for days', the doctor said. 'Doesn't see, doesn't hear, doesn't feel. Absolutely unconscious. Total collapse.'

'Yes, oh, yes, he'll be all right. It's just time, you know. Time and care and patience. Like any other shock – only ten thousand times greater. It's wonderful to see how their memory comes back, slowly, slowly ... You wouldn't believe what man can live through. You wouldn't believe it – it's only flesh and bone, after all, you know.'[1]

The rather animated doctor leading a young reporter through his medical train was used to its sights. The shrapnel cases, amputations, and serious injuries were his primary concern, and he walked past the shock cases without having to intervene. His attitude towards these men embodied the stiff upper lip of military-medical thinking. He did not judge the men for breaking down particularly, but he did frame their illness as a nervous response to intense trauma. The language he uses is remarkably like the terminology familiar to any Victorian medical man. An understanding of nerves, the concept of collapse as a response to an overwhelming situation, and even the chipper optimism that such men would recover with some rest and gentle care in England.[2] Should a soldier not recover, it would be classed as the man's own failure of will or inborn constitution.

The reporter, Jane Anderson, embodies other Victorian tropes of illness in her response to the soldiers. She emphasizes the frailness of the shell-shocked man with his 'slender' veins and his 'nerveless' hands. His helpless pose, passive, almost in prayer, places him as a quiet victim – a sacrifice to the war machine. His vulnerability makes him sympathetic, but it also renders him childlike, if not effeminate.[3] Pity was an emasculating emotion, and injured and disabled men were well aware of that.[4] The doctor leads Anderson through the train looking at his patients, telling stories of heroic surgeries and narrow escapes from Zeppelin attacks. She wonders at how the patients were 'so pitiful and so happy. And I think that they, too, were sometimes filled with wonder.'[5] Not only does Anderson fully accept the doctor's optimistic and heroic portrayal of himself and his work, but she also shares his ideas of shell-shocked soldiers with all of her newspaper readers.

The First World War was not as radically disruptive to theories of mental health as one might assume. And while Anna Loutfi argues that the Boer War started a process where men's nervous disorders were seen as proof of men's failures, these foundations were clearly being laid by narratives of shame and degeneration in the nineteenth century.[6] Pre-war thinking largely shaped medical and military authorities' approaches to shell shock.[7] One can still see Victorian diagnoses like 'neurasthenia' at the forefront of diagnostic debates.[8] And as Mark Humphries argues:

> The realization that specialist treatment had failed to achieve its promise set off a broad discussion within the neurological and psychiatric professions about the nature of nervous illness and its treatability. After much soul searching, most mainstream neurologists and even some psychologists rationalized an explanation that protected their claims to special expertise, falling back on the older argument that nervousness was a heritable trait, linking it to degeneracy.[9]

Works such as Paul Lerner's that study psychiatric trauma from the late nineteenth century through to the 1930s demonstrate how important it is to place wartime psychiatry within its larger contexts, including cultural understandings of mental illness.[10] Tracey Loughran's recent work attempts to place the diagnostic practice of shell shock within its longer medical history by looking at medical journals and contemporary publications on neurology and psychology.[11] Yet the scholarship on shell shock is so robust and impressive that it is easy to imagine that authorities discovered men's mental health for the first time in the trenches of Europe in 1914.[12]

The cultural narratives born out of degeneration fears of the 1880s did not disappear in the crucible of war. Concerns only mounted that a man whose mind broke down was culpable for his illness either through moral failure or weak genetic stock. And this was as true in medical as in lay literature; both doctors and patients alike often viewed shell shock as unmanly.[13] This should come as no surprise as historians emphasize the continuity between Edwardian and wartime masculine values.[14] And more work needs to be done to connect how publicly circulating ideas of manliness related to the actual behaviour and lived experiences of individual men after the war.[15] The war certainly focused attention on military and domestic ideals of masculine endurance and mental stability.[16] As the shell-shocked veteran garnered the most contemporary and historical attention, those whose mental illness was severe enough to be labelled lunatics were largely overlooked. Yet, as Peter Barham notes, men who were sent to asylums during and after the First World War helped cement a wider knowledge of mental illness, and public interest in patients' rights.[17] But the asylums they faced were hardly improvements on their Victorian predecessors; in many ways they were even more crowded and less curative.

It is easy to see the dramatic interventions of early twentieth-century psychiatry and perceive a radical break with previous practices and forms of knowledge. While the Lunacy Act of 1890 undermined psychiatry's jurisdiction and dismantled the system of private asylums, in the decades that followed the profession successfully responded to the challenge. In fact, psychiatrists reimagined themselves as key figures in early treatments of mental disorder, reified in the Mental Treatment Act of 1930. They responded to a potential crisis in their status by expanding voluntary admission for the wealthy, focusing on retaining high-paying patients and decreasing charitable admissions in their institutions.[18] A number of important innovations in the early twentieth century, from the identification of diseases like schizophrenia and tertiary syphilis to the rise of Freud and psychoanalysis, helped mind doctors retain relevance.[19] But there also continued to be a disconnect between cutting-edge medical thinking and lay beliefs, just as there was in the nineteenth century. And even among experts, the tropes of Victorian psychiatry were repeated; in the early twentieth century, talks at the Medico-Legal society still heralded a focus on early treatment and prevention as key to success.[20] This had been the beating heart of Victorian psychiatric thinking. There is no watershed moment in early twentieth-century psychiatry that ends Victorian ways of thinking, and patients admitted in the nineteenth century continued as patients well into the twentieth century. The legacies of Victorian society continued into the twentieth century, though often in their darkest and most cynical forms. Theories of degeneration hardened into eugenics. Somatic theories led to horrific psychosurgeries that may never have been contemplated without late Victorian pessimism about asylum care.

Alfred Fuller was placed under asylum care in October 1867 by his mother. He was twenty-one and suffering his first attack of insanity. The illness came on suddenly, and the young man was apprehended by police in Bath as a wandering lunatic. He was described as always being of a 'weak mind', but his violent delusions came on unexpectedly, and the police found him excitedly swearing and rambling about Napoleon. He was institutionalized and over the decades was a patient at several institutions. In 1927 he was living at the Somerset and Bath Asylum. His medical certificate told a grim story. 'With respect to Mental State he is suffering from Dementia. He is mentally enfeebled, lost, confused, and unable to give any account of himself. He is confined to bed, wet & dirty & resistive to examination.'[21] Fuller spent most of his life in care, entering the system as a young man at the height of Victorian psychiatric philosophy. He lived through the growing fears of degeneration and eugenics with little change to his care or treatment. He became an old man during the Great War, and as soldiers came home ravaged by shell shock, he was confined to bed, unaware of his surroundings or himself. While this book ends in 1914, there was no hard and fast break between Victorian and modern psychiatry for those living in the system.

I do not wish to argue that mental illness exists stripped from time, or that the material circumstances and regimes of care did not change over time. Quite the opposite. Rather, ideas of mental disease are 'glued together by the practices, technologies, and narratives with which it is diagnosed, studied, treated, and represented and by the various interests, institutions, and moral arguments that mobilized these efforts and resources'.[22] Understandings of disease are rooted in specific historical cultures that shift gradually over time. Cutting-edge medical thinking often coexisted with popular ideas from the generation before; and primary care physicians were more unlikely to be up to date on modern research and innovation. This continuity is particularly important in unpacking gendered understandings of men's mental health into the twentieth century.

The brutality of the First World War was long understood as a horrifying, emasculating experience for soldiers. It was difficult to pull untarnished heroism out of the mud and death of the trenches. According to Eric Leed's ground-breaking study on soldier identity, the First World War represented a fundamental break with pre-war masculine identities. Men were alienated from the very loved ones for whom they were fighting.[23] Yet, as more recent scholarship has noted, there was much continuity between Victorian, Edwardian, and early twentieth-century ideals of manhood. As Jessica Meyer notes, men who fought for King and country often embraced a heroic ideal of the soldier-warrior and comrade-in-arms. The war made others yearn for the comforts of home, and their roles as husbands and fathers.[24] This was no less true for disabled veterans who largely accepted that they were supposed to suffer in silence and control their emotions.[25] The cultural purview of the soldier-hero and the paterfamilias survived the war even as new icons emerged. Shell shock would not have proven so challenging for veterans to deal with had they not been shaped by earlier ideals of male mental health and illness.

Notes

1 J. Anderson, 'On the Great White Hospital Train – —Going Home to Die', in F.T. Miller (ed.), *True Stories of the Great War*, vol. 4 (New York, 1917), pp. 321–22.
2 Psychologists who put more emphasis on shell shock as a failure of the will had a less sympathetic approach and would have seen the ill man as culpable in his own breakdown. J. Bourke, *Dismembering the Male: Men's Bodies, Britain and the Great War* (Chicago, 1996), pp. 117–18.

3 D. Serlin, 'Introduction', in K.M. Brian and J.W. Trent Jr, (eds), *Phallacies: Historical Intersections of Disability and Masculinity*, (New York, 2017), p. 9.
4 W. Gagen, 'Remastering the Body, Renegotiating Gender: Physical Disability and Masculinity During the First World War, the Case of J. B. Middlebrook', *European Review of History* 14:4 (2007), p. 537.
5 Anderson, 'On the Great White Hospital Train', p. 332.
6 A. Loutfi, 'Eugenic Nationalism, Biopolitics, and the Masculinization of Hysteria: Historical and Theoretical Reflections', in S. Wendt and P.D. Andersen (eds), *Masculinities and the Nation in the Modern World: Between Hegemony and Marginalization* (New York, 2015), p. 63.
7 T. Loughran, 'A Crisis of Masculinity? Re-writing the History of Shell-Shock and Gender in First World War Britain', *History Compass* 11:9 (2019), p. 730; Loughran, *Shell-Shock and Medical Culture*.
8 Gijswijt-Hofstra and Porter (eds), *Cultures of Neurasthenia*; A.D. Macleod, 'Abrupt Treatments of Hysteria During World War I, 1914–18', *History of Psychiatry* 29:2 (2018), pp. 187–98; W. Jones, 'Psychiatric Battle Casualties: An Intra- and Interwar Comparison', *British Journal of Psychiatry* 178:3 (2001), pp. 242–47.
9 M.O. Humphries, *A Weary Road: Shell Shock in the Canadian Expeditionary Force, 1914–1918* (Toronto, 2018), p. 324.
10 P. Lerner, *Hysterical Men: War, Psychiatry, and the Politics of Trauma in Germany, 1890–1930* (Ithaca, 2003).
11 T. Loughran, 'Hysteria and Neurasthenia in Pre-1914 British Medical Discourse and in Histories of Shell-Shock', *History of Psychiatry* 19:1 (2008), pp. 25–46; T. Loughran, 'Shell Shock, Trauma, and the First World War: The Making of a Diagnosis and Its Histories', *Journal of the History of Medicine and Allied Sciences* 67:1 (2012), pp. 94–119; Loughran, *Shell-Shock and Medical Culture*.
12 Y. Bhattacharjee, 'Shell Shock Revisited: Solving the Puzzle of Blast Trauma', *Science* 319:5862 (2008), pp. 406–8; C. Feudtner, '"Minds the Dead Have Ravished": Shell Shock, History, and the Ecology of Disease-Systems', *History of Science* 31:94 (1993), pp. 377–420; P. Leese, *Shell Shock: Traumatic Neurosis and the British Soldiers of the First World War* (New York, 2002); F. Reid, *Broken Men: Shell Shock, Treatment and Recovery in Britain 1914–30* (New York, 2010); B. Shephard, *A War of Nerves: Soldiers and Psychiatrists in the Twentieth Century* (Boston, 2003).
13 J. Bourke, 'Effeminacy, Ethnicity and the End of Trauma: The Sufferings of "Shell-Shocked" Men in Great Britain and Ireland, 1914–1939', *Journal of Contemporary History* 35:1 (2000), p. 59.

14 G. Mosse, *The Image of Man: The Creation of Modern Masculinity* (New York, 1996), pp. 108–13; Bourke, *Dismembering the Male*, pp. 115–18.
15 M. Roper, 'Between Manliness and Masculinity: The "War Generation" and the Psychology of Fear in Britain, 1914–1950', *Journal of British Studies* 44:2 (2005), p. 345.
16 J. Meyer, *Men of War: Masculinity and the First World War in Britain* (Basingstoke, 2009).
17 P. Barham, *Forgotten Lunatics of the Great War* (New Haven, 2004).
18 Takabayashi, 'Surviving the Lunacy Act of 1890', pp. 249, 258.
19 R. Noll, *American Madness: The Rise and Fall of Dementia Praecox* (Boston, 2011); A. Scull, *Diseases in Civilization: A Cultural History of Insanity* (Princeton, 2015), pp. 290–305; Scull, *Social Order/Mental Disorder*; Shorter, *A History of Psychiatry*, pp. 145–53.
20 Takabayashi, 'Surviving the Lunacy Act of 1890', p. 263.
21 Alfred Fuller, Notice of Admission, 29 October 1867; Medical Statement, Somerset and Bath Asylum, Wells, 8 December 1927, NA, MH 85/7.
22 A. Young, *The Harmony of Illusions Inventing Post-Traumatic Stress Disorder* (Princeton, 1995), p. 6.
23 E. Leed, *No Man's Land: Combat and Identity in World War I* (Cambridge, 1979), p. 4.
24 Meyer, *Men of War*, pp. 2, 6–7.
25 D. Cohen, *The War Come Home: Disabled Veterans in Britain and Germany 1914–1939* (Berkeley, 2001), pp. 144, 189.

Bibliography

Berkshire Record Office
Broadmoor Asylum, Admission records, letters, case notes.

Liverpool Record Office
Diaries of Charles Molyneux, Helena Molyneux, Frederick Molyneux, Henry Hervey Molyneux, Lady Helena Mary Molyneux, Rose Molyneux.

National Archives
Chancery: Petty Bag Office: Commissions and Inquisitions of Lunacy.
Copy of the Annual Reports of the Commissioners in Lunacy to the Lord Chancellor, from the Fourth (1850) to the Fifty-eighth annual report (1904).
General Board of Health, *Papers Relative to Sanitary State of People in England*. Cm 2415, London, 1857–1858.
Journal of Her Majesty's Flag Ship Corvette (1 January 1879–25 October 1879).
Lunacy Commission and Board of Control: Representative Case Papers of Patients.
Registry of Deceased Soldiers, 14th Brigade (1859–1877).
Report of the Royal Commission on the Care and Control of the Feeble Minded, Vol. 8. Cd 4202, London, 1908.
Reports from Committees: Lunacy Law. Vol. 13, 1877.

Wellcome Archive
Baron Franz von Rigal and family. Papers relating to mental illness in the family, c.1911–1920.
Book of Dr F. Parkes Weber, 13 Harley Street.

Glasgow Royal Lunatic Asylum, house surgeon's notes for physician: Male 1856–1895.
Manor House Asylum, later Chiswick House Asylum. Case records, 1870–1925.
'Notes on Insanity with Case Notes from Claybury Asylum.'
Ticehurst House Hospital Papers.

Journals and newspapers

Aberdeen Journal
Advocate: or, Irish Industrial Journal
Athenaeum
Belfast Mercury
Belfast Morning News
Belfast News-Letter
Belgravia: A London Magazine
Berkshire Chronicle
Birmingham Daily Post
Boys of England: A Journal of Sport, Travel, Fun and Instruction for the Youths of All Nations
Boys of England and Jack Harkaway's Journal of Travel, Fun and Instruction
Bradford Bail's Telegraph
Bradford Observer
Brain
Bridport News
Bristol Mercury and Daily Post
British Journal of Inebriety
British Journal of Medicine
British Medical Journal
Bury and Norwich Post
Caledonian Mercury
Cambridge Independent Press
Chelmsford Chronicle
Cheltenham Chronicle
Chepstow Weekly Advertiser
Cheshire Observer
Chester Chronicle
Colburn's United Service Magazine
Cork Constitution
Coventry Evening Telegraph
Cumberland and Westmorland Advertiser, and Penrith Literary Chronicle
Daily Gazette
Daily Mail
Daily News
Daily Post
Daily Telegraph

Derbyshire Times and Chesterfield Herald
Devizes and Wiltshire Gazette
Dewsbury Reporter
Dublin Daily Express
Dublin Daily Nation
Dublin Evening Packet and Correspondent
Dundee Courier
Dundee Evening Post
Dundee People's Journal
Dundee, Perth and Cupar Advertiser
Edinburgh Evening Courant
Edinburgh Evening News
Edinburgh Medical and Surgical Journal
The Enniscorthy News, and County of Wexford Advertiser
The Era
Essex Newsman
Evening Gazette
The Examiner
Exeter and Plymouth Gazette
Exmouth Journal
Fraser's Magazine
Freeman's Journal and Daily Commercial Advertiser
Gentleman's Magazine
Glasgow Evening Post
Glasgow Herald
Gloucester Citizen
Gloucester Journal
Hamilton Advertiser
Hampshire Telegraph and Sussex Chronicle
Hartlepool Northern Daily Mail
Hereford Times
Hertford Mercury
Herts Guardian
Illustrated London News
Illustrated Police News
Inverness Courier
Journal of Mental Science
Journal of Psychological Medicine and Mental Pathology
Kendal Mercury
Lancaster Gazette
The Lancet
Law Journal
The Law Times
Leeds Intelligencer
Leeds Mercury
Leicester Chronicle and the Leicestershire Mercury

Leicestershire Mercury
Leighton Buzzard Observer and Linslade Gazette
Leisure Hour
Liverpool Mail
Liverpool Mercury
Lloyd's Weekly Newspaper
London Daily News
London Evening Standard
London Medical Press and Circular
Londonderry Sentinel
Macmillan's Magazine
Maidstone Telegraph
Manchester Times
Medical Critic and Psychological Journal
Medical News
Merthyr Telegraph, and General Advertiser for the Iron Districts of South Wales
The Monist
Monmouthshire Merlin
Morning Advertiser
Morning Chronicle
Morning Post
Morpeth Herald
Newcastle Guardian and Tyne Mercury
Norfolk News
North London News
North Wales Chronicle
North-Eastern Daily Gazette
Northern Echo
Nottingham Evening Post
Nottingham Journal
Nottinghamshire Guardian
Pall Mall Gazette
Portsmouth Evening News
Preston Guardian
Punch
Renfrewshire Independent
Review of Reviews
Reynolds's Newspaper
Roscommon Messenger
Royal Cornwall Gazette Falmouth Packet, Cornish Weekly News & General Advertiser
Saturday Review
Scotsman
Sheffield & Rotherham Independent
Sheffield Evening Telegraph

Somerset Standard
South Devon Advertiser
South London Chronicle
South Wales Daily News
South Wales Echo
The Spectator
St James's Gazette
Staffordshire Sentinel
Stamford Mercury
The Standard
The Star
Suffolk Chronicle
Sunday Times
Sunderland Daily Echo and Shipping Gazette
The Times
Tipperary Vindicator
Transactions of the Edinburgh Obstetrical Society
Trewman's Exeter Flying Post
Vanity Fair
Waterford Standard
Wells Journal
Western Mail
Western Times
Westminster Review
Westmorland Gazette
Windsor and Eton Express
Worcester Journal
Worcestershire Chronicle
York Herald
Yorkshire Post and Leeds Intelligencer

Digital resources

Bethlem Hospital. Admission Registers, Male Patient Casebooks, Incurable and Criminal Patient Casebooks, Discharge and Death Registers.
The Old Bailey Proceedings Online, 1674–1913.
Oxford Dictionary of National Biography.
UK Parliamentary Papers.

Printed primary sources

Anon. *Fastened-Fellow: A Man's Adventure.* London: E.W. Allen, 1878.
Anon. *The Lancashire Wedding, or Darwin Moralized.* London: Houlston & Wright, 1867.

Anon. *Prudent Marriages and Their Effects on Posterity; or A Father's Advice to his Daughter Against Forming an Alliance with a Plain and Sickly Family*. London: Houlston & Wright, 1858.
the Social Purity Alliance. Armstrong, R.A. and *Our Duty in the Matter of Social Purity: An Address to Young Men*. London: Social Purity Alliance, c. 1885.
Ash, E.L.H. *Mind and Health: The Mental Factor and Suggestion in Treatment, with Special Reference to Neurasthenia and Other Common Nervous Disorders*. London: H.J. Glaisher, 1910.
Bain, A. *The Emotions and the Will*. London: Longmans, Green & Co., 1875.
Ballantyne, R.M. *The Madman and the Pirate*. London: J. Nisbet & Co., 1883.
Barker, J.A. *Secret Book for Men: Containing Necessary Personal and Confidential Light, Instruction, Information, Counsel, and Advice for the Physical, Mental, Moral & Spiritual Weal of Boys, Youths, and Men*. Brighton: publisher unknown, c. 1888.
Barlow, J. *On Man's Power over Himself to Prevent or Control Insanity*. London: William Pickering, 1849.
Beale, L.S. *Our Morality and The Moral Question: Chiefly from the Medical Side*. London: J&A Churchill, 1887.
Benson, A.C. *The House of Quiet: An Autobiography*. London: Murray, 1906.
Benson, E.F. *Our Family Affairs, 1867–1896*. New York: George H. Doran, c. 1921.
Black, A. *Brown and His Friends*. Edinburgh: W.P. Nimmo, 1859.
Booth, W. *In Darkest England and the Way Out*. New York: Funk & Wagnalls, 1890.
Bowack, W.M. *A Lunatic's Writings: Being the Literary Effusions of a Person While under Certification of Insanity*. Edinburgh: James Thin, 1899.
Bradshaw, J.W. *Use and Abuse of Stimulants: On Dipsomania and Its Results, Etc*. 2nd ed. London: G. Philip & Son, 1867.
Brontë, A. *The Tenant of Wildfell Hall*. London: Thomas Hodgson, 1854.
Brooke, E.F. *A Superfluous Woman*. New York: The Cassell Publishing Co., 1894.
Browne, R. *Neurasthenia and Its Treatment by Hypodermic Transfusions*. London: J.A. Churchill, 1894.
Buckle, G.E., ed. *The Letters of Queen Victoria: A Selection from Her Majesty's Correspondence and Journal between the Years 1862 and 1885 v. iii*. London: John Murray, 1928.
Bucknill, J.C. and D.H. Tuke. *A Manual of Psychological Medicine: Containing the History, Nosology, Description, Statistics, Diagnosis, Pathology, and Treatment of Insanity. With an Appendix of Cases*. 2nd edn. London: John Churchill, 1862.
Bucknill, J.C. and D.H. Tuke. *A Manual of Psychological Medicine, Containing the Lunacy Laws*, 4th edn. London: J. & A. Churchill, 1879.
Byrne, T.E.D. *Lunacy and Law, Together with Hints on the Treatment of Idiots*. London: H.K. Lewis, 1864.

Cantlie, J. *Degeneration Amongst Londoners*. London: The Leadenhall Press, 1885.
Chambers, J. *A Mad World and Its Inhabitants*. New York: D. Appleton and Company, 1877.
Clark, D. *Notes on Mental Diseases*. Toronto: Toronto University Medical College, 1892.
Clarke, J.M. *Hysteria and Neurasthenia*. London: John Lane, 1905.
Clouston, J.S. *The Lunatic at Large*. London: The Bodley Head, 1893.
Collins, W. *Armadale*. New York: Harper & Bros, 1866.
———. *Basil*. London: Sampson Low, Son & Co., 1862.
———. *Heart and Science: A Story of the Present Time*, 3 vols. London: Chatto & Windus, 1883.
———. *Man and Wife*, vol. 3. Leipzig: Bernhard Tauchnitz, 1870.
Commission de Lunatico Inquirendo. An Inquiry into the State of Mind of W. F. Windham, Esq., of Fellbrigg Hall, Norfolk. London: W. Oliver, 1861.
Cooper, A. *Syphilis and Pseudo-Syphilis*. London: J. & A. Churchill, 1884.
Couper, C.T. *Reports of Cases Before the High Court and Circuit Courts of Justiciary in Scotland*, vol. 3. Edinburgh: T & T Clark, 1879.
Coverdale, J.H., S.M. Coverdale, and R. Nairn. 'Behind the Mug Shot Grin: Uses of Madness-Talk in Reports of Loughner's Mass Killing.' *Journal of Communication Inquiry* 37, no. 3 (2013): 200–16.
Coxe, J. *Lunacy in Its Relation to the State: A Commentary on the Evidence Taken by the Committee of the House of Commons on Lunacy Law in the Session of 1877*. London: Sampson Low, Marston, Searle & Rivington, 1878.
Cruikshank, G. *The Bottle*. London: Spottiswoode & Shaw, 1847.
Dalkeith, F.S. *How I Cured my Craving for Drink, by One Who Twice Suffered from Delirium Tremens*. Glasgow: James Hedderwick & Sons, 1885.
Davidson, D. *Remembrances of a Religio-maniac: An Autobiography*. Stratford-on-Avon: Shakespeare Press, 1912.
Davidson, J.T. *Wanted, a Man! Manly Talks*. London: Marshall Bros, 1893.
Dickens, C. *The Personal History of David Copperfield*. Boston: Ticknor and Fields, 1867.
Digges, J.R.G. *The Cure of Inebriety: Alcoholism, the Drink and the Tobacco Habit*. London: A.W. Jamieson, 1904.
Dowse, T.S. *The Brain and the Nerves: Their Ailments and Their Exhaustion*. London: Baillière & Co., 1884.
———. *On Brain & Nerve Exhaustion: Neurasthenia, Its nature and Curative Treatment*. London: Baillière & Co., 1887.
Doyle, A.C. *Round the Red Lamp: Being Facts and Fancies of Medical Life*. London: Methuen & Co., 1894.
'Dry Nurse'. *Monomania; [a satire in reference to the trial of McNaughten for the murder of Mr. Drummond]*. London: Saunders and Otley, 1843.
Edwards, W. and B. Harraden. *Two Health-Seekers in Southern California*. Philadelphia: J.B. Lippincott Company, 1896.

Ellis, H. *Sexual Inversion*. Philadelphia: F.A. Davis Co., 1901.
Finneran, J. *Justice: As It Is Administered in Dublin Castle in the Nineteenth Century. The Irish Inquisition: or, Hartfield Lunatic Asylum*. Dublin: privately printed, 1868.
Fleming, M.A. *A Wife's Tragedy*. New York: G.W. Carleton & Co., 1881.
Gilbert, W. *Shirley Hall Asylum; Or, The Memoirs of a Monomaniac*. London: Strahan & Co., 1863.
Gowers, W.R. *Lunacy and Law: An Address on the Prevention of Insanity Delivered before the Medico-Psychological Association of Great Britain and Ireland*. London: J. & A. Churchill, 1903.
Grainger, F.E. *Caged! The Romance of a Lunatic Asylum*. London: Ward, Lock & Co., 1900.
Grand, S. *The Heavenly Twins*. Leipzig: Heinemann and Balestier, 1894.
Granville, J.M. *The Care and Cure of the Insane: Being the Reports of the Lancet Commission on Lunatic Asylums*, vol. 2. London: Hardwicke and Bogue, 1877.
Gustafson, A.C.J. *The Foundation of Death: A Study of the Drink-Question*. London: Kegan Paul & Co., 1884.
Harris, F. *My Life and Loves*, vol. 2. Cimiez, Nice: privately printed, 1922.
Haslam, J. *Illustrations of Madness*. London: G. Hayden, 1810.
——. *Sketches in Bedlam, or, Characteristic Traits of Insanity as Displayed in the Cases of One Hundred and Forty Patients of Both Sexes, Now, or Recently, Confined in New Bethlem*. London: Sherwood, Jones, and Co., 1823.
Head, H. *Syphilis of the Nervous System within Six Years of Infection*. London: John Bale, 1910.
Hewitt, H. *From Harrow School to Herrison House Asylum*. London: C.W. Daniel Company, n. d.
Hobhouse, E. et al. *Health Abroad: A Medical Handbook of Travel*. London: Smith, Elder, & Co., 1899.
Hooper, J.M. *The House of Raby or, Our Lady of Darkness*, vol. 1. London: Chapman and Hall, 1854.
Hovell, D.D. *On Some Conditions of Neurasthenia*. London: J. & A. Churchill, 1886.
Huggard, W.R. and W.G. Lockett. *Davos as Health-Resort: A Handbook*. Davos: Davos Printing Company, 1907.
James, G.L. *Shall I Try Australia? Or, Health, Business, and Pleasure in New South Wales, Forming a Guide to the Australian Colonies for the Emigrant Settler and Business Man*. London: L. U. Gill, 1892.
Kernahan, J.C. *A Literary Gent: A Study in Vanity and Dipsomania*. London: Ward, Lock & Co., 1897.
Lowe, L. *The Bastilles of England: Or, the Lunacy Laws at Work*. London: Crookenden, 1883.
Lytton, R.B. *A Blighted Life: A True Story*. London: London Publishing Office, 1880.
Machan, A. *The Hill of Dreams*. London: E. Grant Richards, 1907.

Mackenzie, H. *The Man of Feeling* [1771]. London: Cassell & Co., 1886.
Macnish, R. *The Anatomy of Drunkenness*. New York: D. Appleton & Co., 1835.
Macpherson, J. *Mental Affections: An Introduction to the Study of Insanity*. London: Macmillan and Co., 1899.
Marryat, F. *A Passing Madness*. London: Nimeguen, 1897.
Mather, M. *Thoughts and Suggestions Relative to the Management of Barony Parochial Board and Poor-House: Together with Hints on Monomania*. Glasgow: printed by John Wright, 1858.
Maudsley, H. *Body and Mind*. London: Macmillan & Co., 1873.
——. *Body and Will*. London: Kegan Paul, 1883.
——. *Physiology and Pathology of the Mind*. London: Macmillan, 1867.
——. *Responsibility in Mental Disease*. New York: Appleton and Company, 1874.
Mayo, T. *Medical Testimony and Evidence in Cases of Lunacy: Being the Croonian Lectures Delivered before the Royal College of Physicians in 1853: With an Essay on the Conditions of Mental Soundness*. London: Parker, 1854.
Merivale, C. *My Experiences in a Lunatic Asylum*. London: Chatto and Windus, 1879.
Mickle, W.J. *General Paralysis of the Insane*. London: H.K. Lewis, 1880.
Miller, F.T., ed. *True Stories of the Great War*, vol. 4, New York: Review of Reviews Company, 1917.
Moore, J.M. *New Zealand for the Emigrant, Invalid, and Tourist*. London: Sampson Low, Marston, Searle, and Rivington, 1890.
Morel, B. *Traité des dégénérescences physiques, intellectuelles et morales de l'espèce humaine et des causes qui produisent ces variétés maladives*. Paris: J.B. Baillière, 1857.
Morgan, J.E. *The Deterioration of Race from the Too Rapid Increase of Great Cities*. London: Longmans, Green, and Co., 1866.
Moseley, W.W. *Twelve Chapters on Nervous or Mind Complaints*. 12th edn. London: Simpkins, Marshall, 1860.
Newcome, H.J. *The Lunatic: Or English Clergymen and Scotch Doctors. An Autobiography*. London: John Pownceby, 1861.
Noble, D. *Elements of Psychological Medicine: An Introduction to the Practical Study of Insanity, Etc.* London: John Churchill, 1853.
Nordau, M. *Degeneration*. London: William Heinemann, 1898.
Nordhoff, C. *California for Health, Pleasure, and Residence: A Book for Travellers and Settlers*. New York: Harper, 1882.
'One of Them.' *Mad Doctors*. London: Swan Sonnenschein & Co., 1890.
Otter, R.H. *Winters Abroad: Some Information Respecting Places Visited by the Author on Account of His Health: Intended for the Use of Invalids*. London: J. Murray, 1882.
Parkin, J. *Notice of the Establishment for the Treatment of Nervous and Mental Maladies*. London: H.W. Martin, 1843.

Peddie, A. *On the Pathology of Delirium Tremens, and Its Treatment, Without Stimulants or Opiates*. Edinburgh: Sutherland and Knox, 1854.

Perceval, J.T. *A Narrative of the Treatment Experienced by a Gentleman, during a State of Mental Derangement; Designed to Explain the Causes and the Nature of Insanity, Etc.* London: Effingham Wilson, 1838.

Philanthropos. *A Voice from the Wilderness: Being A Plea for a Lunatic Asylum for the Middle Classes on Self-Supporting Principles*. London: John Churchill, 1861.

The Philosophy of Insanity, by a Late Inmate of the Glasgow Royal Asylum. London: Houlston & Wright, 1860.

Playfair, W.S. *The Systematic Treatment of Nerve Prostration and Hysteria*. London: Smith, Elder & Company, 1883.

Pope, W.E. *Nervousness: Its Causes, Symptoms, and Cure*, 2nd edn. London: Piper, Stephenson & Spence, 1855.

Public Opinion on Private Lunatic Asylums, Giving an Account of the Frightful Mortality in Them, Disclosed by the Report of the Commissioners in Lunacy. London: W.J. Hurry, 1890.

Rawlings, J.A. *The Greatest Evil of Our Time: An Address to Men*. London: W.G. Wheeler, 1891.

Reade, C. *Hard Cash*. Leipzig: Bernard Tauchnitz, 1864.

———. *It is Never Too Late to Mend: A Matter of Fact Romance*. London: Melbourne, 1911.

———. *The Complete Writings of Charles Reade*, vols 1–14. London: Chatto & Windus, 1895.

———. 'Our Dark Places No. IV.' In *Readiana*. New York: J.W. Lovell Company, 1887.

———. *A Terrible Temptation: A Story of the Day* [1871]. Paris: The Grolier Society, 1900.

Renton, A.W. *The Law of and Practice in Lunacy: With the Lunacy Acts 1890–91*. Edinburgh: W.M. Green & Sons, 1897.

Report of a Special Committee of the Charity Organisation Society on the Education and Care of Idiots, Imbeciles, and Harmless Lunatics, Etc. London: Longmans Green & Co., 1877.

Report, Together with Rules and Regulations of Saughton Hall Private Lunatic Asylum, near Edinburgh. Edinburgh: Balfour and Jack, 1840.

Richardson, J. 'Personal Religion – Papers.' In *The Official Report of the Seventeenth Annual Meeting of the Church Congress Held at Croydon, 1877*. Rev. W. Wilks, ed. Croydon: Jesse W. Ward, 1877.

Ritchie, R.P. *An Inquiry into a Frequent Cause of Insanity in Young Men*. London: Henry Renshaw, 1861.

Rumler. *The Causes, Nature, and Cure of Neurasthenia in General, and of Nervous Disorders of the Generative System in Particular*. 15th edn. Geneva: The Author, 1901.

Rush, B. *An Inquiry into the Effects of Ardent Spirits upon the Human Body and Mind with an Account of the Means of Preventing and of the Remedies for Curing Them*. Exeter: Josiah Richardson, 1819.

S*****R, J. *Ridiculous Fancies: An Allegory. Being the Lucubrations of a Madman.* London: Frederick Arnold, 1872.

Saleeby, C.W. *Parenthood and Race Culture: An Outline of Eugenics.* London: Cassell and Company, 1909.

Savage, G. *Insanity and Allied Neuroses: Practical and Clinical.* 2nd edn. London: Cassell & Company, 1886.

Savill, T.D. *Clinical Lectures on Neurasthenia.* London: Henry J. Glaisher, 1899.

Seymour, E.J. *A Letter to the Right Honourable The Earl of Shaftesbury on the Laws Which Regulate Private Lunatic Asylums.* London: Longman, Brown, Green, Longmans & Roberts, 1859.

Sheppard, E. *Lectures on Madness in its Medical, Legal, and Social Aspects.* London: J. & A. Churchill, 1873.

Spencer, H. *Education: Intellectual, Moral, and Physical.* New York: D. Appleton and Co., 1896.

Spenser, F. *Lucy's Temptation: A Temperance Story for Young Men and Women.* London: R. Culley, 1896.

Strahan, S.A.K. *Marriage and Disease: A Study of Heredity and the More Important Family Degenerations.* London: Kegan Paul, 1892.

——. *Suicide and Insanity: A Physiological and Sociological Study.* London: S. Sonnenschein & Co., 1893.

Swiney, F. *The Bar of Isis, or The Law of the Mother.* London: Open Road Publishing, 1907.

Symonds, J.A. *A Problem in Modern Ethics: Being an Inquiry Into the Phenomenon of Sexual Inversion.* London: publisher unknown, 1896.

Taylor, A.S. *A Manual of Medical Jurisprudence.* Philadelphia: Henry C. Lea's Son & Co., 1880.

——. *The Principles and Practice of Medical Jurisprudence.* London: John Churchill, 1865.

Trollope, A. *He Knew He Was Right*, 3 vols. Leipzig: Bernard Tauchnitz, 1869.

Trotter, T. *An Essay, Medical, Philosophical, and Chemical, On Drunkenness, and Its Effects On The Human Body.* London: T.N. Longman, 1804.

Walker, A.D. *Egypt as a Health Resort, with Medical and Other Hints for Travellers in Syria.* London: J. & A. Churchill, 1873.

Weston, J. *Life in a Lunatic Asylum: An Autobiographical Sketch.* London: Houlston & Wright, 1867.

Wharton, F. *A Treatise on Mental Unsoundness Embracing a General View of Psychological Law.* Philadelphia: Kay & Brother, 1873.

Williamson, W. *Thoughts on Insanity and Its Causes and on the Management of the Insane. To which are Appended Observations on the Report for 1850, of the Lunatic Asylum of the North and East Ridings of Yorkshire.* London: C. Gilpin, 1851.

Wilson, A. *Unfinished Man: A Scientific Analysis of the Psychopath or Human Degenerate.* London: Greening & Co., 1910.

Wilson, G.R. *Drunkenness.* London: Swan Sonnenschein & Co., 1897.

Wilson, W.S. *The Ocean as a Health Resort: A Practical Handbook of the Sea for the Use of Tourists and Health-Seekers.* London: J. & A. Churchill, 1881.
Winslow, F. *On the Incubation of Insanity.* London: S. Highley, 1846.
——. *The Plea of Insanity in Criminal Cases.* London: H. Renshaw, 1843.
Winslow, L.F. *Mad Humanity: Its Forms, Apparent and Obscure.* London: C.A. Pearson, Ltd, 1898.
——. *Manual of Lunacy: A Handbook Relating to the Legal Care and Treatment of the Insane.* London: Smith, Elder & Co. 1874.
——. *Recollections of Forty Years.* London: John Ouseley, 1910.
Worcester, S. *Insanity and Its Treatment: Lectures on the Treatment of Insanity and Kindred Nervous Diseases.* New York: Boericke & Tafel, 1882.
Wynter, A. *The Borderlands of Insanity.* London: Henry Renshaw, 1877.
Yates, E. 'Mr. Wilkie Collins in Gloucester Place.' In *Celebrities at Home, Third Series.* 145–56. London: Office of 'The World', 1879.

Secondary sources

Adair, R., J. Melling, and B. Forsythe. 'Migration, Family Structure and Pauper Lunacy in Victorian England: Admissions to the Devon County Pauper Lunatic Asylum, 1845–1900.' *Continuity and Change* 12 no. 3 (1997): 373–401.
Adams, J. *Healing with Water: English Spas and the Water Cure, 1840–1960.* Manchester: Manchester University Press, 2015.
Adityanjee, Y.A., D. Theodoridis Aderibigbe, W. Victor, and R. Vieweg. 'Dementia Praecox to Schizophrenia: The First 100 Years.' *Psychiatry and Clinical Neurosciences* 53, no. 4 (1999): 437–48.
Ainsley, J.N. '"Some Mysterious Agency": Women, Violent Crime, and the Insanity Acquittal in the Victorian Courtroom.' *Canadian Journal of History* 35, no. 1 (2000): 37–56.
Alberti, F.B., ed. *Medicine, Emotion, and Disease, 1700–1950.* Basingstoke: Palgrave Macmillan, 2006.
Andrews, J. *The History of Bethlem.* London: Routledge, 1997.
——. *'They're in the Trade ... of Lunacy/They "Cannot Interfere"– They Say': The Scottish Lunacy Commissioners and Lunacy Reform in Nineteenth-Century Scotland.* London: Wellcome Institute for the History of Medicine, 1998.
Andrews, J., A. Briggs, R. Porter, P. Tucker, and K. Waddington. *The History of Bethlem.* Abingdon: Routledge, 1997.
Andrews, J. and A. Digby, eds. *Sex and Seclusion, Class and Custody: Perspectives on Gender and Class in the History of British and Irish Psychiatry.* Amsterdam: Rodopi, 2004.
Appignanesi, L. *Mad, Bad and Sad: The History of Women and the Mind Doctors from 1800 to the Present.* London: Virago, 2008.

Arieno, M.A. *Victorian Lunatics: A Social Epidemiology of Mental Illness in Mid-Nineteenth-Century England*. Selinsgrove: Susquehanna University Press, 1989.
Augstein, H.F. 'J.C. Prichard's Concept of Moral Insanity: A Medical Theory on the Corruption of Human Nature', *Medical History* 40, no. 3 (1996): 311–43.
Bacopoulos-Viau, A. and A. Fauvel. 'The Patient's Turn: Roy Porter and Psychiatry's Tales, Thirty Years On.' *Medical History* 60, no. 1 (2016): 1–18.
Bailey, J. *Unquiet Lives: Marriage and Marriage Breakdown in England 1660–1800*. Cambridge: Cambridge University Press, 2003.
Bailey, P. 'Adventures in Space: Victorian Railway Erotics, or Taking Alienation for a Ride.' *Journal of Victorian Culture* 9, no. 1 (2004): 1–21.
Bailey, V. *'This Rash Act': Suicide Across the Life Cycle in the Victorian City*. Stanford: Stanford University Press, 1998.
Barfoot, M. and A.W. Beveridge. 'Madness at the Crossroads: John Home's Letters from the Royal Edinburgh Asylum, 1886–1887.' *Psychological Medicine* 20 (1990): 263–84.
Barham, P. *Forgotten Lunatics of the Great War*. New Haven: Yale University Press, 2004.
Barrow, R.J. 'Rape on the Railway: Women, Safety, and Moral Panic in Victorian Newspapers.' *Journal of Victorian Culture* 20, no. 3 (2015): 341–56.
Bartlett, P. 'The Asylum, the Workhouse, and the Voice of the Insane Poor in 19th-Century England.' *International Journal of Law and Psychiatry* 21, no. 4 (1998): 421–32.
———. *The Poor Law of Lunacy: The Administration of Pauper Lunatics in Mid-Nineteenth-Century England*. London: Leicester University Press, 1999.
Bartlett, P. and D. Wright, eds. *Outside the Walls of the Asylum: The History of Care in the Community 1750–2000*. London: Bloomsbury Publishing, 1999.
Bater, P. 'The Tukes' Asylum in Chiswick.' *Brentford and Chiswick Local History Journal* 14 (2005): 7.
Baur, N. and J. Melling. 'Dressing and Addressing the Mental Patient: The Uses of Clothing in the Admission, Care and Employment of Residents in English Provincial Mental Hospitals, c. 1860–1960.' *Textile History* 45, no. 2 (2014): 145–70.
Begiato, J. 'Between Poise and Power: Embodied Manliness in Eighteenth- and Nineteenth-Century British Culture.' *Transactions of the Royal Historical Society* 26 (2016): 125–47.
———. *Manliness in Britain, 1760–1900: Bodies, Emotion, and Material Culture*. Manchester: Manchester University Press, 2020.
Beveridge, A. '*Britain's Siberia*: Mary Coutts's Account of the Asylum System.' *Journal of the Royal College of the Physicians of Edinburgh* 35, no. 2 (2005): 175–81.

———. 'Life in the Asylum: Patients' Letters from Morningside, 1873–1908.' *History of Psychiatry* 9, no. 36 (1998): 431–69.
———. 'Voices of the Mad: Patients' Letters from the Royal Edinburgh Asylum, 1873–1908.' *Psychological Medicine* 27, no. 4 (1997), 899–908.
Bhattacharjee, Y. 'Shell Shock Revisited: Solving the Puzzle of Blast Trauma.' *Science* 319, no. 5862 (2008): 406–8.
Bivins, R. and J. Pickstone, eds. *Medicine, Madness and Social History: Essays in Honour of Roy Porter*. Basingstoke: Palgrave Macmillan, 2007.
Bland, L. *Banishing the Beast: Feminism, Sex and Morality*. London: Tauris Parke, 2002.
Boddice, R. 'The Manly Mind? Revisiting the Victorian "Sex in Brain" Debate.' *Gender & History* 23, no. 3 (2011): 321–40.
———. *The Science of Sympathy: Morality, Evolution, and Victorian Civilization*. Baltimore: University of Illinois Press, 2016.
Bonea, A., M. Dickson, S. Shuttleworth, and J. Wallis. *Anxious Times: Medicine and Modernity in Nineteenth-Century Britain*. Pittsburgh: University of Pittsburgh Press, 2019.
Bonnell, M. 'The Legacy of Sarah Grand's *The Heavenly Twins*: A Review Essay.' *English Literature in Transition* 36, no. 4 (1993): 467–78.
Borsay, A. *Disabled Children: Contested Caring, 1850–1979*. London: Taylor & Francis Group, 2012.
Bourke, J. *Dismembering the Male: Men's Bodies, Britain and the Great War*. Chicago: University of Chicago Press, 1996.
———. 'Effeminacy, Ethnicity and the End of Trauma: The Sufferings of "Shell-Shocked" Men in Great Britain and Ireland, 1914–1939.' *Journal of Contemporary History* 35, no. 1 (2000): 57–69.
Bourrier, K. *The Measure of Manliness: Disability and Masculinity in the Mid-Victorian Novel*. Ann Arbor: University of Michigan Press, 2015.
Boyd, K. *Manliness and the Boys' Story Paper in Britain: A Cultural History, 1855–1940*. Basingstoke: Palgrave Macmillan, 2003.
Boyle, T. *Black Swine in the Sewers of Hampstead: Beneath the Surface of Victorian Sensationalism*. New York: Viking Press, 1989.
Brian, K.M. and J.W. Trent Jr, eds. *Phallacies: Historical Intersections of Disability and Masculinity*. New York: Oxford University Press, 2017.
Brodie, J.F. and M. Redfield, eds. *High Anxieties: Cultural Studies in Addiction*. Berkeley: University of California Press, 2002.
Brown, T.E. 'Dance of the Dialectic? Some Reflections (Polemic and Otherwise) on the Present State of Nineteenth-Century Asylum Studies.' *Canadian Bulletin of Medical History* 11, no. 2 (1994): 267–95.
Buckton, O.S. *Secret Selves: Confession and Same Sex Desire in Victorian Autobiography*. Chapel Hill: University of North Carolina Press, 1998.
Busfield, J. 'The Female Malady? Men, Women and Madness in Nineteenth Century Britain.' *Sociology* 28, no. 1 (1994): 259–77.
———. *Men, Women and Madness: Understanding Gender and Mental Disorder*. Basingstoke: Palgrave Macmillan, 1996.

Bynum, W.F. 'Alcoholism and Degeneration in 19th Century European Medicine and Psychiatry.' *British Journal of Addiction* 79, no. 4 (1984): 59–70.

Bynum, W.F. and M. Neve. 'Hamlet on the Couch: Hamlet Is a Kind of Touchstone by Which to Measure Changing Opinion – Psychiatric and Otherwise – about Madness.' *American Scientist* 74, no. 4 (1986): 390–96.

Bynum, W.F., R. Porter, and M. Shepherd, eds. *The Anatomy of Madness: Essays in the History of Psychiatry*, 2 vols. London: Tavistock, 1985.

Byrne, K. *Tuberculosis and the Victorian Literary Imagination*. Cambridge: Cambridge University Press, 2011.

Campana, J. *The Pain of Reformation: Spenser, Vulnerability, and the Ethics of Masculinity*. New York: Fordham University Press, 2012.

Capp, B. 'The Double Standard Revisited: Plebeian Women and Male Sexual Reputation in Early Modern England.' *Past & Present* 162, no. 1 (1999): 70–100.

Carnes, M.C. and C. Griffen (eds). *Meanings for Manhood: Constructions of Masculinity in Victorian America*. Chicago: University of Chicago Press, 1990.

Casey, C. 'Common Misperceptions: The Press and Victorian Views of Crime.' *Journal of Interdisciplinary History* 41, no. 3 (2011): 367–91.

Chaney, S. '"No 'Sane' Person Would Have Any Idea": Patients' Involvement in Late Nineteenth-Century British Asylum Psychiatry.' *Medical History* 60, no. 1 (2016): 37–53.

Chase, K. and M. Levenson. *The Spectacle of Intimacy: A Public Life for the Victorian Family*. Princeton: Princeton University Press, 2000.

Cherry, S. *Medical Services and the Hospitals in Britain, 1860–1939*. Cambridge: Cambridge University Press, 1996.

Chesler, P. *Women and Madness*. Garden City: Doubleday and Co., 1972.

Cocks, H.G. 'Making the Sodomite Speak: Voices of the Accused in English Sodomy Trials, c. 1800–98.' *Gender & History* 18, no. 1 (2006): 87–107.

Cocks, H.G. and M. Houlbrook, eds. *Palgrave Advances in the Modern History of Sexuality*. Houndmills: Palgrave, 2006.

Codell, C.K. 'Infantile Hysteria and Infantile Sexuality in Late Nineteenth-Century German-Language Medical Literature.' *Medical History* 27, no. 2 (1983): 186–96.

Cohen, D. *Family Secrets: The Things We Tried to Hide*. New York: Penguin, 2013.

———. *The War Come Home: Disabled Veterans in Britain and Germany 1914–1939*. Berkeley: University of California Press, 2001.

Cohen, M. and T. Hitchcock, eds. *English Masculinities 1660–1800*. London: Longman, 1999.

Cohen, S. *Folk Devils and Moral Panics*. New York: Routledge, 2011.

Coleborne, C. 'Families, Patients and Emotions: Asylums for the Insane in Colonial Australia and New Zealand, c. 1880–1910.' *Social History of Medicine* 19, no. 3 (2006): 425–42.

———. *Madness in the Family: Insanity and Institutions in the Australasian Colonial World, 1860–1914*. Basingstoke: Palgrave Macmillan, 2010.
———. 'White Men and Weak Masculinity: Men in the Public Asylums in Victoria, Australia, and New Zealand, 1860s–1900s.' *History of Psychiatry* 25, no. 4 (2014): 468–76.
———. *Why Talk About Madness? Bringing History into the Conversation*. Basingstoke: Palgrave Macmillan, 2020.
Coleborne, C. and D. MacKinnon, eds. *Madness in Australia: Histories, Heritage and the Asylum*. St Lucia: University of Queensland Press, 2003.
Colella, S. *Charlotte Riddell's City Novels and Victorian Business: Narrating Capitalism*. New York: Routledge, 2016.
Cook, M. *Narratives of Enclosure in Detective Fiction: The Locked Room Mystery*. London: Palgrave Macmillan, 2011.
Cooke, A.C. *Moral Panics, Mental Illness Stigma, and the Deinstitutionalization Movement in American Popular Culture*. Basingstoke: Palgrave Macmillan, 2017.
Cox, C. *Negotiating Insanity in the Southeast of Ireland, 1820–1900*. Manchester: Manchester University Press, 2018.
Critchley, M and E.A. Critchley. *John Hughlings Jackson: Father of English Neurology*. Oxford: Oxford University Press, 1998.
Crozier, A. 'What was Tropical about Tropical Neurasthenia? The Utility of the Diagnosis in the Management of British East Africa.' *Journal of the History of Medicine and Allied Sciences* 64, no. 4 (2009): 518–48.
Crozier, I. 'Nineteenth-Century Psychiatric Writing about Homosexuality before Havelock Ellis: The Missing Story.' *Journal of the History of Medicine and Allied Sciences* 63, no. 1 (2008): 65–102.
———. 'Pillow Talk: Credibility, Trust and the Sexological Case History.' *History of Science* 46, no. 4 (2008): 375–404.
Curtis, L.P. *Jack the Ripper and the London Press*. New Haven: Yale University Press, 2001.
Darby, R. 'Pathologizing Male Sexuality: Lallemand, Spermatorrhea, and the Rise of Circumcision.' *Journal of the History of Medicine and Allied Sciences* 60, no. 3 (2005): 283–319.
Davidoff, L. *Worlds Between: Historical Perspectives on Gender and Class*. Cambridge: Cambridge University Press, 1995.
Davidson, R. and L.A. Hall, eds. *Sex, Sin and Suffering: Venereal Disease and European Society since 1870*. Abingdon: Routledge, 2001.
Davis, G. *'The Cruel Madness of Love': Sex, Syphilis and Psychiatry in Scotland, 1880–1930*. Amsterdam: Rodopi, 2008.
———. 'The Most Deadly Disease of Asylumdom: General Paralysis of the Insane and Scottish Psychiatry, c.1840–1940.' *Journal of the Royal College of Physicians of Edinburgh* 42, no. 3 (2012): 266–73.
Degerman, D. '"Am I Mad?": The Windham Case and Victorian Resistance to Psychiatry.' *History of Psychiatry* 30, no. 4 (2019): 457–68.
Delap, L., B. Griffin, and A. Wills, eds. *The Politics of Domestic Authority in Britain since 1800*. London: Palgrave Macmillan, 2009.

Deslandes, P. 'Curing Mind and Body in the Heart of the Canadian Rockies: Empire, Sexual Scandal and the Reclamation of Masculinity, 1880s–1920s.' *Gender & History* 21, no. 2 (2009): 358–79.
Digby, A. *Madness, Morality and Medicine: A Study of the York Retreat 1796–1914*. Cambridge: Cambridge University Press, 1985.
Dixon, J., 'Havelock Ellis and John Addington Symonds, *Sexual Inversion* (1897).' *Victorian Review* 35, no. 1 (2009): 72–77.
du Plessis, R. 'A Hermeneutic Analysis of Delusion Content from the Casebooks of the Grahamstown Lunatic Asylum, 1890–1907.' *South African Journal of Psychiatry* 25 (2019): 1–7.
Dudink, S., K. Hagemann, and A. Clark, eds. *Representing Masculinity: Male Citizenship in Modern Western Culture*. Houndmills: Palgrave Macmillan, 2007.
Dudink, S., K. Hagemann, and J. Tosh, eds. *Masculinities in Politics and War: Gendering Modern History*. Manchester: Manchester University Press, 2004.
Dunnage, J. 'The Work of Cesare Lombroso and its Reception: Further Contexts and Perspectives.' *Crime, History & Societies* 22, no. 2 (2018): 5–8.
Durbach, N. *Spectacle of Deformity: Freak Shows and Modern British Culture*. Berkeley: University of California Press, 2010.
Eastoe, S. *Idiocy, Imbecility and Insanity in Victorian Society: Caterham Asylum, 1867–1911*. Houndmills: Palgrave Macmillan, 2020.
Eigen, J. 'Lesion of the Will: Medical Resolve and Criminal Responsibility in Victorian Insanity Trials.' *Law & Society Review* 33, no. 2 (1999): 425–59.
———. *Mad-Doctors in the Dock: Defending the Diagnosis, 1760–1913*. Baltimore: Johns Hopkins University Press, 2016.
———. *Unconscious Crime: Mental Absence and Criminal Responsibility in Victorian London*. Baltimore: Johns Hopkins University Press, 2003.
———. *Witnessing Insanity: Madness and Mad-Doctors in the English Court*. New Haven: Yale University Press, 1995.
Ellis, H. *Masculinity and Science in Britain, 1831–1918*. London: Palgrave Macmillan, 2017.
———. 'This Starting, Feverish Heart: Matthew Arnold and the Problem of Manliness.' *Critical Survey* 20, no. 3 (2008): 97–115.
———. 'Thomas Arnold, Christian Manliness and the Problem of Boyhood.' *Journal of Victorian Culture* 19, no. 4 (2014): 425–41.
Emsley, C. *Hard Men: Violence in England since 1750*. London: Hambledon, 2005.
———. 'Violent Crime in England in 1919: Post-war Anxieties and Press Narratives.' *Continuity and Change* 23, no. 1 (2008), 173–95.
Fabrega Jr, H. 'The Culture and History of Psychiatric Stigma in Early Modern and Modern Western Societies: A Review of Recent Literature.' *Comprehensive Psychiatry* 32, no. 2 (1991): 97–119.

Farquharson, L. 'A "Scottish Poor Law of Lunacy"? Poor Law, Lunacy Law and Scotland's Parochial Asylums.' *History of Psychiatry* 28, no. 1 (2017): 15–28.

Fennell, P. *Treatment Without Consent: Law, Psychiatry and the Treatment of Mentally Disordered People Since 1845*. London: Routledge, 1996.

Feudtner, C. '"Minds the Dead Have Ravished": Shell Shock, History, and the Ecology of Disease-Systems.' *History of Science* 31, no. 94 (1993): 377–420.

Fichman, M. and J.E. Keelan. 'Resister's Logic: The Anti-Vaccination Arguments of Alfred Russel Wallace and Their Role in the Debates over Compulsory Vaccination in England, 1870–1907.' *Studies in History and Philosophy of Biological and Biomedical Sciences* 38, no. 3 (2007): 585–607.

Finlayson, G. *The Seventh Earl of Shaftesbury, 1801–1885*. Vancouver: Regent College Publishing, 1981.

Finnane, M. 'Asylums, Families, and the State.' *History Workshop* 20 (1985): 134–48.

———. *Insanity and the Insane in Post-Famine Ireland*. London: Croom Helm, 1981.

Foyster, E. *Marital Violence: An English Family History, 1660–1857*. Cambridge: Cambridge University Press, 2005.

Franklin, B. 'Hospital – Heritage – Home: Reconstructing the Nineteenth Century Lunatic Asylum.' *Housing, Theory and Society* 19 (2002): 170–84.

Frawley, M. *Invalidism and Identity in Nineteenth-Century Britain*. Chicago: University of Chicago Press, 2004.

Gabriele, A. *Reading Popular Culture in Victorian Print: Belgravia and Sensationalism*. New York: Palgrave Macmillan, 2009.

Gagen, W. 'Remastering the Body, Renegotiating Gender: Physical Disability and Masculinity During the First World War, the Case of J. B. Middlebrook.' *European Review of History* 14, no. 4 (2007): 525–41.

Garland, D. 'On the Concept of Moral Panic.' *Media Culture* 4, no. 1 (2008): 9–30.

Garrigan, K.O., ed. *Victorian Scandals: Representations of Gender and Class*. Athens: University of Ohio Press, 1992.

Garton, S. *Medicine and Madness: A Social History of Insanity in New South Wales, 1880–1940*. Kensington: University of South Wales Press, 1988.

Gijswijt-Hofstra, M. and R. Porter, eds. *Cultures of Neurasthenia from Beard to the First World War*. Amsterdam: Rodopi, 2001.

Gilbert, A.N. 'Masturbation and Insanity: Henry Maudsley and the Ideology of Sexual Repression.' *Albion: A Quarterly Journal Concerned with British Studies* 12, no. 3 (1980): 268–82.

Gilbert, S. and S. Gubar. *The Madwoman in the Attic: The Woman Writer and the Nineteenth Century Literary Imagination*. New Haven: Yale University Press, 2000.

Glover-Thomas, N. *Reconstructing Mental Health Law and Policy*. London: Butterworths, 2002.

Godfrey, B.S., C. Emsley, and G. Dunstall, eds. *Comparative Histories of Crime*. London: Routledge, 2011.
Godfrey, E. *Masculinity, Crime and Self-Defence in Victorian Literature*. Basingstoke: Palgrave, 2011.
Goldhill, S. *A Very Queer Family Indeed: Sex, Religion and the Bensons in Victorian Britain*. Chicago: University of Chicago Press, 2016.
Goldsmith, S. 'Nostalgia, Homesickness and Emotional Formation on the Eighteenth-Century Grand Tour.' *Cultural and Social History* 15, no. 3 (2018): 333–60.
Goldstein, J. 'The Uses of Male Hysteria: Medical and Literary Discourse in Nineteenth-Century France.' *Representations* 34 (1991): 134–65.
Gomory, T., D. Cohen, and S.A. Kirk. 'Madness or Mental Illness? Revisiting Historians of Psychiatry.' *Current Psychology* 32, no. 2 (2013): 119–35.
Goodman, H. 'Mad Men: Borderlines of Insanity, Masculinity and Emotion in Victorian Literature and Culture.' PhD Dissertation, University of London, Royal Holloway College, 2015.
———. 'Madness in Marriage: Erotomania and Marital Rape in *He Knew He Was Right* and *The Forsyte Saga*.' *Victorian Network* 4, no. 2 (2012): 47–71.
Grandy, C. 'Cultural History's Absent Audience.' *Cultural and Social History* 16, no. 5 (2019): 643–63.
Griffin, B. 'Hegemonic Masculinity as a Historical Problem.' *Gender & History* 30, no. 2 (2018): 377–400.
———. *The Politics of Gender in Victorian Britain: Masculinity, Political Culture and the Struggle for Women's Rights*. Cambridge: Cambridge University Press, 2012.
Haley, B. *The Healthy Body and Victorian Culture*. Cambridge: Harvard University Press, 1978.
Hall, L.A. 'Forbidden by God, Despised by Men: Masturbation, Medical Warnings, Moral Panic, and Manhood in Great Britain, 1850–1950.' *Journal of the History of Sexuality* 2, no. 3 (1992): 365–87.
———. '"It was Affecting the Medical Profession": The History of Masturbatory Insanity Revisited.' *Pedagogia Historica* 39, no. 6 (2003): 685–99.
Halliday, E. 'Themes in Scottish Asylum Culture: The Hospitalisation of the Scottish Asylum 1880–1914.' PhD Dissertation, University of Stirling, 2003.
Hamlett, J. *At Home in the Institution: Material Life in Asylums, Lodging Houses and Schools in Victorian and Edwardian England*. London: Palgrave Macmillan, 2014.
Hands, T. 'Sobering Up the Magdalenes' Drunken Sisters: The Institutional Treatment of "Female Drunken Pests" in Scotland, 1900–15.' *Social History of Alcohol and Drugs* 27, no. 1 (2013): 62–81.
Hanley, A.R. *Medicine, Knowledge and Venereal Diseases in England, 1886–1916*. Basingstoke: Palgrave Macmillan, 2017.
Härmänmaa, M. and C. Nissen, eds. *Decadence, Degeneration, and the End: Studies in the European Fin de Siècle*. Houndmills: Palgrave Macmillan, 2014.

Harvey, K. and A. Shepard. 'What Have Historians Done with Masculinity? Reflections on Five Centuries of British History, Circa 1500–1950.' *Journal of British Studies* 44, no. 2 (2005): 274–80.

Hawkins, M. 'Durkheim's Sociology and Theories of Degeneration.' *Economy and Society* 28, no. 1 (1999): 118–37.

Hervey, N. 'Advocacy or Folly: The Alleged Lunatics' Friend Society, 1845–1863.' *Medical History* 30 (1986): 245–75.

Hewitt, J. *Institutionalizing Gender: Madness, the Family, and Psychiatric Power in Nineteenth-Century France*. Ithaca: Cornell University Press, 2020.

Hewitt, M., ed. *An Age of Equipoise: Reassessing Mid-Victorian Britain*. Aldershot: Ashgate, 2001.

Hickman, C. *Therapeutic Landscapes: A History of English Hospital Gardens since 1800*. Manchester: Manchester University Press, 2013.

Hide, L. *Gender and Class in English Asylums, 1890–1914*. Basingstoke: Palgrave Macmillan, 2014.

Higginbotham, A.R. '"Sin of the Age": Infanticide and Illegitimacy in Victorian London.' *Victorian Studies* 32, no. 3 (1989): 319–37.

Honaker, L. '"One Man to Rely On": Long John Silver and the Shifting Character of Victorian Boys' Fiction.' *Journal of Narrative Theory* 34, no. 1 (2004): 27–53.

Honigsbaum, M. *A History of the Great Influenza Pandemics: Death, Panic and Hysteria, 1830–1920*. New York: I.B. Tauris, 2013.

Hoolihan, C. 'Health and Travel in Nineteenth-Century Rome.' *Journal of the History of Medicine and Allied Sciences* 44 (1989): 462–85.

Horden, P. and R. Smith, eds. *The Locus of Care: Families, Communities, Institutions, and the Provision of Welfare since Antiquity*. London: Routledge, 1998.

Houston, R.A. 'Asylums: The Historical Perspective Before, During, and After.' *The Lancet Psychiatry* 7, no. 4 (2020): 354–62.

——. 'Madness and Gender in the Long Eighteenth Century.' *Social History* 27, no. 3 (2002): 309–32.

——. 'Rights and Wrongs in the Confinement of the Mentally Incapable in Eighteenth-Century Scotland.' *Continuity and Change* 18, no. 3 (2003): 373–94.

Huertas, R. 'Another History for Another Psychiatry: The Patient's View.' *Culture & History Digital Journal* 2, no. 1 (2013): 1–20.

Hughes, W. *The Maniac in the Cellar: Sensation Novels of the 1860s*. Princeton: Princeton University Press, 1980.

Humphries, M.O. *A Weary Road: Shell Shock in the Canadian Expeditionary Force, 1914–1918*. Toronto: University of Toronto Press, 2018.

Hunt, A. 'The Great Masturbation Panic and the Discourses of Moral Regulation in Nineteenth- and Early Twentieth-Century Britain.' *Journal of the History of Sexuality* 8, no. 4 (1998): 575–615.

Hunt, G., C. Mellor, and J. Turner. 'Wretched, Hatless and Miserably Clad: Women and the Inebriate Reformatories from 1900–1913.' *British Journal of Sociology* 40, no. 2 (1989): 244–70.

Hunter, R.A. and I. Macalpine. *Psychiatry for the Poor: 1881 Colney Hatch Asylum-Friern Hospital 1973*. Folkestone: Dawsons of Pall Mall, 1974.

Hurley, K. 'Hereditary Taint and Cultural Contagion: The Social Etiology of Fin-de-Siècle Degeneration Theory.' *Nineteenth-Century Contexts* 14, no. 2 (1990): 193–214.

Hurn, J. 'The History of General Paralysis of the Insane in Britain, 1830 to 1950.' PhD Dissertation, University College London, 1998.

Ifill, H. *Creating Character: Theories of Nature and Nurture in Victorian Sensation Fiction*. Manchester: Manchester University Press, 2018.

Jackson, M. *The Borderland of Imbecility: Medicine, Society and the Fabrication of the Feeble Mind in Late Victorian and Edwardian England*. Manchester: Manchester University Press, 2000.

Jacyna, L.S. and S.T. Casper, eds. *The Neurological Patient in History*. Rochester: University of Rochester Press, 2012.

Jann, R. 'Darwin and the Anthropologists: Sexual Selection and its Discontents.' *Victorian Studies* 37, no. 2 (1994): 287–306.

Jay, M. *The Air Loom Gang: The Strange and True Story of James Tilly Mathews and His Visionary Madness*. New York: Bantam Press, 2003.

Jennings, E. *Curing the Colonizers: Hydrotherapy, Climatology, and French Colonial Spas*. Durham: Duke University Press, 2006.

Johnston, H., ed. *Punishment and Control in Historical Perspectives*. Houndmills: Palgrave Macmillan, 2008.

Jones, K. 'Robert Gardiner Hill and the Non-Restraint Movement.' *Canadian Journal of Psychiatry* 29, no. 2 (1984): 121–24.

———. 'The Windham Case: The Enquiry Held in London in 1861 into the State of Mind of William Frederick Windham, Heir to the Felbrigg Estate.' *British Journal of Psychiatry* 119, no. 551 (1971): 425–33.

Jones, W. 'Psychiatric Battle Casualties: An Intra- and Interwar Comparison.' *British Journal of Psychiatry* 178, no. 3 (2001): 242–47.

Jordan, A. *Love Well the Hour: The Life of Lady Colin Campbell*. Leicester: Matador, 2010.

Kain, J. *Insanity and Immigration Control in New Zealand and Australia, 1860–1930*. Basingstoke: Palgrave Macmillan, 2019.

———. 'The Ne'er-Do-Well: Representing the Dysfunctional Migrant Mind, New Zealand 1850–1910.' *Studies in the Literary Imagination* 48, no. 1 (2015): 75–92.

Kavka, M. 'Ill but Manly: Male Hysteria in Late Nineteenth-Century Medical Discourse.' *Nineteenth Century Prose* 25, no. 1 (1998): 116–39.

Kelm, M. 'Women, Families and the Provincial Hospital for the Insane, British Columbia, 1905–1915.' *Journal of Family History* 19, no. 2 (1994): 177–93.

Kennaway, J. 'The Piano Plague: The Nineteenth-Century Medical Critique of Female Musical Education.' *Gesnerus* 68, no. 1 (2011): 26–40.

Kilday, A.M. *A History of Infanticide in Britain c. 1600 to the Present*. Houndmills: Palgrave Macmillan, 2013.

King, H. *The Disease of Virgins: Green Sickness, Chlorosis and the Problems of Puberty*. London: Routledge, 2004.
Knowles, T. and S. Trowbridge, eds. *Insanity and the Lunatic Asylum in the Nineteenth Century*. London: Pickering & Chatto, 2015.
Kromm, J. 'Olivia Furiosa: Maniacal Women from Richardson to Wollstonecraft.' *Eighteenth-Century Fiction* 16, no. 3 (2004): 343–72.
Kushner, H.I. 'Suicide, Gender, and the Fear of Modernity in Nineteenth-Century Medical and Social Thought.' *Journal of Social History* 26, no. 2 (1993): 461–90.
Labrum, B. 'Looking Beyond the Asylum: Gender and the Process of Committal in Auckland, 1870–1910.' *New Zealand Journal of History* 26 (1992): 125–44.
Laing, O. *The Trip to Echo Spring: On Writers and Drinking*. New York: Picador, 2014.
Large, D.C. *The Grand Spas of Central Europe: A History of Intrigue, Politics, Art and Healing*. Lanham: Rowman & Littlefield, 2015.
Lawrence, C. 'Degeneration under the Microscope at the Fin de Siècle.' *Annals of Science* 66, no. 4 (2009): 455–71.
Le Francois, B., R. Menzies, and G. Reaume, eds. *Mad Matters: A Critical Reader in Canadian Mad Studies*. Toronto: Canadian Scholars' Press, 2013.
Lee, Y.S. *Masculinity and the English Working Class: Studies in Victorian Autobiography and Fiction*. London: Routledge, 2007.
Leed, E. *No Man's Land: Combat and Identity in World War I*. Cambridge: Cambridge University Press, 1979.
Leese, P. *Shell Shock: Traumatic Neurosis and the British Soldiers of the First World War*. New York: Palgrave Macmillan, 2002.
Lens, C.E., I.M. Daey Ouwens, A.T.L. Fiolet, A. Ott, P.J. Koehler, and W.M.A. Verhoeven. 'The Clinical Spectrum of General Paralysis of the Insane: A Historical Cohort Study.' *European Psychiatry* 30:S1 (2015): 1.
Lerner, P. *Hysterical Men: War, Psychiatry, and the Politics of Trauma in Germany, 1890–1930*. Ithaca: Cornell University Press, 2003.
Levine-Clark, M. 'Dysfunctional Domesticity: Female Insanity and Family Relationships Among the West Riding Poor in the Mid-Nineteenth Century.' *Journal of Family History* 25, no. 3 (2000): 341–61.
——. *Unemployment, Welfare, and Masculine Citizenship: 'So Much Honest Poverty' in Britain, 1870–1930*. New York: Palgrave Macmillan, 2015.
Liggins, E. 'Prostitution and Social Purity in the 1880s and 1890s.' *Critical Survey* 15, no. 3 (2003): 39–55.
——. 'Writing Against the "Husband-Fiend": Syphilis and Male Sexual Vice in the New Woman Novel', *Women's Writing* 7, no. 2 (2000): 175–95.
Loeb, L. 'Doctors and Patent Medicines in Modern Britain: Professionalism and Consumerism.' *Albion: A Quarterly Journal Concerned with British Studies* 33, no. 3 (2001): 404–25.
Logan, P.M. *Nerves and Narratives: A Cultural History of Hysteria in Nineteenth-Century British Prose*. Berkeley: University of California Press, 1997.

Long, V. *Destigmatising Mental Illness? Professional Politics and Public Education in Britain, 1870–1970*. Manchester: Manchester University Press, 2014.

Loughran, T. 'A Crisis of Masculinity? Re-writing the History of Shell-Shock and Gender in First World War Britain.' *History Compass* 11, no. 9 (2019): 727–38.

———. 'Hysteria and Neurasthenia in Pre-1914 British Medical Discourse and in Histories of Shell-Shock.' *History of Psychiatry* 19, no. 1 (2008): 25–46.

———. *Shell-Shock and Medical Culture in First World War Britain*. Cambridge: Cambridge University Press, 2017.

———. 'Shell Shock, Trauma, and the First World War: The Making of a Diagnosis and Its Histories.' *Journal of the History of Medicine and Allied Sciences* 67, no. 1 (2012): 94–119.

Luckin, B. 'Revisiting the Idea of Degeneration in Urban Britain, 1830–1900.' *Urban History* 33, no. 2 (2006): 234–52.

Machann, C. *Masculinity in Four Victorian Epics: A Darwinist Reading*. London: Taylor & Francis, 2010.

MacKenzie, C. *Psychiatry for the Rich: A History of Ticehurst Private Asylum 1792–1917*. London: Routledge, 1993.

Macleod, A.D. 'Abrupt Treatments of Hysteria During World War I, 1914–18.' *History of Psychiatry* 29, no. 2 (2018): 187–98.

Malcolm, E. and G. Jones, eds. *Medicine, Disease, and the State in Ireland, 1650–1940*. Cork: Cork University Press, 1999.

Mandler, P. 'The Problem with Cultural History.' *Cultural and Social History* 1, no. 1 (2004): 94–117.

Marland, H. *Dangerous Motherhood: Insanity and Childbirth in Victorian Britain*. Houndmills: Palgrave Macmillan, 2004.

Marland, H. and J. Adams. 'Hydropathy at Home: The Water Cure and Domestic Healing in Mid-Nineteenth-Century Britain.' *Bulletin of the History of Medicine* 83, no. 3 (2009): 499–529.

Mason, D. *Secret Vice: Masturbation in Victorian Fiction and Medical Culture*. Manchester: Manchester University Press, 2013.

Masters, B. *The Life of E.F. Benson*. London: Chatto & Windus, 1991.

Mauger, A. '"Confinement of the Higher Orders": The Social Role of Private Lunatic Asylums in Ireland, c. 1820–60.' *Journal of the History of Medicine and Allied Sciences* 67, no. 2 (2012): 281–317.

———. *The Cost of Insanity in Nineteenth-Century Ireland: Public, Voluntary and Private Asylum Care*. Basingstoke and New York: Palgrave Macmillan, 2018.

Maunder, A. and G. Moore, eds. *Victorian Crime, Madness and Sensation*. London: Routledge, 2004.

McCandless, P. '"Curses of Civilization": Insanity and Drunkenness in Victorian Britain.' *British Journal of Addiction* 79, no. 4 (1984): 49–58.

———. 'Dangerous to Themselves and Others: The Victorian Debate over the Prevention of Wrongful Confinement.' *Journal of British Studies* 23, no. 1 (1983): 84–104.

———. 'Liberty and Lunacy: The Victorians and Wrongful Confinement.' *Journal of Social History* 11, no. 3 (1978): 366–86.
McCarthy, A. 'Migration and Madness at Sea: The Nineteenth- and Early Twentieth-Century Voyage to New Zealand.' *Social History of Medicine* 28, no. 4 (2015): 706–24.
McCormack, M. *The Independent Man: Citizenship and Gender Politics in Georgian England*. Manchester: Manchester University Press, 2005.
McDonagh, P. *Idiocy: A Cultural History*. Liverpool: Liverpool University Press, 2008.
McLaren, A. *Impotence: A Cultural History*. Chicago: University of Chicago Press, 2007.
Melling, J. 'Family Matters? Psychiatry, Kinship and Domestic Responses to Insanity in Nineteenth-Century England.' *History of Psychiatry* 18, no. 2 (2007): 247–54.
Melling, J. and B. Forsythe, eds. *Insanity, Institutions, and Society, 1800–1914: A Social History of Madness in Comparative Perspective*. London: Routledge, 1999.
———. *The Politics of Madness: The State, Insanity, and Society in England, 1845–1914*. London: Routledge, 2006.
Meyer, J. *Men of War: Masculinity and the First World War in Britain*. Basingstoke: Palgrave, 2009.
Micale, M. 'Charcot and the Idea of Hysteria in the Male: Gender, Mental Science, and Mental Diagnosis in Late Nineteenth-Century France.' *Medical History* 34, no. 4 (1990): 363–411.
Micale, M. and P. Lerner, eds. *Traumatic Pasts: History, Psychiatry, and Trauma in the Modern Age, 1870–1930*. Cambridge: Cambridge University Press, 2001.
Michael, P. *Care and Treatment of the Mentally Ill in North Wales, 1800–2000*. Cardiff: University of Wales Press, 2003.
Middleton, J. 'The Cock of the School: A Cultural History of Playground Violence in Britain, 1880–1940.' *Journal of British Studies* 52, no. 4 (2013): 887–907.
Milne-Smith, A. 'Shattered Minds: Madmen on the Railways, 1860–1880.' *Journal of Victorian Culture* 21, no. 1 (2016): 21–39.
———. 'Work and Madness: Overworked Men and Fears of Degeneration, 1860s–1910s.' *Journal of Victorian Culture* 24, no. 2 (2019): 159–78.
Mindham, R.H.S. 'The West Riding of Yorkshire Pauper Lunatic Asylum at Wakefield, 1814–1995.' *British Journal of Psychiatry* 217, no. 3 (2020): 534.
Mitchinson, W. 'Gender and Insanity as Characteristics of the Insane: A Nineteenth-Century Case.' *Canadian Bulletin of Medical History* 4 (1987): 99–117.
———. 'Hysteria and Insanity in Women: A Nineteenth-Century Canadian Perspective.' *Journal of Canadian Studies* 21, no. 3 (1986): 87–105.
Moran, R. *Knowing Right from Wrong: The Insanity Defense of Daniel McNaughtan*. New York: Free Press, 1981.

Mosse, G. *The Image of Man: The Creation of Modern Masculinity*. New York: Oxford University Press, 1996.
Müller-Wille, S. and C. Brandt, eds. *Heredity Explored: Between Public Domain and Experimental Science, 1850–1930*. Cambridge: The MIT Press, 2016.
Murat, L. *The Man Who Thought He Was Napoleon: Toward a Political History of Madness*. D. Dusinberre, trans. Chicago: University of Chicago Press, 2014.
Nash, D. and A. Kilday. *Cultures of Shame: Exploring Crime and Morality in Britain 1600–1900*. London: Palgrave Macmillan, 2010.
Neill, D. 'Merchants, Malaria and Manliness: A Patient's Experience of Tropical Disease.' *Journal of Imperial and Commonwealth History* 46, no. 2 (2018): 203–25.
Niessen, O.C. *Aristocracy, Temperance and Social Reform: The Life of Lady Henry Somerset*. London: Tauris Academic Studies, 2007.
Noll, R. *American Madness: The Rise and Fall of Dementia Praecox*. Boston: Harvard University Press, 2011.
Nye, R.A. *Crime, Madness, & Politics in Modern France: The Medical Concept of National Decline*. Princeton: Princeton University Press, 1984.
O'Ceallaigh Ritschel, N. *Bernard Shaw, W. T. Stead, and the New Journalism: Whitechapel, Parnell, Titanic, and the Great War*. New York: Palgrave Macmillan, 2017.
Oberhelman, D.D. 'Trollope's Insanity Defense: Narrative Alienation in *He Knew He Was Right*.' *Studies in English Literature, 1500–1900* 35, no. 4 (1995): 789–806.
Odden, K.M. '"Able and Intelligent Medical Men Meeting Together:" The Victorian Railway Crash, Medical Jurisprudence, and the Rise of Medical Authority.' *Journal of Victorian Culture* 8, no. 1 (2003): 33–54.
Olsen, M.R. 'The Founding of the Hospital for the Insane Poor, Denbigh.' *Transactions of Denbigh Historical Society* 23 (1974): 193–217.
Oppenheim, J. *'Shattered Nerves': Doctors, Patients, and Depression in Victorian England*. New York: Oxford University Press, 1991.
Owen, A. *The Darkened Room: Women, Power and Spiritualism in Late Victorian England*. Philadelphia: University of Pennsylvania Press, 1990.
Pantelidou, M. and A.K. Demetriades. 'The Enigmatic Figure of Dr Henry Maudsley (1835–1918).' *Journal of Medical Biography* 22, no. 3 (2014): 180–88.
Parry-Jones, W.L. 'English Private Madhouses in the Eighteenth and Nineteenth Centuries.' *Proceedings of the Royal Society of Medicine* 66, no. 7 (1973): 659–64.
——. *The Trade in Lunacy: A Study of Private Madhouses in England in the Eighteenth and Nineteenth Centuries*. Toronto: University of Toronto Press, 1972.
Parsons, J. and R. Hehold, eds. *The Victorian Male Body*. Edinburgh: Edinburgh University Press, 2017.

Pearlston, K. 'Male Violence, Marital Unity, and the History of the Interspousal Tort Immunity.' *Journal of Legal History* 36, no. 3 (2015): 260–98.
Pedlar, V. *'The Most Dreadful Visitation': Male Madness in Victorian Fiction.* Liverpool: Liverpool University Press, 2006.
Pick, D. *Faces of Degeneration: A European Disorder, c. 1848–1918.* Cambridge: Cambridge University Press, 1989.
Pinfold, J. 'Horse Racing and the Upper Classes in the Nineteenth Century.' *Sport in History* 28, no. 3 (2008): 414–30.
Pionke, A.D. and D.T. Millstein, eds. *Victorian Secrecy: Economies of Knowledge and Concealment.* Aldershot: Ashgate Publishing, Ltd, 2010.
Pittard, C. '"Cheap, Healthful Literature": The *Strand* Magazine, Fictions of Crime, and Purified Reading Communities.' *Victorian Periodicals Review* 40, no. 1 (2007): 1–23.
Porter, R. *Mind-Forg'd Manacles: A History of Madness in England from the Restoration to the Regency.* London: Athlone, 1987.
———. 'The Patient's View: Doing Medical History from Below.' *Theory and Society* 14, no. 2 (1985): 175–98.
Porter, R. and A. Wear, eds. *Problems and Methods in the History of Medicine.* New York: Croom Helm, 1987.
Porter, R. and D. Wright, eds. *The Confinement of the Insane: International Perspectives, 1800–1965.* Cambridge: Cambridge University Press, 2003.
Porter, R., H. Nicholson, and B. Bennett, eds. *Women, Madness, and Spiritualism: Georgina Weldon and Louisa Lowe.* London: Routledge, 2016.
Porter, T.M. *Genetics in the Madhouse: The Unknown History of Human Heredity.* Princeton: Princeton University Press, 2018.
Prestwich, P. 'Female Alcoholism in Paris, 1870–1920: The Response of Psychiatrists and of Families.' *History of Psychiatry* 14, no. 3 (2003): 321–36.
Prior, P. *Madness and Murder: Gender, Crime and Mental Disorder in Nineteenth-Century Ireland.* Dublin: Irish Academic Press, 2008.
Rawling, K. 'Visualising Mental Illness: Gender, Medicine and Visual Media, c1850–1910.' PhD Dissertation, University of London, Royal Holloway College, 2011.
Ray, L. 'Models of Madness in Victorian Asylum Practice.' *European Journal of Sociology* 22, no. 2 (1981): 229–64.
Reaume, G. *Remembrance of Patients Past: Patient Life at the Toronto Hospital for the Insane, 1870–1940.* Toronto: University of Toronto Press, 2000.
Reid, F. *Broken Men: Shell Shock, Treatment and Recovery in Britain 1914–30.* New York: Bloomsbury Academic, 2010.
Reiss, B. *Theaters of Madness: Insane Asylums and Nineteenth-Century American Culture.* Chicago: University of Chicago Press, 2008.
Richards, S.F. '"That Doctor and His Heartless, Bloodless Science!": Disembodied Rational Masculinity in Victorian American Culture.' *Nineteenth-Century Contexts* 36, no. 4 (2014): 347–61.

Richardson, A. and C. Willis, eds. *The New Woman in Fiction and Fact: Fin-de-Siècle Feminisms*. Houndmills: Palgrave Macmillan, 2001.

Rimke, H. 'From Sinners to Degenerates: The Medicalization of Morality in the 19th Century.' *History of the Human Sciences* 15, no. 1 (2002): 59–88.

Rodrick, A. 'Melodrama and Natural Science: Reading the "Greenwich Murder" in the Mid-Century Periodical Press.' *Victorian Periodicals Review* 50, no. 1 (2017): 66–99.

Roper, M. 'Between Manliness and Masculinity: The "War Generation" and the Psychology of Fear in Britain, 1914–1950.' *Journal of British Studies* 44, no. 2 (2005): 343–62.

———. 'Slipping Out of View: Subjectivity and Emotion in Gender History.' *History Workshop Journal* 59 (2005): 57–72.

Roper, M. and J. Tosh, eds. *Manful Assertions: Masculinities in Britain since 1800*. London: Routledge, 1991.

Rosenberg, C. 'Contested Boundaries: Psychiatry, Disease, and Diagnosis.' *Perspectives in Biology and Medicine* 49, no. 3 (2006): 407–24.

Rosenberg, C. and J. Golden, eds. *Framing Disease: Studies in Cultural History*. New Brunswick: Rutgers University Press, 1992.

———. 'The Tyranny of Diagnosis: Specific Entities and Individual Experience.' *Milbank Quarterly* 80, no. 2 (2002): 237–60.

Rothery, M. and H. French, eds. *Making Men: The Formation of Elite Male Identities in England c. 1660–1900: Sourcebook*. Basingstoke: Palgrave Macmillan, 2012.

Rowbotham, J. and K. Stevenson, eds. *Criminal Conversations: Victorian Crimes, Social Panic, and Moral Outrage*. Columbus: Ohio State University Press, 2005.

Rowbotham, J., K. Stevenson, and S. Pegg. *Crime News in Modern Britain: Press Reporting and Responsibility, 1820–2010*. Houndmills: Palgrave Macmillan, 2013.

Rowland, M. 'Shame and Futile Masculinity: Feeling Backwards in Henry Mackenzie's *Man of Feeling*.' *Eighteenth-Century Fiction* 31, no. 3 (2019): 529–48.

Saucier, R. and D. Wright. 'Madness in the Archives: Anonymity, Ethics, and Mental Health Research.' *Journal of the Canadian Historical Association* 23, no. 2 (2012): 81–82.

Schuster, D.G. *Neurasthenic Nation: America's Search for Health, Happiness, and Comfort, 1869–1920*. New Brunswick: Rutgers University Press, 2011.

Schwieso, J.J. '"Religious Fanaticism" and Wrongful Confinement in Victorian England: The Affair of Louisa Nottidge.' *Social History of Medicine* 9, no. 2 (1996): 159–74.

Scull, A., ed. *Cultural Sociology of Mental Illness*. Los Angeles: Sage Reference, 2014.

Scull, A. *Diseases in Civilization: A Cultural History of Insanity*. Princeton: Princeton University Press, 2015.

———. *Hysteria: The Disturbing History*. Oxford: Oxford University Press, 2011.

———. *Madhouses, Mad-Doctors, and Madmen: The Social History of Psychiatry in the Victorian Era*. Philadelphia: University of Pennsylvania Press, 2015.

———. *Madness in Civilization: A Cultural History of Insanity, from the Bible to Freud, from the Madhouse to Modern Medicine*. Princeton: Princeton University Press, 2015.

———. *Museums of Madness: The Social Organization of Insanity in Nineteenth-Century England*. New York: St. Martin's Press, 1979.

———. *Social Order/Mental Disorder: Anglo-American Psychiatry in Historical Perspective*. Berkeley: University of California Press, 1989.

Scull, A., C. MacKenzie, and N. Hervey. *Masters of Bedlam: The Transformation of the Mad-Doctoring Trade*. Princeton: Princeton University Press, 2014.

Secord, J. *Visions of Science: Books and Readers at the Dawn of the Victorian Age*. Chicago: University of Chicago Press, 2014.

Sedgwick, E. *Epistemology of the Closet*. Berkeley: University of California Press, 2008.

Seidman, S. 'The Power of Desire and the Danger of Pleasure: Victorian Sexuality Reconsidered.' *Journal of Social History* 24, no. 1 (1990): 47–67.

Shattock, J., ed. *Journalism and the Periodical Press in Nineteenth-Century Britain*. Cambridge: Cambridge University Press, 2017.

Shaw, C. 'Liberalizing Paternalism? Men and the 1891 Slander of Women Act.' Unpublished paper.

Shepard, A. *Meanings of Manhood in Early Modern England*. Oxford: Oxford University Press, 2003.

Shephard, B. *A War of Nerves: Soldiers and Psychiatrists in the Twentieth Century*. Boston: Harvard University Press, 2003.

Shepherd, A. *Institutionalizing the Insane in Nineteenth-Century England*. London: Pickering & Chatto, 2014.

Shepherd, A. and D. Wright. 'Madness, Suicide and the Victorian Asylum: Attempted Self-Murder in the Age of Non-Restraint.' *Medical History* 46, no. 2 (2002): 175–96.

Shepherd, J. '"I Am Not Very Well I Feel Nearly Mad When I Think of You": Male Jealousy, Murder and Broadmoor in Late-Victorian Britain.' *Social History of Medicine* 30, no. 2 (2017): 277–98.

———. 'Life for the Families of the Victorian Criminally Insane.' *Historical Journal* 63, no. 3 (2020): 603–32.

———. '"One of the Best Fathers until He Went Out of His Mind": Paternal Child-Murder, 1864–1900.' *Journal of Victorian Culture* 18, no. 1 (2013): 17–35.

———. 'Victorian Madmen: Broadmoor, Masculinity and the Experiences of the Criminally Insane, 1863–1900.' PhD Dissertation, Queen Mary University of London, 2013.

Shiman, L.L. *Crusade against Drink in Victorian England.* London: Macmillan Press, 1988.
Shorter, E. *A History of Psychiatry: From the Era of the Asylum to the Age of Prozac.* New York: John Wiley & Sons, Inc., 1997.
———. *From Paralysis to Fatigue: A History of Psychosomatic Illness in the Modern Era.* New York: The Free Press, 1992.
Showalter, E. *The Female Malady: Women, Madness, and English Culture, 1830–1980.* New York: Penguin Books, 1985.
Siena, K., ed. *Sins of the Flesh: Responding to Sexual Disease in Early Modern Europe.* Toronto: Centre for Reformation and Renaissance Studies, 2005.
Silverman, D.L. *Art Nouveau in Fin-de-Siecle France: Politics, Psychology, and Style.* Berkeley: University of California Press, 1989.
Slijkhuis, J. and H. Oosterhuis. '"Paralysed with Fears and Worries": Neurasthenia as a Gender-Specific Disease of Civilization.' *History of Psychiatry* 24, no. 1 (2013): 79–93.
Small, H. *Love's Madness: Medicine, the Novel, and Female Insanity, 1800–1865.* Oxford: Clarendon Press, 1996.
Smith, A. *Victorian Demons: Medicine, Masculinity and the Gothic at the Fin-de-Siècle.* Manchester: Manchester University Press, 2004.
Smith, C. and J. Giggs, eds. *Location and Stigma: Contemporary Perspectives on Mental Health Care.* Boston: Unwin Hyman, 1988.
Smith, E.J. 'Class, Health and the Proposed British Anthropometric Survey of 1904.' *Social History of Medicine* 28, no. 2 (2015): 308–29.
Smith, L. *Cure, Comfort and Safe Custody: Public Lunatic Asylums in Early Nineteenth-Century England.* London: Bloomsbury Publishing, 1999.
———. '"Your Very Thankful Inmate": Discovering the Patients of an Early County Lunatic Asylum.' *Social History of Medicine* 21, no. 2 (2008): 237–52.
Smith, R. *Trial by Medicine: Insanity and Responsibility in Victorian Trials.* Edinburgh: Edinburgh University Press, 1981.
———. 'The Victorian Controversy about the Insanity Defence.' *Journal of the Royal Society of Medicine* 81 (1988): 70–73.
Soares, C. 'The Path to Reform? Problematic Treatments and Patient Experience in Nineteenth-Century Female Inebriate Institutions.' *Cultural & Social History* 12, no. 3 (2015): 411–29.
Spierenburg, P., ed. *Men and Violence: Gender, Honour, and Rituals in Modern Europe and America.* Columbus: Ohio State University Press, 1998.
Spongberg, M. *Feminizing Venereal Disease: The Body of the Prostitute in Nineteenth-Century Medical Discourse.* New York: New York University Press, 1997.
Springhall, J. *Youth, Popular Culture and Moral Panics: Penny Gaffs to Gangsta-rap, 1830–1996.* New York: St. Martin's Press, 1998.
Stearns, P. *Shame: A Brief History.* Champaign: University of Illinois Press, 2017.

Stearns, P. and C. Stearns. 'Emotionology: Clarifying the History of Emotions and Emotional Standards.' *American Historical Review* 90, no. 4 (1985): 813–36.
Stengers, J. and A. Van Neck. *Masturbation: The History of a Great Terror.* Translated by K.A. Hoffmann. New York: Palgrave, 2001.
Stephens, E. 'Pathologizing Leaky Male Bodies: Spermatorrhea in Nineteenth-Century British Medicine and Popular Anatomical Museums.' *Journal of the History of Sexuality* 17, no. 3 (2008): 421–38.
Stevens, M. *Broadmoor Revealed: Victorian Crime and the Lunatic Asylum.* Barnsley: Pen and Sword, 2013.
Steward, J.R. 'Moral Economies and Commercial Imperatives: Food, Diets and Spas in Central Europe: 1800–1914.' *Journal of Tourism History* 4, no. 2 (2012): 181–203.
Stiles, A. *Popular Fiction and Brain Science in the Late Nineteenth Century.* Cambridge: Cambridge University Press, 2011.
Stoler, A.L. 'Colonial Archives and the Arts of Governance.' *Archival Science* 2 (2002): 87–109.
Sussman, H. *Victorian Masculinities: Manhood and Masculine Poetics in Early Victorian Literature and Art.* Cambridge: Cambridge University Press, 1995.
Sutton, E. *Aubrey Beardsley and British Wagnerism in the 1890s.* Oxford: Oxford University Press, 2001.
Suzuki, A. *Madness at Home: The Psychiatrist, the Patient, and the Family in England, 1820–1860.* Berkeley: University of California Press, 2006.
———. 'The Politics and Ideology of Non-Restraint: The Case of the Hanwell Asylum.' *Medical History* 39 (1995): 1–17.
Swartz, S. 'Asylum Case Records: Fact and Fiction.' *Rethinking History* 22, no. 3 (2018): 289–301.
Takabayashi, A. 'Surviving the Lunacy Act of 1890: English Psychiatrists and Professional Development during the Early Twentieth Century.' *Medical History* 61, no. 2 (2017): 246–69.
Tankard, A. 'Emasculation, Eugenics and the Consumptive Voyeur in *The Portrait of a Lady* (1881) and *The Story of a Nobody* (1893).' *Critical Survey* 20, no. 3 (2008): 61–78.
Taylor, J.R.B. *Hospital and Asylum Architecture in England, 1840–1914: Building for Health Care.* London: Mansell, 1991.
Tobia, P. 'The Patients of the Bristol Lunatic Asylum in the Nineteenth Century, 1861–1900.' PhD Dissertation, University of the West of England, 2017.
Tomes, N. *The Art of Asylum Keeping: Thomas Story Kirkbride and the Origins of American Psychiatry.* Philadelphia: University of Pennsylvania Press, 1994.
Tomkins, A. *Medical Misadventure in an Age of Professionalisation, 1780–1890.* Manchester: Manchester University Press, 2017.

Topp, L. 'Single Rooms, Seclusion and the Non-Restraint Movement in British Asylums, 1838–1844.' *Social History of Medicine* 31, no. 4 (2018): 754–73.
Topp, L., J.E. Moran, and J. Andrews. *Madness, Architecture and the Built Environment: Psychiatric Spaces in Historical Context*. New York: Routledge, 2007.
Torrey, E.F. and J. Miller. *The Invisible Plague: The Rise of Mental Illness from 1750 to the Present*. New Brunswick: Rutgers University Press, 2007.
Tosh, J. *A Man's Place: Masculinity and the Middle-Class Home in Victorian England*. New Haven: Yale University Press, 1999.
——. *Manliness and Masculinities in Nineteenth-Century Britain*. Harlow: Pearson Education, 2005.
——.'Masculinities in an Industrializing Society: Britain, 1800–1914.' *Journal of British Studies* 44, no. 2 (2005): 330–42.
Townsend, J. '"Unreliable Observations": Medical Practitioners and Venereal Disease Patient Narratives in Victorian Britain.' *Nineteenth-Century Gender Studies* 9, no. 2 (2013): 1–17.
Trotter, D. 'A Media Theory Approach to Representations of "Nervous Illness" in the Long Nineteenth Century.' *Journal of Victorian Culture* 24, no. 2 (2019): 146–58.
Turner, D. *Fashioning Adultery: Gender, Sex and Civility in England, 1660–1740*. Cambridge: Cambridge University Press, 2002.
Turner, T. 'Rich and Mad in Victorian England.' *Psychological Medicine* 19, no. 1 (1989): 29–44.
Unsworth, C. 'Law and Lunacy in Psychiatry's "Golden Age."' *Oxford Journal of Legal Studies* 13, no. 4 (1993): 479–507.
Upchurch, C. *Before Wilde: Sex Between Men in Britain's Age of Reform*. Berkeley: University of California Press, 2013.
——. 'Full-Text Databases and Historical Research: Cautionary Results from a Ten-Year Study.' *Journal of Social History* 46, no. 1 (2012): 89–105.
Ussher, J.M. *Women's Madness: Misogyny or Mental Illness?* Amherst: University of Massachusetts Press, 1992.
Valverde, M. '"Slavery from Within": The Invention of Alcoholism and the Question of Free Will.' *Social History* 22, no. 3 (1997): 251–68.
Vernon, J. *Distant Strangers: How Britain Became Modern*. Berkeley: University of California Press, 2014.
Vleugels, A. *Narratives of Drunkenness: Belgium, 1830–1914*. New York: Routledge, 2015.
Walkowitz, J.R. *City of Dreadful Delight: Narratives of Sexual Danger in Late-Victorian London*. Chicago: University of Chicago Press, 1992.
——. 'Jack the Ripper and the Myth of Male Violence.' *Feminist Studies* 8, no. 3 (1982): 542–74.
Waller, J. '"The Illusion of an Explanation": The Concept of Hereditary Disease, 1770–1870.' *Journal of the History of Medicine and Allied Sciences* 57, no. 4 (2002): 410–48.

Wallis, J. 'A Home or a Gaol? Scandal, Secrecy, and the St James's Inebriate Home for Women.' *Social History of Medicine* 31, no. 4 (2018): 774–95.
——. *Investigating the Body in the Victorian Asylum: Doctors, Patients, and Practices*. Basingstoke: Palgrave Macmillan, 2017.
——. 'Looking Back: This Fascinating and Fatal Disease.' *The Psychologist* 25, no. 10 (2012): 790–91.
Walsh, B. *Domestic Murder in Nineteenth-Century England: Literary and Cultural Representations*. London: Routledge, 2016.
Walton, S. *Guilty but Insane: Mind and Law in Golden Age Detective Fiction*. Oxford: Oxford University Press, 2015.
Ward, O. 'John Langdon Down: The Man and the Message.' *Down Syndrome Research and Practice* 6, no. 1 (1999): 19–24.
Wear, A., ed. *Medicine in Society: Historical Essays*. Cambridge: Cambridge University Press, 1992.
Wear, A., J. Geyer-Kordesch, and R. French, eds. *Doctors and Ethics: The Earlier Historical Settings of Professional Ethics*. Amsterdam: Rodopi, 1993.
Weeks, J. *Coming Out: Homosexual Politics in Britain from the Nineteenth Century to the Present*. London: Quartet Books, 1977.
——. *Sexuality and Its Discontents: Meanings, Myths, & Modern Sexualities*. London: Routledge & K. Paul, 1985.
Welsh, A. *George Eliot and Blackmail*. Cambridge: Harvard University Press, 1985.
Wendt, S. and P.D. Andersen, eds. *Masculinities and the Nation in the Modern World: Between Hegemony and Marginalization*. New York: Palgrave Macmillan, 2015.
White, S. 'The Insanity Defense in England and Wales Since 1843.' *Annals of the American Academy of Political and Social Science* 477, no. 1 (1985): 43–57.
Wiener, M.J. 'Judges v. Jurors: Courtroom Tensions in Murder Trials and the Law of Criminal Responsibility in Nineteenth-Century England.' *Law and History Review* 17, no. 3 (1999): 467–506.
——. *Men of Blood: Violence, Manliness, and Criminal Justice in Victorian England*. Cambridge: Cambridge University Press, 2004.
Wiesenthal, C. *Figuring Madness in Nineteenth-Century Fiction*. Houndmills: Palgrave Macmillan, 1997.
Wilde, S. 'The Elephants in the Doctor–Patient Relationship: Patients' Clinical Interactions and the Changing Surgical Landscape of the 1890s.' *Health and History* 9, no. 1 (2007): 2–27.
Williams, K. *Get Me a Murder a Day! A History of Mass Communications in Britain*. London: Bloomsbury Academic, 1997.
Wilson, P.K. 'Eighteenth-Century "Monsters" and Nineteenth-Century "Freaks": Reading the Maternally Marked Child.' *Literature and Medicine* 21, no. 1 (2002): 1–25.
Wise, S. *Inconvenient People: Lunacy, Liberty and the Mad-Doctors in Victorian England*. Berkeley: Counterpoint, 2013.

Wood, A.D. '"The Fashionable Diseases": Women's Complaints and their Treatment in Nineteenth-Century America.' *Journal of Interdisciplinary History* 4, no. 1 (1973): 25–52.

Wood, J.C. *Violence and Crime in Nineteenth Century England: The Shadow of Our Refinement*. London: Routledge, 2004.

Wright, D. 'Getting Out of the Asylum: Understanding the Confinement of the Insane in the Nineteenth Century.' *Social History of Medicine* 10, no. 1 (1997): 137–55.

———. *Mental Disability in Victorian England: The Earlswood Asylum, 1847–1901*. Oxford: Clarendon Press, 2001.

Wright, D. and A. Digby. *From Idiocy to Mental Deficiency: Historical Perspectives on People with Learning Disabilities*. London: Routledge, 1996.

Wynter, R. '"Good in All Respects": Appearance and Dress at Staffordshire County Lunatic Asylum, 1818–54.' *History of Psychiatry* 22, no. 1 (2011): 40–57.

Yeazell, R.B., ed. *Sex, Politics, and Science in the Nineteenth-Century Novel*. Baltimore: Johns Hopkins University Press, 1986.

Young, A. *The Harmony of Illusions Inventing Post-Traumatic Stress Disorder*. Princeton: Princeton University Press, 1995.

Zieger, S. *The Mediated Mind: Affect, Ephemera and Consumerism in the Nineteenth Century*. New York: Fordham University Press, 2018.

Index

accident 43, 68, 69, 100, 126, 233
acts of parliament
    Contagious Diseases Acts 52n33, 248
    County Asylums Act 24
    Criminal Law Amendment Act 137n118
    Dangerous Lunatic Act (1838) 232
    Habitual Criminals Act (1869) 256n78
    Irish Lunatic Asylums for the Poor Act (1817) 24
    Lunacy Scotland Act (1857) 24
    Lunacy Act (1845) 6, 21
    Lunacy Act (1890) 87n3, 93n84, 148, 265
    Lunacy Asylum and Pauper Lunatics Act (1845) 21
    Mental Treatment Act (1930) 24, 265
    Prevention of Crimes Act (1871) 256n78
    Slander of Women Act 176n79
    Vaccination Acts 51n33
    Vagrancy Act (1898) 137n118
advice
    legal 210
    literature 225
    medical 61, 69, 70, 75, 76, 77, 78, 85, 86, 104, 128, 227, 236
    patient 35

After Care Association 211
alcohol 11, 33, 101, 107–12, 129, 132n48, 132n50, 132n53, 133n55, 133n63, 133n65, 146, 152–54, 157, 170, 197, 222, 228–34, 246, 246n72, 261n175 *see also* liquor, drunk, drink
alienist vi, 3, 6, 7, 76, 123, 226, 247 *see* doctor
alleged lunatic 141, 143, 146, 156, 157, 203
Alleged Lunatics' Friend Society 43, 143, 144, 145, 146, 148, 151
army 66, 95n108, 105, 188, 190, 201, 216n76 *see also* military
asylums x, 1, 6–7, 9–12, ch. 1, 59–62, 65–67, 70–76, 78–87, 88n8, 89–90n18, 89n20, 89n27, 90n30, 95n108, 99, 100, 103, 104, 106, 109, 111, 117–19, 123, 124, 128–29, 146–48, 150, 154–60, 161, 170, 171n7, 171n10, 200, 202, 204, 206, 207, 209, 210, 211, 221, 222, 225, 227, 230, 233–34, 236, 240, 242, 243, 246, 266, 175n71, 183, 184, 185, 191, 193, 200, 202, 204, 206–10, 221, 222, 225, 227,

304 *Index*

230, 233–34, 236, 240, 242, 243, 266
admissions 10, 26, 29–30, 32–33, 38, 39, 40, 43, 46, 47, 79, 90n30, 104, 106, 111, 114, 118, 121, 124, 126, 135n97, 138n147, 158, 218n116, 218n119, 225, 226, 244, 245, 246, 265
Baldovan Asylum 118
Bethlem Asylum 1, 9, 19n55, 22, 30, 32, 38, 41, 111, 245–46
Bethnal House Asylum 118, 134n72, 245
Blacklands House 45
Brislington House Asylum 33, 118
Bristol Asylum 41, 229
Broadmoor Asylum 9, 19n55, 22, 37, 81, 89n25, 89n26, 150–51, 174n59, 186, 204, 208, 209, 210, 215n54, 220n147, 233
Camberwell House 42
Claybury Asylum 136n103
Clifton Hall Asylum 238
Colney Hatch Asylum 27, 230
Crichton Royal Asylum 126
criminal 10, 24, 25, 203, 234
county/pauper 9, 10, 22–24, 27, 28, 29, 35, 85, 104, 105, 120, 142
Durham Asylum 44, 45
Earlswood Asylum 85
Fisherton House Asylum 208
Glasgow Royal Lunatic Asylum 9, 10, 19n55, 22, 34–35, 38, 39, 40, 111, 118, 234, 239, 240, 242
Grove Hall Asylum 243
Hanwell Asylum 46, 246
Hampshire County Lunatic Asylum 208
Hayes Park Asylum 144
Holloway Sanitorium 51n29, 101

Kent Asylum 46, 192
Leicester Borough Asylum 207
London Sick Asylum 78
Macclesfield Asylum 231
Manor House Asylum 9, 19n56, 22, 32, 33, 63, 64, 78, 136n110, 106, 114, 116, 120, 121, 126, 156, 157, 243, 245
Moorcroft House 152–53
Morningside Asylum 10
Murray's Asylum 128
North Wales Lunatic Asylum 83, 96n137
Northamptonshire Asylum 231
Northampton State Lunatic Hospital 135n97
Northumberland House 45
Peckham House 41
private 9, 12, 22, 23, 24, 27, 29, 33, 39, 42, 62, 63, 72, 75, 79, 104, 118, 131n24, 142, 146, 147, 152, 169, 173n47, 176n77, 265
Richmond Asylum 124
Royal Albert Hospital 85
Royal Edinburgh Asylum 31
Somerset and Bath Asylum 266
St Andrew's Hospital 170
St Thomas's Hospital 214n36
Sussex and Brandenburgh House asylums 72
Ticehurst Asylum 9, 27, 49n9, 158, 178n115
West Riding lunatic Asylum 35
York Asylum 135n97
York Retreat 47
attendant 32, 40–47, 57n123, 65, 66, 74, 76, 78, 89n18, 89n26, 158, 207, 208, 209, 225, 231
autobiography 77, 126

bath 46
beast, bestial, etc. 2, 3, 5, 39, 85, 98, 103, 106, 114, 146, 183, 190, 195, 197, 198, 238

Index

boarders, boarding out 33, 48n3, 71–72, 87n2, 101, 197
body, bodies 2, 9, 67, 113, 117, 122, 160, 223, 228, 236, 237, 238, 241, 248, 251, 261n175
breadwinner 60, 86, 104
brothel 124, 250
business 40, 63, 70, 74, 101, 104, 169, 240, 242, 245–46

case history 9, 116, 119, 128, 156–60, 245
case studies
  Captain Childe 144–45
  Reverend H.J. Dodwell 149–52, 174n55, 175n67, n71
  Earl of Eldon 67–68
  George Fordham 207–9
  Charles Merivale 156–60
  Henry Meux 11, 69–71
  Charles Molyneux 68–71
  Evan Roberts 83–84
  Laurence Ruck 152–56
  George Gilbert Scott 167–70
  George Grant Suttie 126–28
  John Tierney 205–07
  William Windham 160–67
casebook 32, 33, 35, 46, 106, 114, 115, 158, 243
causes of insanity *see* madness
certification of lunacy 10, 12, 27, 30, 33, 40, 64, 67, 69–71, 73–74, 79–80, 89n18, 96n130, 101, 110, 126–27, 138n145, 140–43, 147–48, 151, 155–57, 159–60, 168–69, 171, 177, 204, 266
Chancery 10, 74, 162, 170
  cases 12, 20n59, 60, 68–70, 89n17, 179n128, 181n167
  court 62, 142, 149, 153, 155, 157, 160, 167–69
  patients 72, 93n80
childhood 122, 125
children 28, 30, 37, 38, 70, 73, 84, 99, 101, 114, 116, 117, 122, 125, 126, 128, 129, 152, 153, 158, 163, 164, 168, 169, 186, 188, 190, 192, 205, 223, 225, 227, 230, 234, 235, 239, 245, 247, 248–51
civilization 13, 221, 223, 224, 228, 231, 232, 238, 240, 241, 244, 247, 252
city 228, 240
class 2, 4, 22–23, 26, 28, 33, 60, 112, 142, 222, 228, 235, 252
  middle-class 9, 13, 29, 55n84, 56n105, 61, 65, 76, 77, 78, 99, 117, 160, 224, 228, 235–36, 239, 240, 246, 248, 251
  upper-class 9, 25, 61, 76, 99, 239, 248
  working-class 10, 12, 13, 28, 35, 37, 48, 56n105, 65, 84, 127, 165, 187, 228, 235–36, 251
community care 71
congenital 25, 85, 123, 124, 224, 233, 239, 249
control 2, 5, 8, 11, 23, 27, 28, 35, 36, 37, 38, 47, 55n84, 60, 61, 67, 79, 80, 81, 82, 86, 98, 99, 100, 101, 103, 104, 108–14, 122–25, 127–29, 130n14, 134n76, 140, 143, 144, 152–56, 161, 163, 164, 165, 170, 183, 184, 187, 193, 205, 206, 209, 210, 224, 232, 236, 240, 250, 267
crime 80, 116, 122, 142, 175n71, 185, 186, 188, 193, 194, 197, 199, 200, 228, 231, 232, 233, 235, 250
  arson 45, 233, 257n80
  assault 43, 44, 45, 46, 149, 192, 194, 195, 257n80
  fraud 149, 257n80
  sexual offence 128, 257n80
  theft 235, 257n80

criminal insanity 201–10
cure 3, 6, 13, 25, 26, 29, 37, 47, 76, 77, 78, 79, 117, 118, 124, 129, 145, 184, 193, 198, 215n54, 225, 232, 246

dangerous 22, 27, 37, 38, 39, 40, 44, 63, 64, 66, 80, 81, 83, 111, 118, 121, 124, 125, 150, 154, 159, 164, 185, 188, 189, 191, 193, 195, 198, 206, 207, 209, 212n5, 222, 223, 228, 231, 233, 234, 236, 239, 242, 244
Darwin, Charles 94n96
Darwinian 129
death 3, 13, 20n60, 26, 40, 42, 43, 44, 45, 46, 55n96, 58n129, 66, 67, 68, 69, 70, 77, 83, 84, 85, 89n18, 91n43, 91n52, 96n127, 103, 111, 134n68, 137n118, 151, 167, 170, 191, 200, 201, 202, 203, 204, 206, 207, 227, 230, 233, 234, 238, 240, 242, 245, 249, 250, 260n152, 260n153, 267
degeneration 5, 8, 13, 115, 164, ch. 6, 264, 265, 266
delirium tremens 110, 111, 132n53, 133n65, 193, 197, 231, 256n69
delusion 3, 14, 32, 34, 35, 38, 39, 40, 42, 43, 44, 63, 66, 73, 74, 83, 90n30, 106, 109, 112, 114, 115, 116, 120, 121, 136n110, 144, 145, 147, 148, 149, 153, 154, 155, 156, 157, 158, 159, 163, 178n115, 191, 193, 197, 205, 207, 209, 210, 233, 242, 243, 245, 256n72, 266
diagnosis 4, 5, 7, 8, 13, 27, 28, 36, 90n30, 99, 100, 102, 110, 140, 141, 142, 151, 155, 158, 159, 160, 163, 170, 180n140, 211, 223, 236, 237, 241, 242, 244, 245, 247, 258n104, 258n110
epilepsy 40, 44, 46, 57n129, 62, 69, 72, 78, 136n103, 159, 233, 245
feeble-minded 230, 255n52
General Paralysis of the Insane 13, 223, 241–47, 249, 251, 252, 261n170
hysteria 76, 121, 122, 157, 193, 237
hypochondria 94n96, 158, 159, 160, 178n109
idiocy 7, 22, 85, 99, 106, 163, 248, 249
imbecile 106, 118, 232
mania 33, 44, 45, 64, 83, 106, 111, 121, 132n47, 154, 190, 197
melancholia 2, 73, 74, 84, 104, 116, 121, 124, 178n109, 245
misdiagnosis 147, 154, 157
monomania 146, 227, 239, 245
moral insanity 163, 166, 179n132, 180n139
neurasthenia 13, 122, 157, 159, 221, 222, 228, 236–37, 242, 252, 258n110, 264
paralysis 66, 78, 90n30, 163, 234, 242, 243, 245
divorce 129, 248
doctors 14, 21, 31, 38, 46, 62, 67, 73, 75, 76, 78, 79, 84, 96n127, 100, 105, 106, 110, 118, 120, 123, 124, 126, 127, 128, 131n24, 136n110, 138n151, 152, 155, 157, 159, 160, 168, 169, 189, 191, 197, 207, 208, 229, 230, 234, 237–39, 246, 250, 251, 263, 264 *see also* alienist, neurologist, psychiatrist, physician

George Beard 237
Charles Bucknill 163, 236
John Conolly 47, 153
Thomas Stretch Dowse 77, 78, 240, 242
William Richard Gowers 72–73
Henry Maudsley 107, 119, 132n51, 159, 203, 226, 232, 240, 241, 246, 261n170
William Julius Mickle 236, 243, 258n104
Thomas Mayo 163, 180n140
William Orange 209, 234, 235
William Evans Pope 237
Rumler 123, 221
George Savage 123, 247
Edward J. Seymour 178
Edgar Sheppard 101–02
Forbes Benignus Winslow 179n132, 224
Lyttleton S. Forbes Winslow 24, 72, 150, 154, 162, 163, 174n63, 175n66, 182n173, 203, 207, 209, 224
domestic 185, 187, 192, 193, 235, 265
violence 187–94, 213n19
drink/drinking 110, 111, 112, 118, 132n53, 138n147, 153, 154, 156, 169, 229, 230, 231, 234, 235, 244
dipsomania 132n53, 133n62
drunk 4, 10, 13, 32, 107, 108, 109, 133n56, 154, 202, 228–29, 233, 238, 240
inebriate 80, 128, 154, 176n78, 197
drugs 107

eccentric 3, 12, 63, 64, 66, 142, 161, 165, 206
effeminate 2, 5, 103, 106, 119, 120, 128, 264
emasculate 5, 13, 47, 99, 100, 113, 120, 122, 264, 267

emotion 2, 3, 8, 9, 11, 38, 39, 60, 61, 99, 102, 103, 122, 125, 126, 154, 158, 164, 185, 199, 202, 233, 239, 264, 267
anger 28, 32, 98, 99, 151, 154, 189, 199, 206
anxiety 8, 13, 63, 66, 156, 194, 237, 238, 240, 252
depression 38, 40, 81, 94n96
despair 39, 59, 102, 197, 231
fear 1, 35, 37, 38, 40, 99, 102, 103, 106, 111, 114, 116, 117, 119, 121, 122, 156, 184, 185, 187, 194, 196, 198, 201, 211, 223, 229, 232, 235, 237, 238
fury 59, 193, 200
grief 103, 109, 129
joy 3
pity 184, 264
rage 32, 39, 126, 199
sadness 231
excess 34, 98, 101, 108, 109, 112, 116, 120, 123, 129, 152, 153, 154, 166, 169, 199, 221, 223, 230, 241, 244, 245, 246, 251, 261n170, 261n180
exercise 70, 76, 82, 116, 162, 228
eugenics 222, 229, 230, 248, 261n186

failure 28, 40, 48, 56n105, 62, 68, 72, 78, 82, 99, 100, 101, 104, 108, 110, 116, 122, 123, 132n48, 150, 151, 158, 163, 229, 236, 263, 264, 265, 267n1
fall 62, 232, 233
family 3, 7, 9, 10, 11, 12, 14, 18n50, 23–28, 30–33, 35, 37–40, 47, 56n105, 59–63, 65–73, 75–87, 89n18, 90n27, 95n112, 96n127, 99, 101–06, 109, 128, 131n42,

140–44, 146, 148, 152, 155–56, 161–65, 167–70, 187–90, 192–94, 200, 206, 211n2, 224, 225, 230, 232, 233, 234, 236, 238, 248, 250, 251, 252
  family history 120, 138n147, 218n119, 223, 229, 232, 235, 239
feminist 5, 26, 248, 249, 261n186, 266

genetics 129, 224, 265
genius 16n30, 160
gentleman 36, 74, 105, 120, 150, 152, 156, 157, 161, 165, 168, 197, 221
gossip 84, 157, 159

homosexual 122–29, 137n118
horse 105
hydrotherapy 76, 79
  hydropathy 76

illness viii, 7, 9, 10, 12, 27, 31, 32, 36, 39, 62, 63, 67, 69, 71, 75, 76, 77, 79, 91n52, 99, 100, 106, 107, 108, 111, 112, 116, 117, 120, 121, 124, 136n103, 143, 156, 157, 159, 160, 190, 171n7, 178n117, 197, 200, 211, 223, 224, 225, 228, 229, 233, 235, 240, 241, 245, 246, 247–51
impotence 114, 120
infanticide 186, 217n103, 213n23
inheritance 151, 160, 165, 211n2, 221, 222, 223–28, 230, 231, 233, 239, 241, 244, 247, 248, 249, 251, 252, 263, 264, 265, 266, 267
  of wealth, property 70, 131n24 *see also* family history
injury 44, 68, 90n40, 107, 128, 189, 236

institutionalization 22, 23, 25, 27, 29, 30, 36, 40, 48, 50n16, 64, 67, 101, 103, 104, 157, 187, 251
intemperance 108, 112, 122, 155, 230
Ireland 24, 50n19, 60, 206, 232
  Dublin 124
  Irish 6, 232, 250

liquor 109, 110
Lunacy Law Reform Association 143, 148, 151 *see also* alcohol
lunacy reform 3, 48n2, 148, 229
luxury 27, 29, 239

madness
  boundaries of 12, 63, 64, 73, 80, 96n127, 150, 153, 157–61, 187, 204
  causes 98, 100, 107, 111, 112, 118, 165n66, 194, 197, 221, 236–40, 251
  hereditary nature of 13, 151, 155, 164, 222, 224–28, 230, 232, 239
  masculinity 2, 5–6, 8, 13, 98, 103, 184, 186, 199
  shame 11, 12, 99–100, 101–07, 140, 170
  theories of xiii, 3–4, 7
  women and 4, 5–6, 12, 13, 21, 25–26, 39, 40, 59–61, 76, 82, 86, 96n127, 100, 108–09, 112, 118, 145, 148, 171, 183, 186, 224, 225, 227, 236–37, 244
manhood 2, 5, 8, 11, 12, 95n113, 99, 103, 113, 141, 165, 167, 171, 221, 222, 228, 230, 239, 241, 242, 246, 252, 267
manly 36, 37, 76, 99, 103, 105, 108, 112, 120, 127, 128, 162, 197, 224, 236, 265
manslaughter 42, 43

Index

marriage 70, 82, 110, 116, 120, 145, 153, 155, 159, 161, 162, 166, 173n47, 193, 233, 249, 250
masturbation 117–22, 123, 124, 126, 134n72, 136n103, 136n110, 137n116, 250
onanism 120, 121, 123
media 8, 12, 23, 80, 145, 148, 156, 161, 168, 181n162, ch. 5
newspaper 6, 10, 22, 37, 41, 69, 70, 71, 72, 82, 84, 88n9, 146, 147, 179n125, ch. 5, 248, 264
memoirs 9, 22, 34, 110, 142, 157, 229
military 3, 25, 36, 106, 111, 144, 222, 236, 263, 264, 265
modern life 195, 198, 221, 222, 235, 236, 237, 239, 252
modern civilization 241
modernity 5, 53n53, 240
moral failure 100, 129, 163, 229, 265
moral treatment 3, 21, 25, 48, 48n2
murder 35, 38, 41, 55n83, 80, 81, 109, 149, 184, 185, 186, 188, 191, 194, 195, 197, 201, 204, 205, 206, 207, 208, 257n80

nerves or nervous system 62, 78, 103, 108, 119, 120, 122, 189, 198, 228, 235, 237, 240, 242, 263
nervous disorder or diseases 30, 74, 75, 77, 157–58, 235–37, 240, 258, 263, 264
nervous temperament 77, 227
nervousness 71, 74, 76, 158, 238
neurologist 72, 264
novels
Anne Brontë, *The Tenant of Wildfell Hall* 109

Emma Brooke, *A Superfluous Woman* 249–50
Wilkie Collins, *Armadale* 76, *Basil* 238–39, *Heart and Science* 103, *Man and Wife* 109–10
Charles Dickens, *The Personal History of David Copperfield* 73–74
Sarah Grand, *The Heavenly Twins* 249
F.E. Grainger, *Caged! The Romance of a Lunatic Asylum* 111
Coulson Kernahan, *A Literary Gent* 110
Charles Reade, *Hard Cash* 146, *It is Never Too Late to Mend* 102–03, *A Terrible* Temptation 59, 62
Anthony Trollope, *He Knew he was Right* 98

overwork 77, 107, 114, 121, 159, 168, 169, 232, 236–40, 241, 242, 246, 251

patriarch 31, 67, 80, 88n8, 101, 104, 109, 143, 148, 152
pauper 10, 21, 22, 23, 24, 28, 29, 30, 35, 38, 41, 46, 71, 72, 85, 104, 113, 118, 142, 148, 207, 228, 234
perversion 113, 114, 122, 123, 136n110, 250
phrenology 160
physician *see* doctor
Poor Law 28, 50n19, 79, 83
poverty 104, 108, 186, 199, 222, 228, 229, 255n52
prison 35, 44, 83, 93n84, 102, 123, 126, 128, 129, 203, 204, 232, 233, 236
gaol 24
jail 80

privacy viii, 61, 68, 71, 150, 156, 157, 187, 198
 private x, 17n32, 24, 25, 48, 63, 65, 68, 69, 74, 77, 79–86, 87, 92n70, 106, 114, 125, 137n118, 140, 141, 142, 144, 146, 153, 168, 170, 194
prostitution 52n33, 134n78, 152, 153, 248
psychiatrist 237, 265
puerperal insanity 186, 217n103

railway 78, 164, 165, 166, 180n148, 194–96, 198
religion 98, 206
 religious 3, 35, 108, 121, 122, 123, 125, 128, 158, 159, 160, 178n109, 191, 225, 229, 236
Royal Commission on Venereal Disease 248
reputation 48n2, 78, 95n113, 112, 140, 143, 153, 155, 156, 157, 159, 161, 163, 167, 168, 169, 170, 176n81

same-sex desire *see* homosexual
scandal 66, 72, 78, 82, 85, 140, 147, 167, 185, 188
Scotland 24, 71, 92n64, 127, 137n118, 225, 256n77
secret 59, 61, 67, 68, 88n12, 99, 106, 117, 121, 122, 131n42, 140, 141, 144, 149, 157, 175n75, 191, 195, 249, 250
seizure 69, 158, 159
self-control 2, 3, 5, 8, 36, 37, 82, 103, 108, 112, 122, 123, 125, 130n14, 144, 153, 163, 206, 209, 224
sensation 6, 12, 61, 82, 96n127, 97n139, 108, 109, 131n42, 140, 146, 147, 161, ch. 5, 229, 249

sex 8, 11, 101, 112, 118, 121–3, 125–26, 134n77, 222, 227, 247, 248, 249, 250–51
sexual deviance or excess 16n30, 101, 112–17, 120, 123–24, 127, 129, 137n128, 223, 244, 245, 261n170, 261n180 *see also* masturbation
shell shock 6, 263–67
ship 111, 114, 121, 194, 196–8, 216n76
sin 117, 121, 122, 137n118, 149, 250
single care 11, 71–75, 82, 92n70
somatic 102, 226, 266
spa 76, 77, 79, 94n94
stigma viii, 3, 4, 11–12, 23, 27, 29, 34, 35, 55n96, 79, 83, 89n27, 99, 100, 101–02, 104, 106–07, 140, 157, 170, 184, 185, 187, 192, 201, 211, 215n52, 229, 233, 241
Strahan, Samuel 226–27
suicide 10, 39, 40, 45, 57n127, 95n108, 103, 158, 159, 193, 234
 self-murder 39
syphilis 114, 139, 244, 245–50, 252, 265

travel 11, 30, 33, 60, 61, 66, 68, 75–79, 93n88, 95n108, 95n112, 103, 126, 168, 169, 194, 195, 196, 197, 251
treatment 1, 3, 4, 6, 10, 11, 22, 25, 27, 29, 32, 33, 36, 47, 59, 60–62, 66, 231, 245, 246, 247, 264
 early treatment 13, 227, 265, 266
trial 10, 35, 36, 38, 42, 64, 68, 69, 70, 71, 73, 75, 89n26, 128, 141, 145, 146, 149, 150, 153, 155, 156, 160–64, 167, 169, 170, 175n74,

179n128, 185, 202, 203, 204, 205, 207, 208, 233, 248, 256n69, 257n80

urban 13, 194, 227, 228, 235, 238, 240

venereal disease 116, 248
vice 107, 108, 112, 122, 128, 134n72, 118n118, 137n128, 166, 203, 249
violence 4, 5, 11, 12, 14n5, 12, 23, 32, 33, 37–47, 55n83, 55n84, 61, 79–81, 82, 115, 126, 151, ch. 5, 248, 256n72
von Rigal family 250–51

Wales 24, 71, 83–84, 87n2, 89n23
wandering lunatic 83, 266

Weldon, Georgiana 51n26, 182n173
will (legal document) 70, 71, 91n56, 208
will (willpower) 23, 27, 31, 62, 69, 86, 100, 108, 109, 112, 132n48, 141, 158, 161, 206, 236, 248, 263, 267n2, 137n118
workhouse 24, 28, 30, 43, 46, 48, 50n19, 87n2, 90n27, 104, 207
wrongful certification 141, 160, 171, 182n173
    confinement 27, 93n84, 142, 143, 145, 147, 148, 151, 152, 159, 162, 170, 171, 172n12, 185, 186, 200

EU authorised representative for GPSR:
Easy Access System Europe, Mustamäe tee 50,
10621 Tallinn, Estonia
gpsr.requests@easproject.com